W9-AEF-152

NURSING PHOTOBOOK™

Working with Orthopedic Patients

NURSING82 BOOKS
INTERMED COMMUNICATIONS, INC.
SPRINGHOUSE, PENNSYLVANIA

4-29-82

***NURSING82* BOOKS**

NURSING PHOTOBOOK™ SERIES
Providing Respiratory Care
Managing I.V. Therapy
Dealing with Emergencies
Giving Medications
Assessing Your Patients
Using Monitors
Providing Early Mobility
Giving Cardiac Care
Performing GI Procedures
Implementing Urologic Procedures
Controlling Infection
Ensuring Intensive Care
Coping with Neurologic Disorders
Caring for Surgical Patients
Working with Orthopedic Patients
Nursing Pediatric Patients
Helping Geriatric Patients
Attending Ob/Gyn Patients
Aiding Ambulatory Patients
Carrying Out Special Procedures

NURSING SKILLBOOK® SERIES
Reading EKGs Correctly
Dealing with Death and Dying
Managing Diabetics Properly
Assessing Vital Functions Accurately
Helping Cancer Patients Effectively
Giving Cardiovascular Drugs Safely
Giving Emergency Care Competently
Monitoring Fluid and Electrolytes Precisely
Documenting Patient Care Responsibly
Combatting Cardiovascular Diseases Skillfully
Coping with Neurologic Problems Proficiently
Using Crisis Intervention Wisely
Nursing Critically Ill Patients Confidently

NURSE'S REFERENCE LIBRARY™
Diseases
Diagnostics

***Nursing82* DRUG HANDBOOK™**

PROFESSIONAL GUIDE TO DRUGS™

NURSING PHOTOBOOK™ Series

PUBLISHER
Eugene W. Jackson

EDITORIAL DIRECTOR
Jean Robinson

CLINICAL DIRECTOR
Barbara McVan, RN

ART DIRECTOR
Lisa A. Gilde

Intermed Communications Book Division

DIRECTOR
Timothy B. King

DIRECTOR, RESEARCH
Elizabeth O'Brien

DIRECTOR, PRODUCTION AND PURCHASING
Bacil Guiley

Staff for this volume

EDITOR
Patricia K. Lawson

SENIOR CLINICAL EDITOR
Paulette J. Strauch, RN

CLINICAL EDITOR
Carol H. Best, RN, CNRN

ASSOCIATE EDITOR
Paul Vigna, Jr.

SPECIAL ASSIGNMENTS EDITOR
Patricia R. Urosevich

PHOTOGRAPHER
Paul A. Cohen

ASSOCIATE DESIGNERS
Linda Jovinelly Franklin
Scott M. Stephens
Carol Stickles

ASSISTANT PHOTOGRAPHER
Thomas Staudenmayer

EDITORIAL/GRAPHIC COORDINATOR
Doreen K. Stowers

CLINICAL/GRAPHIC COORDINATOR
Evelyn M. James

COPY EDITOR
Sharyl D. Wolf

EDITORIAL STAFF ASSISTANT
Cynthia A. O'Connell

PHOTOGRAPHY ASSISTANT
Frank Margeson

ART PRODUCTION MANAGER
Robert Perry

ARTISTS
Virginia Crawford
Diane Fox
Robert H. Renn
Sandra Simms
Louise Stamper
Joan Walsh
Robert Walsh
Ron Yablon

RESEARCHER
Vonda Heller

TYPOGRAPHY MANAGER
David C. Kosten

TYPOGRAPHY ASSISTANTS
Janice Haber
Ethel Halle
Diane Paluba
Nancy Wirs

PRODUCTION MANAGERS
Wilbur D. Davidson
Robert L. Dean, Jr.

PRODUCTION ASSISTANT
Donald G. Knauss

ILLUSTRATORS
Dimitrios Bastas
John Dougherty
Russell Farrell
Jean Gardner
Ralph Giguere
Robert Jackson
Bob Jones
Don Kruzinski
Polly Krumbhaar Lewis
Earl Parker
Dennis Schofield
Bud Yingling

SERIES GRAPHIC DESIGNER
John C. Isely

COVER PHOTO
Photographic Illustrations

Clinical consultants for this volume

Jane Farrell, RN, BS
Orthopedic Clinician
Bellin Memorial Hospital
Green Bay, Wisc.

Ella Ryan-Meloni, RN, BSN
Head Nurse
Hospital of the University of Pennsylvania
Philadelphia, Pa.

010482

Library of Congress Cataloging in Publication Data

Main entry under title:

Working with orthopedic patients.

(Nursing photobook)
"Nursing82 books."
Bibliography: p.
1. Orthopedic Nursing. I. Intermed Communications, Inc.
II. Series.
RD753.W67 610.73'677 82-2979
ISBN 0-916730-44-1 AACR2

Contents

Contributors

At the time of original publication, these contributors held the following positions.

Patricia L. Botic is a clinician/clinical nurse specialist in the intermediate spinal cord injury/neurosurgery and neurology units at Thomas Jefferson University Hospital, Philadelphia. She earned a nursing diploma at St. Francis General Hospital School of Nursing, Pittsburgh, and a BSN degree at the University of Pittsburgh. Ms. Botic also holds an MSN degree from the University of Maryland Baltimore Professional Schools, Baltimore.

Jane Farrell, an advisor for this PHOTOBOOK, is an orthopedic clinician at Bellin Memorial Hospital in Green Bay, Wisconsin. She is a diploma graduate of St. Mary's Hospital School of Nursing in Milwaukee and holds a BS degree in human adaptability from the University of Wisconsin-Green Bay's College of Human Biology. Ms. Farrell is a member of the American Nurses' Association and the National Association of Orthopedic Nurses.

Mary N. Moore is content coordinator of undergraduate adult health and illness at the University of Pennsylvania, Philadelphia. She earned an AB Nursing degree at Bates College, Lewistown, Maine, and an MAEd at Saint Joseph's University in Philadelphia. Ms. Moore also holds an MSN degree from Philadelphia's University of Pennsylvania, and is a doctoral candidate for a DNS degree there. She is a member of the American Nurses' Association and Sigma Theta Tau.

Madeline T. Pozzi is a staff nurse at Philadelphia's Hospital of the University of Pennsylvania. A BSN degree graduate of West Chester (Pa.) State College, Ms. Pozzi is an MSN degree candidate at the University of Pennsylvania, Philadelphia. She is a member of the National Association of Orthopedic Nurses.

Letitia Ann Prosock is a primary nurse at Thomas Jefferson University Hospital in Philadelphia. A member of the National Association of Orthopedic Nurses, Ms. Prosock earned a nursing diploma at Methodist Hospital School of Nursing, Philadelphia.

Dennis G. Ross is assistant professor of nursing at Castleton (Vt.) State College. He earned an AS degree at Cuyahoga Community College, Cleveland, a BSN degree at the University of Cincinnati, and an MSN degree at the University of California, San Francisco. He is a member of the American Nurses' Association, the National League for Nursing, the National Association of Orthopedic Nurses, the Association of Operating Room Nurses, Inc., Sigma Theta Tau, the Vermont State Nurses' Association, and the Rutland County Nurses' Association. Mr. Ross is also a member of the editorial board of the ORTHOPEDIC NURSES ASSOCIATION JOURNAL.

Ella Ryan-Meloni, an advisor for this PHOTOBOOK, is a head nurse at the Hospital of the University of Pennsylvania, Philadelphia. She is a diploma graduate of the Hospital of the University of Pennsylvania School of Nursing and a BSN degree graduate of Villanova (Pa.) University. She holds memberships in the American Nurses' Association and the Pennsylvania Nurses' Association.

Alice Stahl-Poyss is an evening staff-development instructor at the Hospital of the University of Pennsylvania in Philadelphia. She earned a nursing diploma at the Hospital of the University of Pennsylvania School of Nursing, and a BSN degree at Holy Family College, Philadelphia. She is an MSN degree candidate at the University of Pennsylvania, Philadelphia.

Deborah Moorehead Thorpe is an orthopedic clinical nurse specialist at Saint Francis Hospital in Tulsa, Oklahoma. She holds a BSN degree from Illinois Wesleyan University, Bloomington, Illinois, and an MSN degree from Boston University. She is a member of the National Association of Orthopedic Nurses, the American Nurses' Association, the National League for Nursing, and Sigma Theta Tau.

Introduction

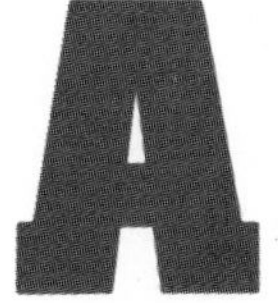

re you ready to explore the field of orthopedics? Perhaps you've always avoided your hospital's orthopedics unit. Maybe you felt you needed an engineering course to understand the equipment involved. If so, your feeling's not unusual. But, this book can help you approach orthopedic patients more confidently.

First, to help identify and treat your patient's orthopedic problem, establish a firm foundation in anatomy and physiology. In the first section of this book, you'll find vivid anatomical illustrations, accompanied by concise explanatory text. You'll also find detailed information on orthopedic disorders, with step-by-step instructions for performing a comprehensive orthopedic assessment.

Understanding anatomy and physiology *starts* you on the right track. But, the real key to caring for orthopedic patients rests on your grasping a few basic principles that apply to all these patients, whether they're in casts, traction, or recovering from surgery. Consider yourself well on the right track if you provide: frequent neurovascular assessments, to detect and prevent nerve and blood vessel damage; maintenance of injury-site immobilization, to allow bone and tissue repair; conscientious skin care, to prevent skin breakdown at points of contact with orthopedic and other equipment; and proper positioning, exercise, and early ambulation, to prevent immobilization complications. Master these principles with the help of the guidelines you'll find throughout the book.

Of course, you must also cope with specific equipment, such as splints, casts, slings, immobilizers, and traction setups. That's where our detailed section on dealing with immobilization devices can help. If you're not familiar with the newest casting materials, if you don't know the difference between skin and skeletal traction, and if you're not sure when to use a temporary splint instead of a long-term splint, look for the answers in this section.

In addition to these standard forms of immobilization, new surgical treatment alternatives are continually being developed. For example, internal and external fixation immobilize a fracture without immobilizing an entire limb, the way a cast or traction might. And for a fracture that won't heal, surgical implantation of electrical bone-stimulation equipment may be the answer. For a severely degenerated joint, the doctor may perform total hip or knee replacement. We'll discuss all of these procedures in the detailed way necessary for your complete understanding.

What can you do to prevent immobility and other orthopedic complications? The last section of the book focuses on this problem. There, you'll find exercises your patient can perform for greater strength and mobility, as well as positioning aids that will reduce skin breakdown and nerve damage. We'll also show you how to use ambulation aids to promote early mobility.

Are you beginning to feel more confident about orthopedics already? Then, read on. By the time you finish this book, you'll have mastered orthopedic basics. Study it, and the skills will be at your fingertips, for use in your day-to-day nursing care.

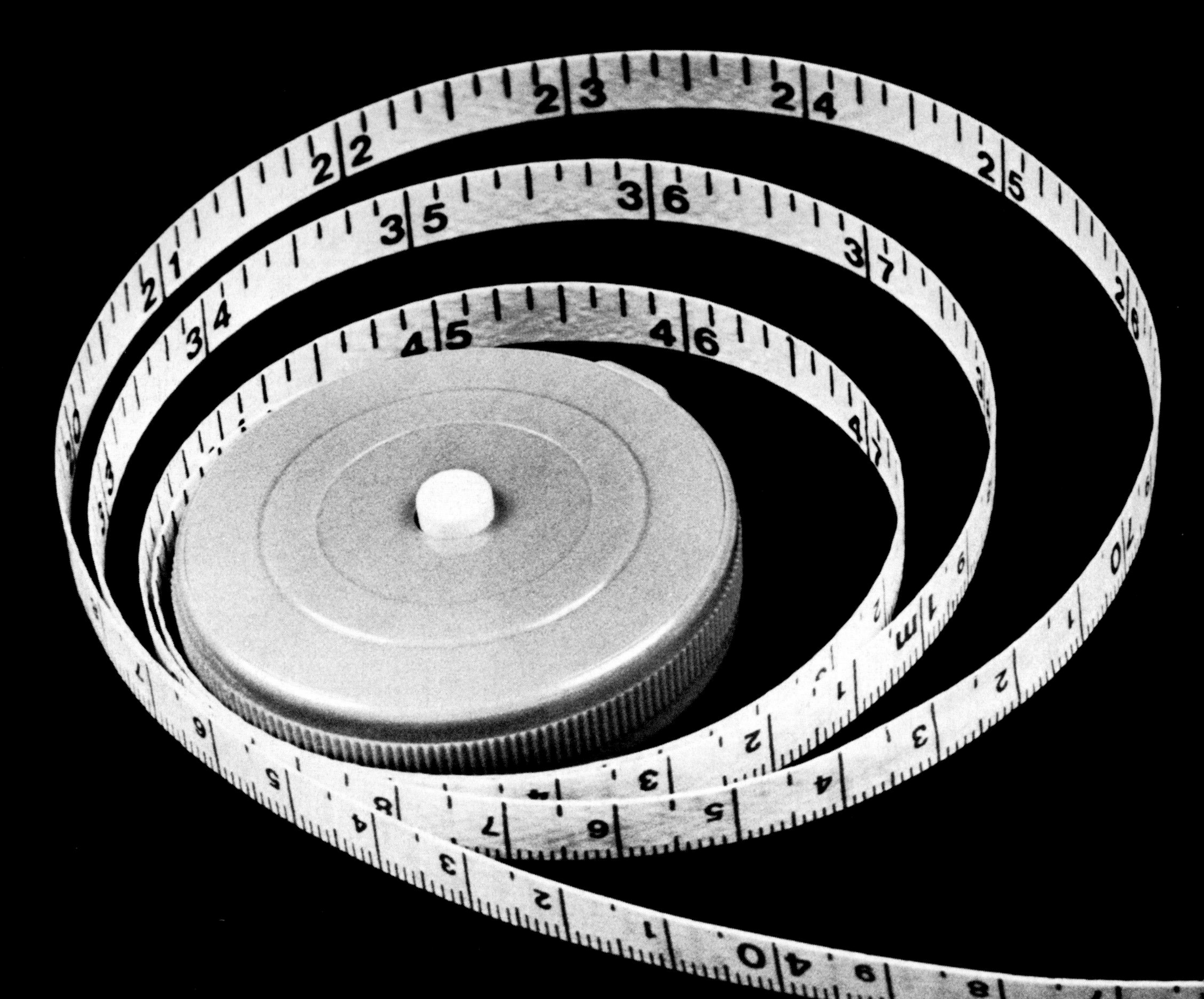

Identifying Orthopedic Disorders

Anatomy and physiology

Assessment

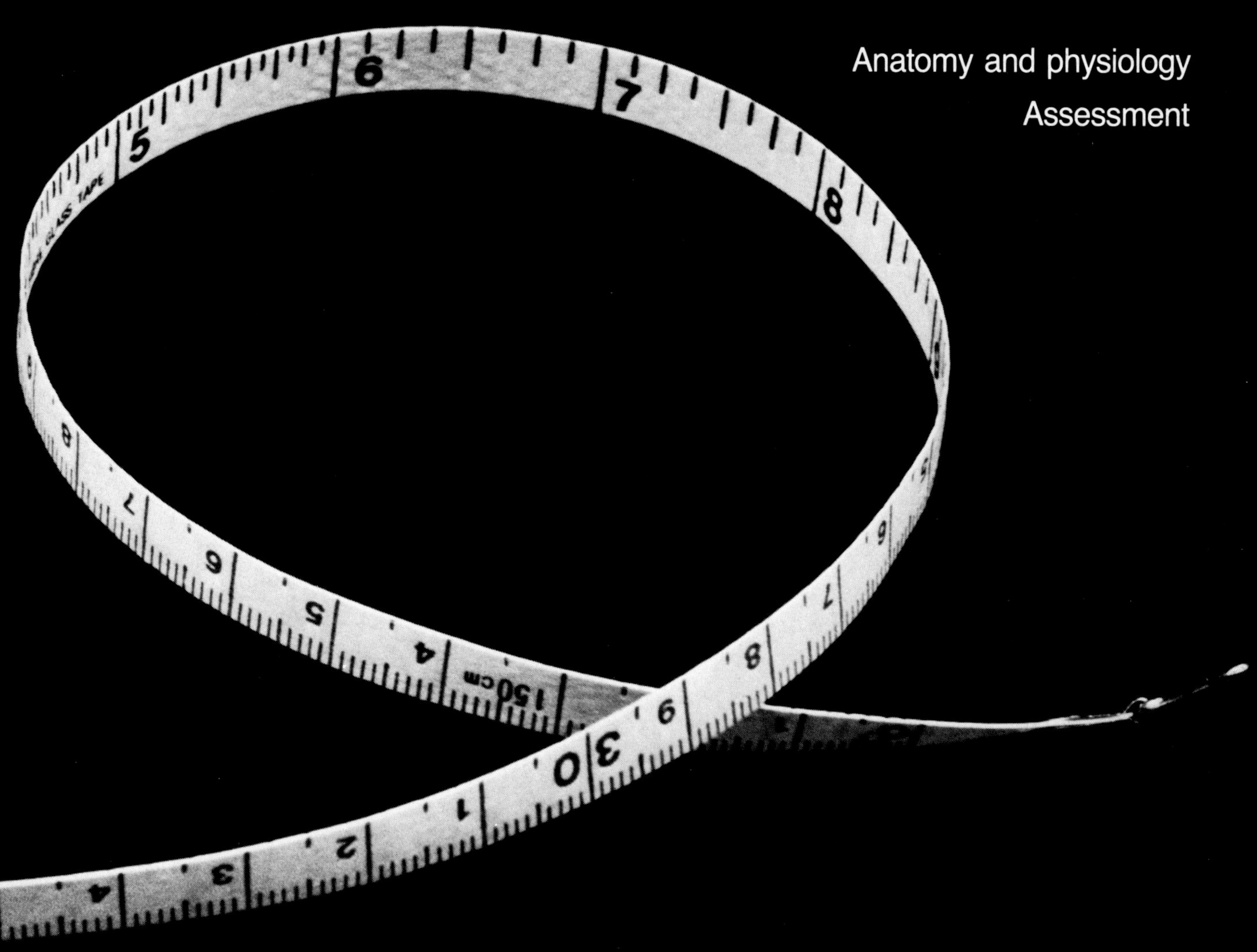

Anatomy and physiology

You probably studied the musculoskeletal system thoroughly during your nursing education. But, do you recall the various ways muscles contract to produce movement? Or the six types of synovial joints? Unless you're an orthopedic nursing specialist, you probably don't. To refresh your memory, we'll quickly review musculoskeletal anatomy and physiology.

Study the text and illustrated charts on the following pages. Then, you'll be better prepared to assess and care for any orthopedic problems.

Understanding the musculoskeletal system

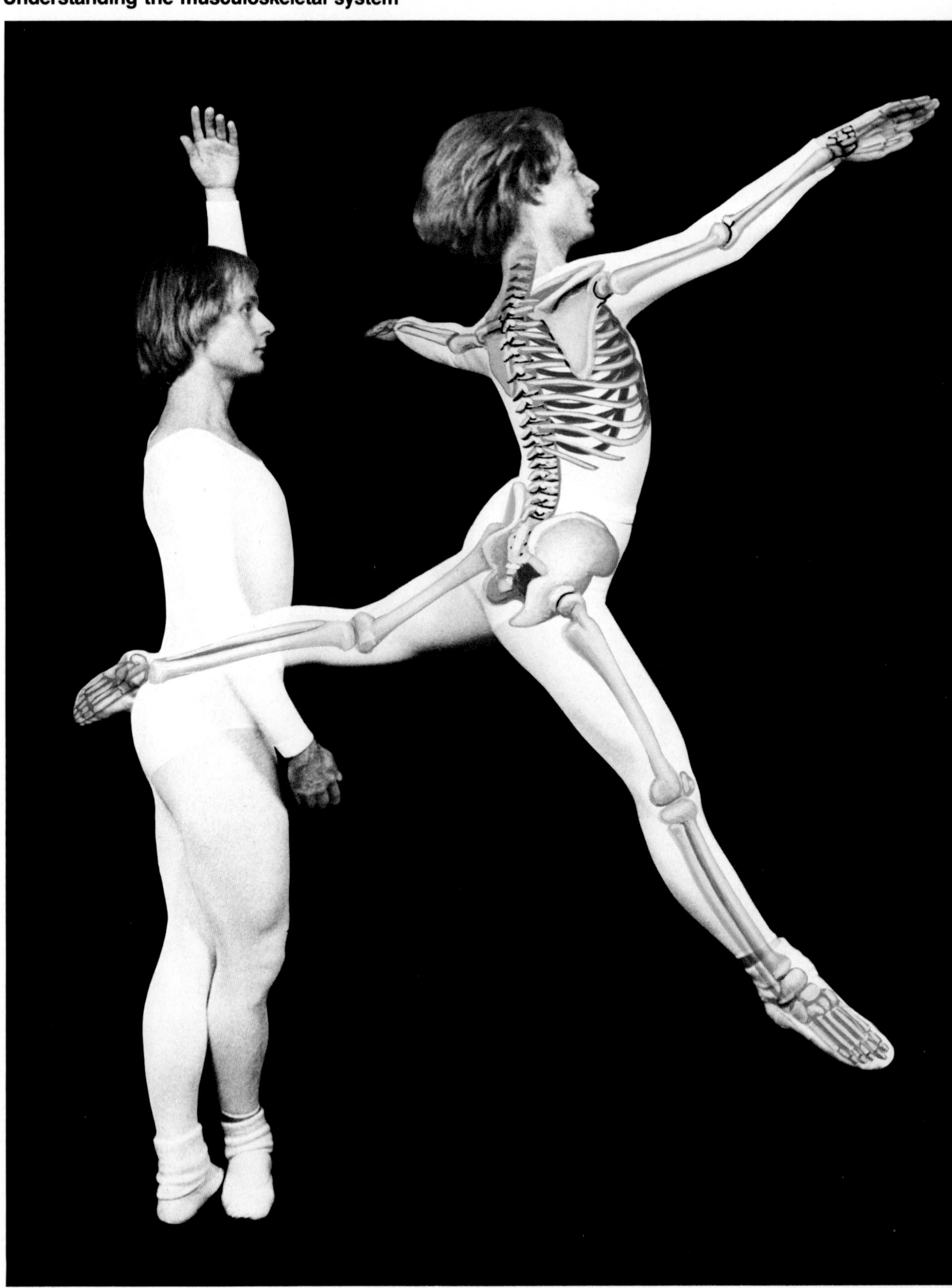

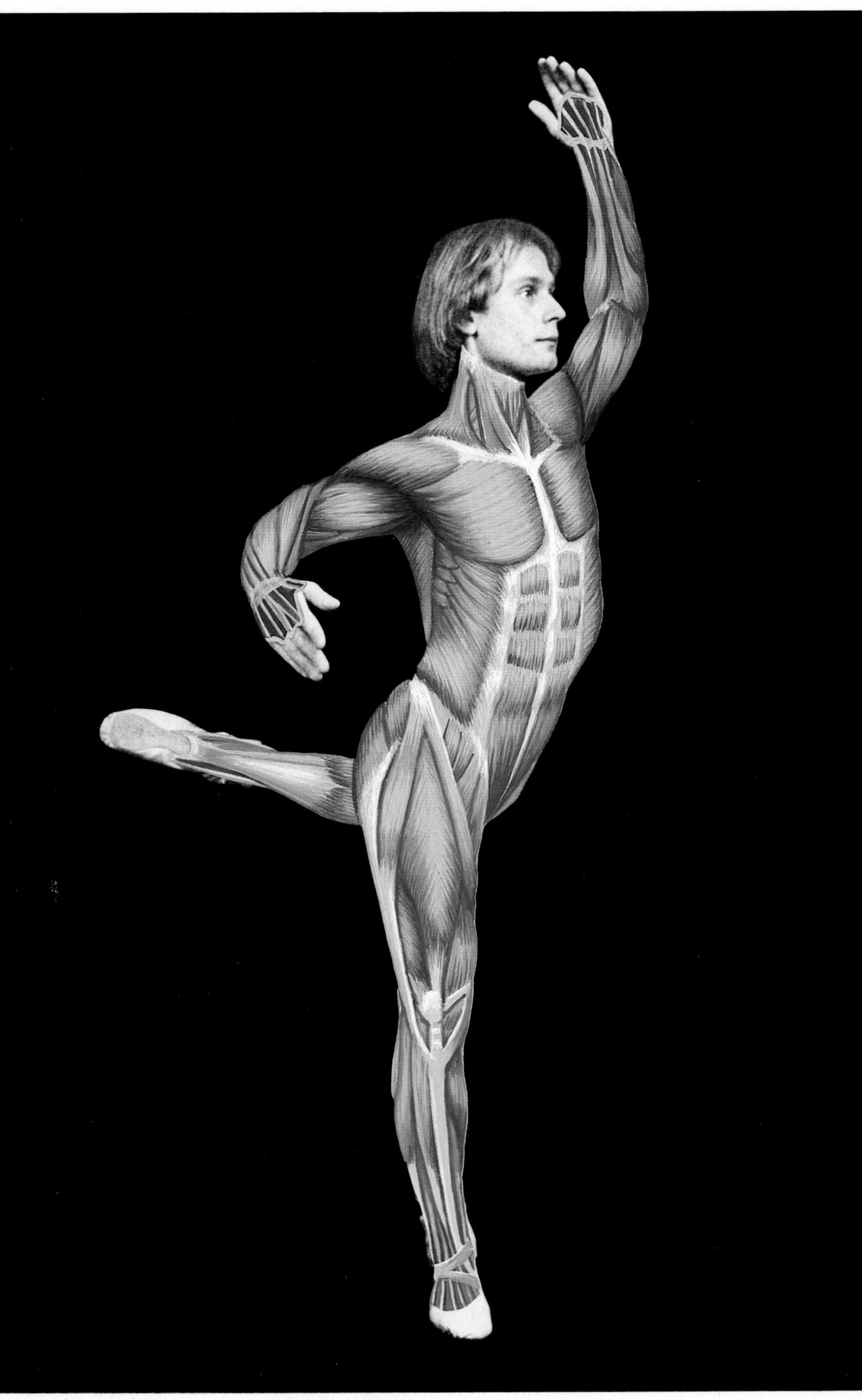

A person's musculoskeletal system provides both support and movement for his body. Standing erect, walking, and running all depend on musculoskeletal development and coordination.

The musculoskeletal system includes 206 bones, which are connected at joints. The joints are held together by ligaments and cushioned by cartilage. Tendons attach muscles to the bones.

To understand the system better, study the following illustrated explanation.

Bones: The body's framework

The bones serve as the body's framework or skeleton. The human skeleton consists of two main divisions: axial (the body's upright structure), and appendicular (the body's appendages). Eighty bones make up the axial skeleton, which includes the skull, vertebral column, and ribs. The appendicular skeleton includes 126 bones which form the arms, hips, and legs.

The skeletal system features four major bone types. Their names reflect their shapes: *long* (for example, the femur), *short* (for example, the carpals), *flat* (for example, the scapulae), and *irregular* (for example, the vertebrae).

Included among the irregular bones are sesamoid and wormian bones. Sesamoid bones, such as the patellae, occur in conjunction with tendons at points in the body where considerable pressure occurs. Wormian bones occur in cranial sutures.

In addition to providing support and allowing movement, bones perform three essential functions:

- They protect a person's vital organs, such as his brain, heart, and lungs.
- They store calcium and release it to the bloodstream, according to body requirements.
- They manufacture new blood cells in the red bone marrow.

How is an individual bone structured? A bone contains both nonliving and living components, organized in groupings called haversian systems (see illustration on following page). In each system, rigid material forms in layers called lamellae, creating the bone's matrix. Between these layers are small spaces, called lacunae, that house living cells. Tissue fluid circulates through this rigid, calcified material to the bone cells by way of microscopic passageways called canaliculi. The tissue fluid supplies food and oxygen and removes cell wastes.

Anatomy and physiology

Understanding the musculoskeletal system continued

The fluid is routed to the canaliculi from the haversian canal, a small vessel located at the center of each cylindrical lamella. The haversian canal, in turn, receives fluid from Volkmann's canal, a channel that communicates with the periosteum at the bone's surface. The periosteum is a vascularized membrane layer that covers the bone, except at joint surfaces.

Bone tissue formation, called osteogenesis, is a continuous process. Tissue formation occurs outside the bone, while tissue destruction (resorption) begins inside the bone and moves outward. In childhood and adolescence, growth outpaces disintegration. During early adulthood, the two processes balance each other. However, between age 35 and 40, bone resorption begins to overtake the body's tissue production, hollowing out and weakening bone structure. This deterioration makes aging bones more vulnerable to damage from any stress, such as bending or impact.

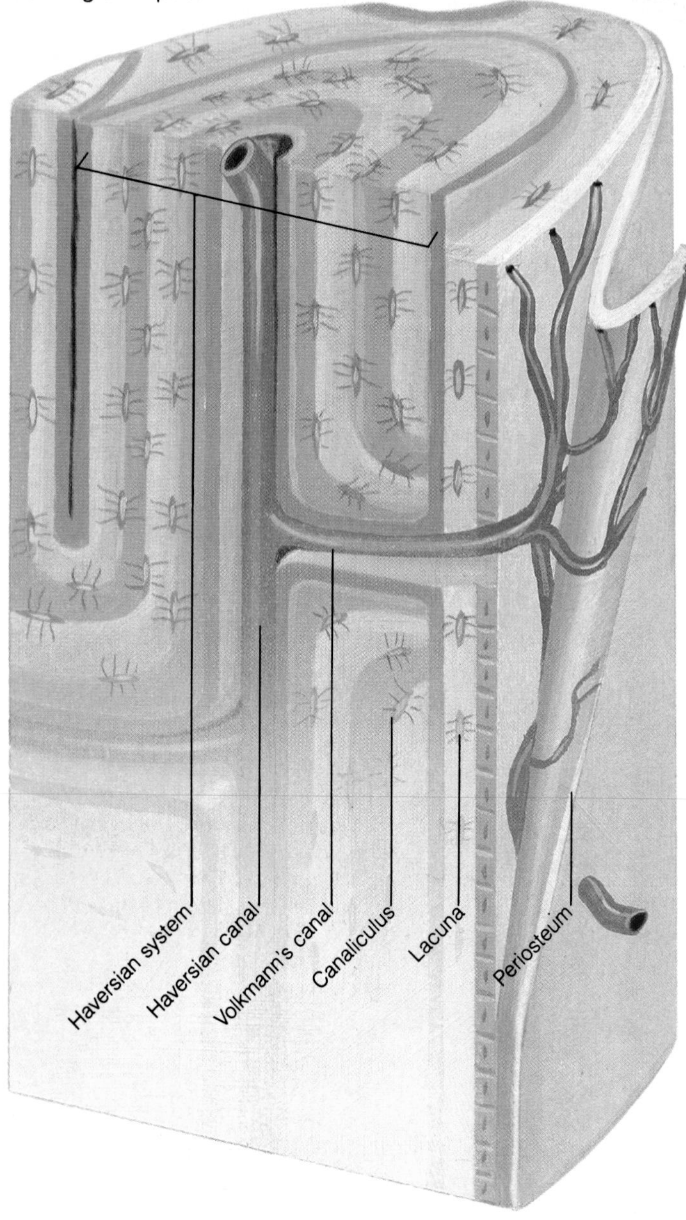

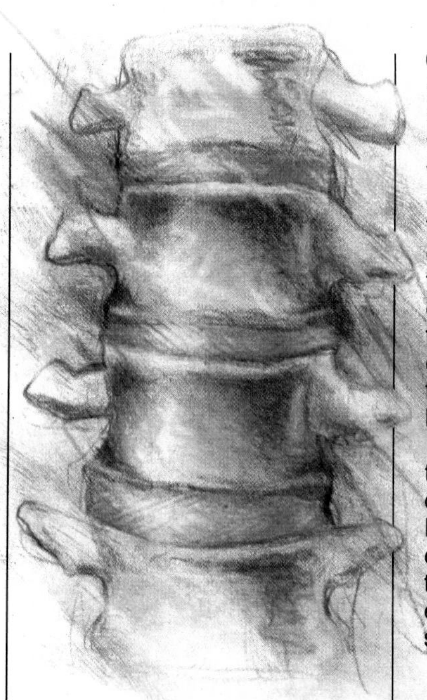

Cartilage: Three types

Cartilage contains a firm gel substance in its matrix, which gives it more flexibility than bone. Cartilage is avascular, so nutrient tissue fluids reach its cells (called chondrocytes) by diffusing through the matrix gel from capillaries in the cartilage's fibrous covering (perichondrium), or from the synovial fluid (for cartilage covering a bone's joint surface).

The musculoskeletal system contains three types of cartilage (see illustrations). **Fibrocartilage** has the greatest tensile strength of the three. It occurs in the intervertebral discs and in the symphysis pubis.

Elastic cartilage possesses firmness and elasticity. It occurs in the external ear and the eustachian tube.

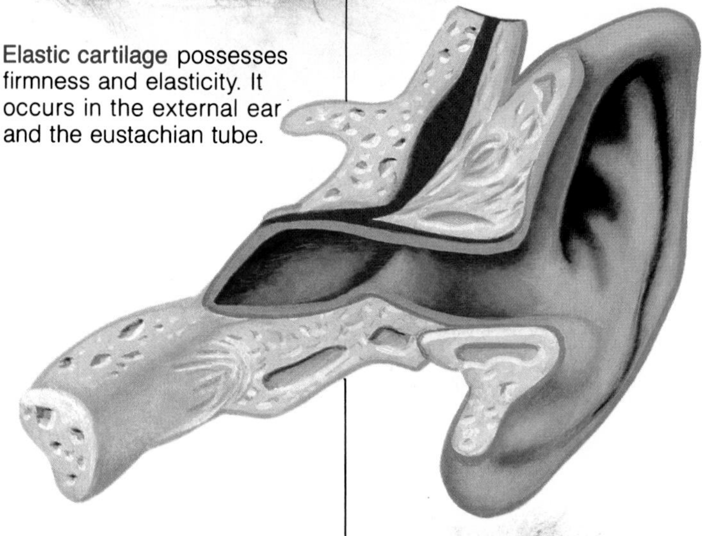

Hyaline cartilage, the most common cartilage type, is firm, yet slightly flexible. It cushions most of the joints to help soften any impact. Hyaline cartilage also occurs in part of the nasal septum, the larynx, the trachea, and the bronchial rings.

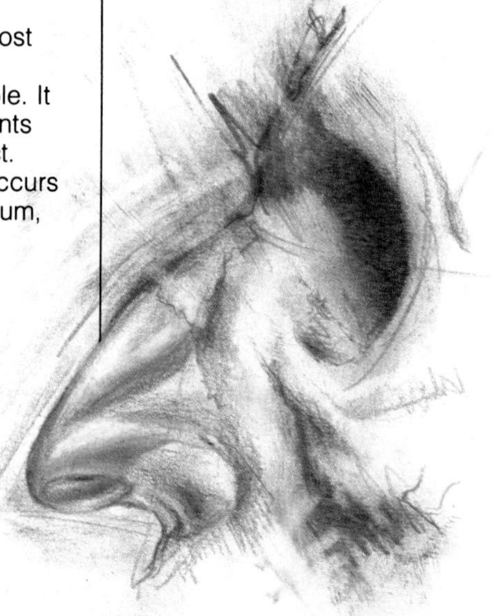

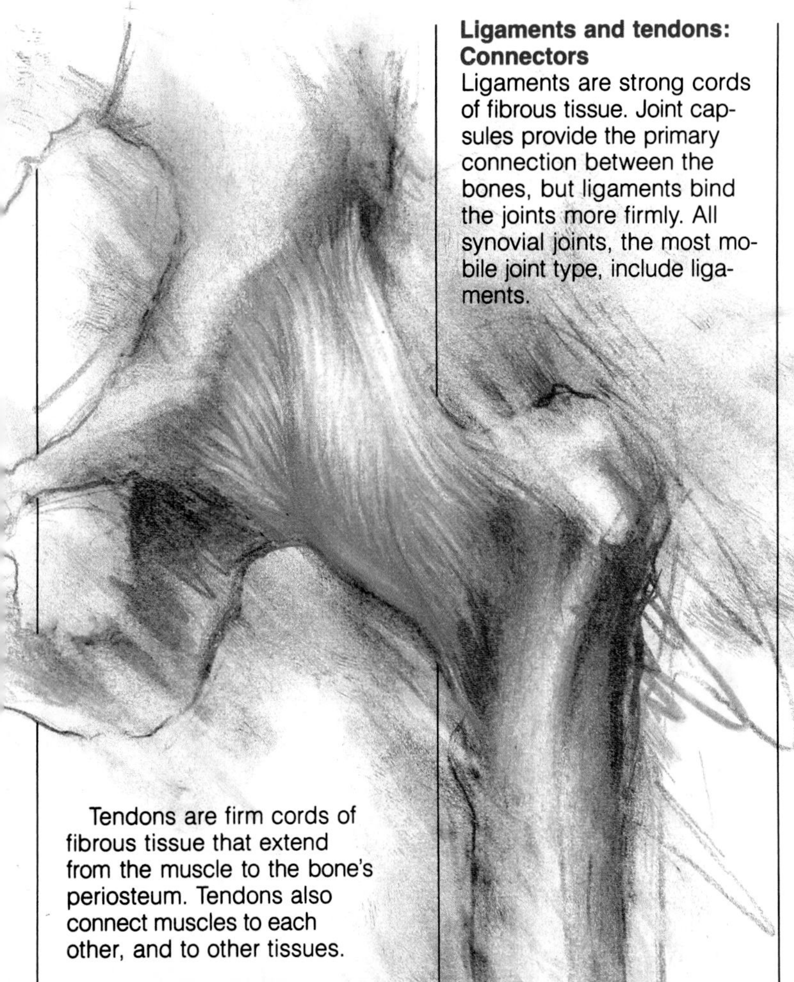

Ligaments and tendons: Connectors

Ligaments are strong cords of fibrous tissue. Joint capsules provide the primary connection between the bones, but ligaments bind the joints more firmly. All synovial joints, the most mobile joint type, include ligaments.

Tendons are firm cords of fibrous tissue that extend from the muscle to the bone's periosteum. Tendons also connect muscles to each other, and to other tissues.

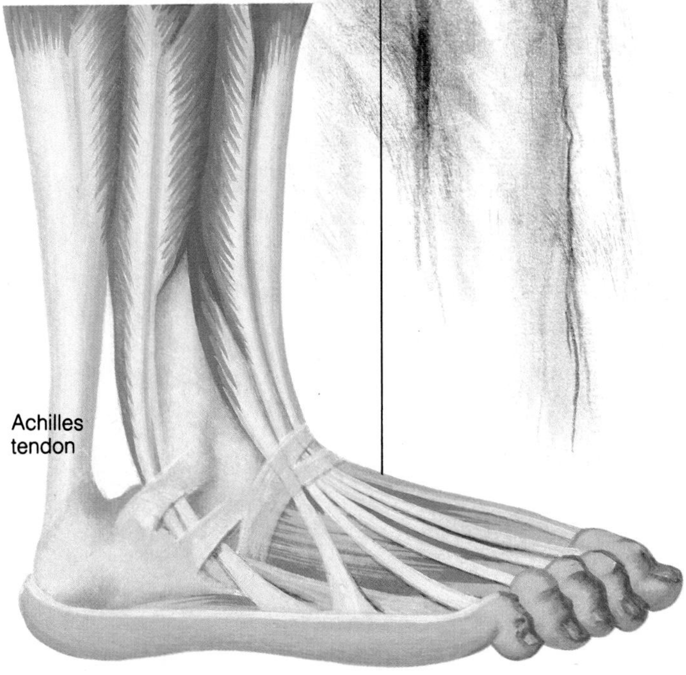

Achilles tendon

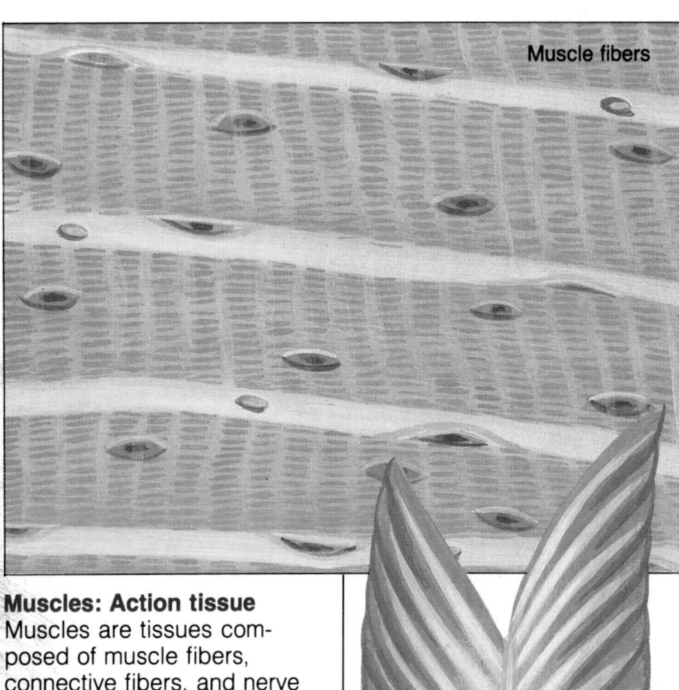

Muscles: Action tissue

Muscles are tissues composed of muscle fibers, connective fibers, and nerve fibers. They vary in size, shape, and arrangement, ranging from miniature strands, such as the stapedius muscle of the middle ear, to large masses, such as the gluteus maximus in the buttocks.

Muscles can be long and tapered, short and blunt, triangular, quadrilateral, or irregular.

Muscle fiber arrangement varies. In some muscles, the fibers run parallel to the muscle's long axis. In others, the fibers are oblique and bipennate, like the feathers of a quill pen. In a third type, fibers curve out from a narrow attachment at the muscle's end to form a triangle.

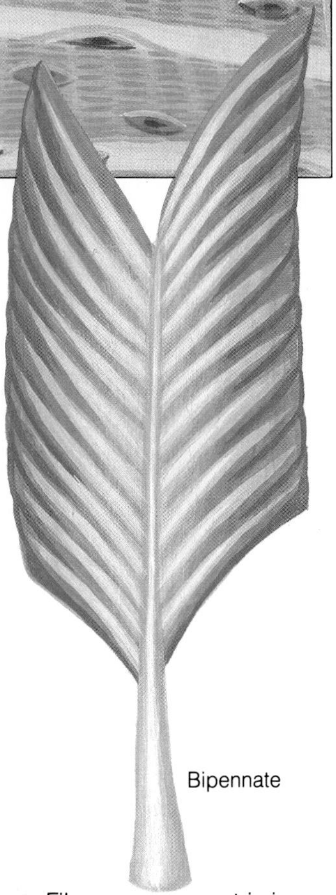

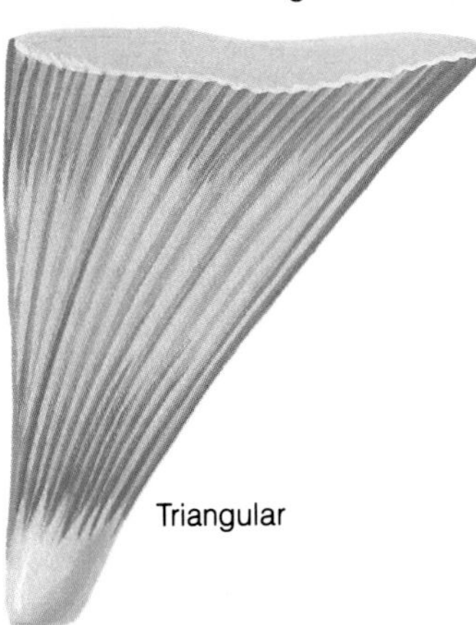

Bipennate

Fiber arrangement is important because of its relationship to a muscle's function. For example, a bipennate muscle can produce stronger contractions than other muscle types.

The muscles and skeleton work together to perform movement. The muscles contract to move bones, while the joints allow this movement to occur. For details, read the following pages.

Anatomy and physiology

Learning about joints

Joints are points of *articulation* (connection) between bones. Most joints allow movement between bones, permitting activities such as grasping and running. Others join bones firmly together, permitting little or no movement. The body's three basic joint types (fibrous, cartilaginous, and synovial) are shown in the first line of boxes. The next six boxes show different types of synovial joints.

Fibrous joints, composed of fibrous tissue, tightly connect the articular surfaces of two bones. Two types of fibrous joints exist: the suture and the syndesmosis. Sutures, which permit no movement, occur only in the skull. They unite rigid pieces of the skull to form a protective covering for the brain. A syndesmosis permits minimal movement between bones; for example, in the distal tibiofibular joint (see illustration).

Cartilaginous joints connect two bones with cartilage, allowing only slight movement. The pubic bone juncture is an example.

Synovial joints, the most common joint type, have the most complex structure and permit maximum mobility. These joints include: (a) joint capsule, (b) synovial membrane, (c) articular cartilage, and (d) synovial cavity.

B
A
C
D
C

Synovial gliding joints allow only limited motion—back and forth or sideways. Gliding joints occur between most carpal and metacarpal bones of the hand.

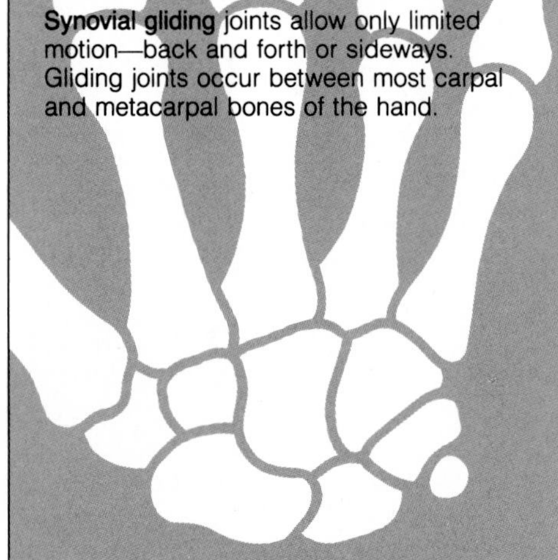

Synovial condyloid (ellipsoidal) joints allow movement in two perpendicular planes (biaxial movement). In this type of joint, an oval-shaped condyle (rounded projection on a bone) fits into an elliptical socket. An example is the juncture between the radius and the carpal bones in the wrist.

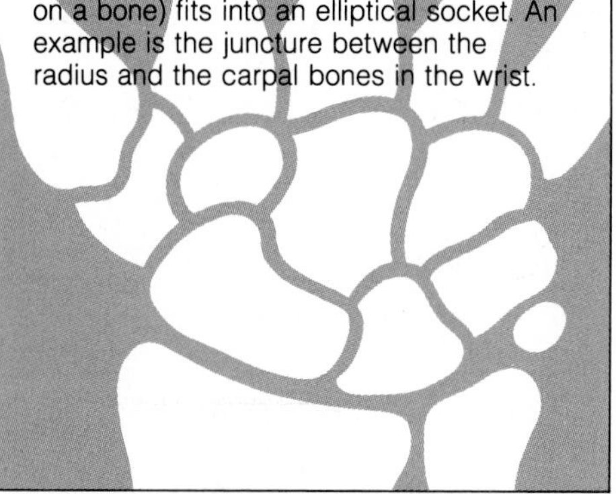

Synovial saddle joints also allow biaxial movement. The name's derived from the saddle-shaped surfaces of the articulating bones. An example is the juncture between the thumb's metacarpal bone and the wrist's trapezium carpal bone.

Synovial pivot joints permit one bone to pivot on its axis in the arch of a second bone. A person's body has two of these joints: between the first two cervical vertebrae (the atlas and the axis, shown here) and between the proximal ends of the radius and the ulna (the two forearm bones).

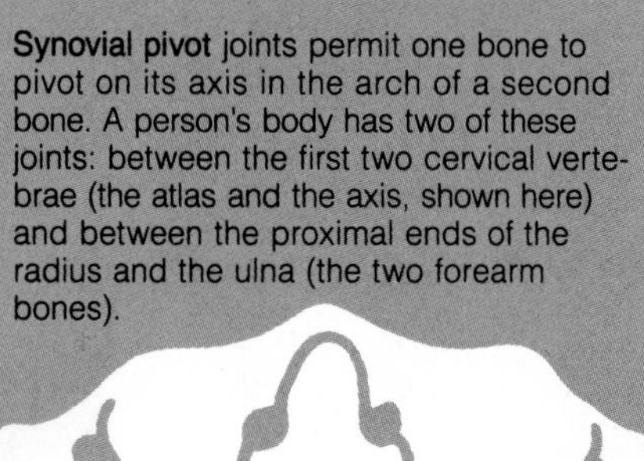

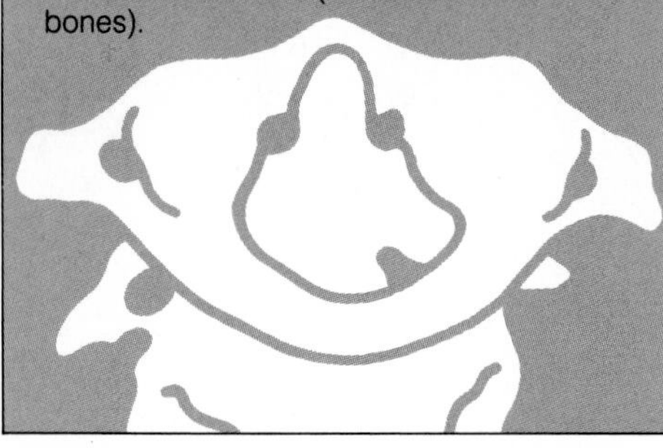

Synovial hinge joints work like hinges on a door. The elbow's one example of this kind of joint.

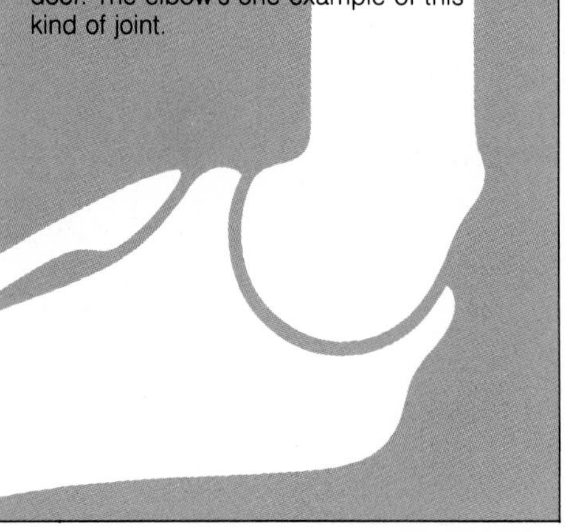

Synovial ball-and-socket joints permit the greatest range of motion. In these joints, the ball-shaped head of one bone fits into the concave socket of another bone. An example is the hip joint.

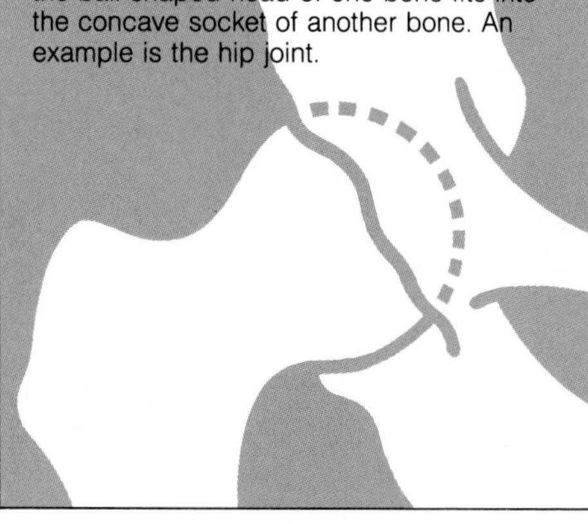

Understanding skeletal muscle movement

As you know, skeletal muscles contract to control a person's posture, help maintain his normal body temperature, and initiate movement. To contract, all skeletal muscles require some form of stimulation, either internal, from motor neurons; or external, from stimuli such as electricity, heat, or injury.

Skeletal muscles usually retain some of their tautness, even at rest. This muscle tone, prompted by nerve impulses from the spinal cord, helps maintain body posture. Muscles also contract in the following eight ways, most of which produce movement:

- *Isotonic* contractions shorten muscle length while maintaining muscle tension, generating movement.
- *Isometric* contractions tighten a muscle by increasing muscle tension without shortening the muscle. Although isometric contractions produce no direct movement, most body movements involve a combination of isometric and isotonic contractions.
- *Twitch* contractions are quick, jerky reactions to a single stimulus. Following the stimulation, the muscle shortens for a fraction of a second. After it reaches its shortest point, the muscle relaxes and returns to normal size. The entire contraction usually lasts less than a tenth of a second.
- *Tetanic contractions* are serial, continuous contractions, in which individual contractions can't be distinguished. They occur in response to a bombardment of the muscle by rapid, successive stimuli. If the excessive stimulation ceases abruptly, the incomplete tetanic contractions may convert to a normal contraction.
- *Treppe (or staircase) phenomenon* is a series of increasingly stronger twitch contractions occuring in response to repeated stimuli of constant intensity. After a period of repeated contractions, however, the relaxation phase of the muscle contraction diminishes and eventually disappears, leaving the muscle partially contracted. This phenomenon has a practical application in an athlete's warm-up exercises.
- *Fasciculation* is an abnormal contraction visible through the skin as a slight ripple. It occurs after motor neuron destruction, from spontaneous neural impulses transmitted by the dying nerve fibers.
- *Fibrillation,* an abnormal contraction in which individual fibers contract in an unsynchronized way, produces muscle flutter but no effective movement. It occurs in denervated muscle fibers after motor neurons have been destroyed.
- *Convulsions* are abnormal, violent, rhythmic contractions and relaxations of muscle groups.

Performing movement

To perform a particular movement, skeletal muscles sheathing two adjacent bones exert pull on those bones. To do so, some muscles will contract isometrically and some will contract isotonically. The degree of contraction necessary depends on the strength required to carry out the movement.

Skeletal muscles almost always work in a group. *Prime mover* muscles initiate bone movement, *antagonist* muscles relax during movement, and *synergist* muscles either directly assist prime movers or steady another part of the participating muscle-bone system to allow for more effective movement.

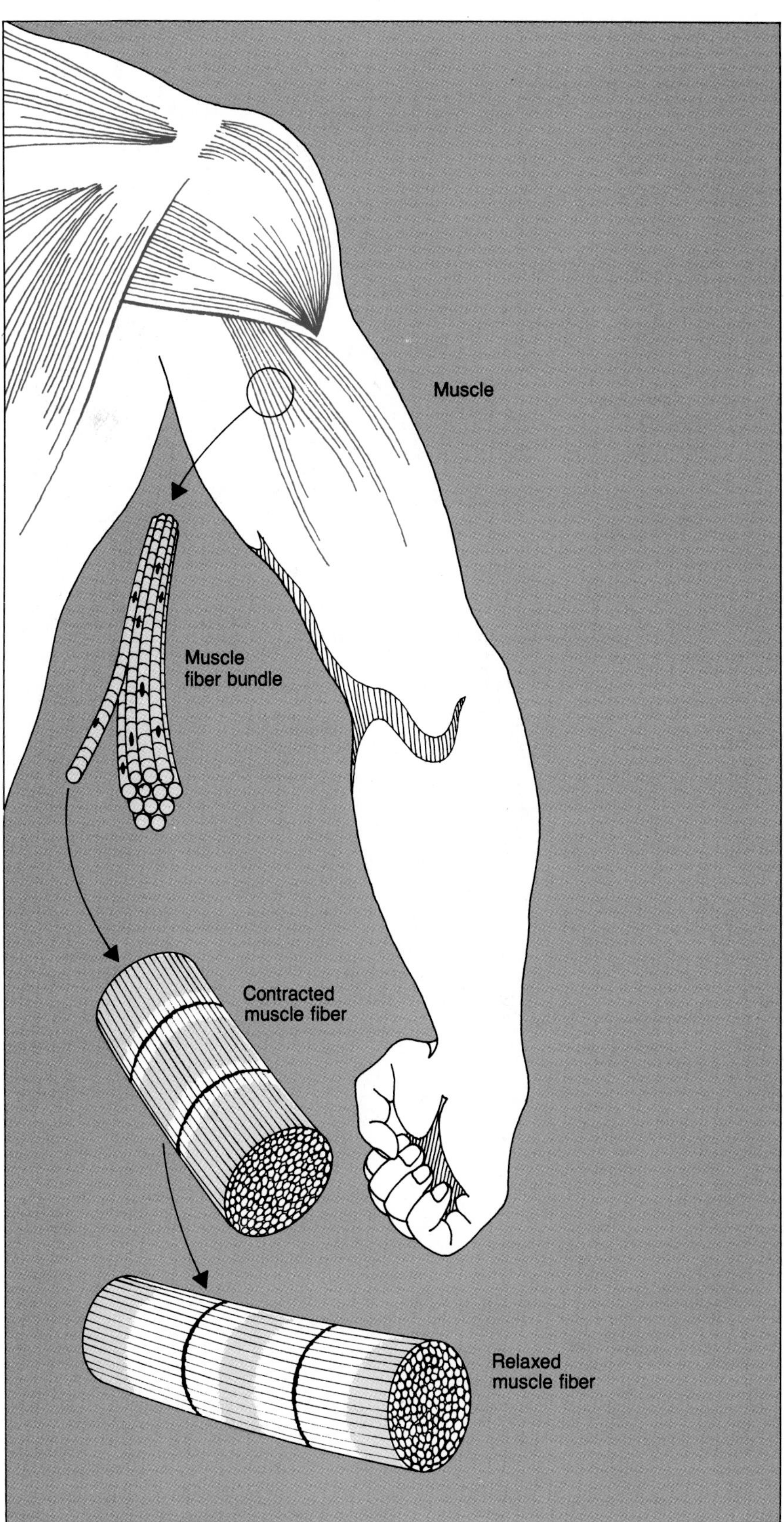

Anatomy and physiology

Reviewing joint movement

Muscle contractions move a person's bones at the joints. Are you familiar with the different kinds of joint movement? If not, review the following terms:

Flexion *decreases* the angle between the anterior surfaces of articulating bones. Bending your head forward is a common example of this movement.

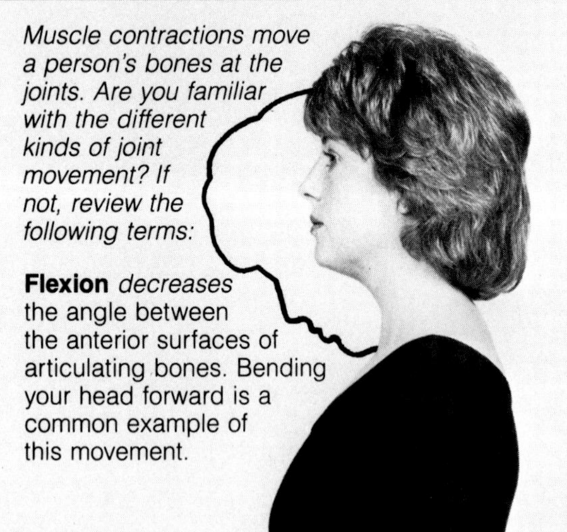

Abduction, when seen from the front, moves a bone in the appendicular skeleton *away* from the body's midline. Spreading your arms outward at the shoulder demonstrates this movement. For parts of extremities, this term refers to movement of the *part* away from the *extremity's* axial line.

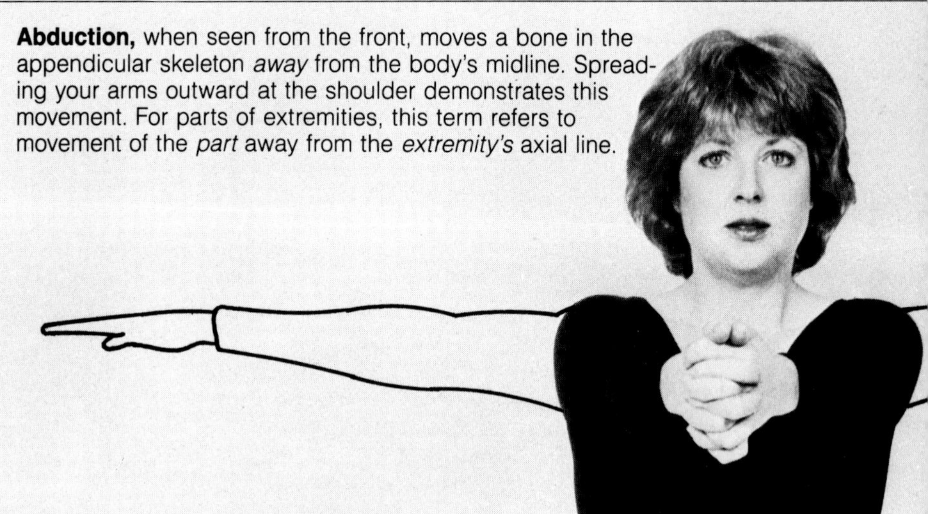

Extension *increases* the angle between the anterior surfaces of articulating bones. Extension returns a body part from the flexed position to its original (neutral) anatomical position. Straightening your head after flexion is a common example of this movement.

Hyperextension continues the act of extension beyond the original anatomical position; for example, when you look up toward the ceiling.

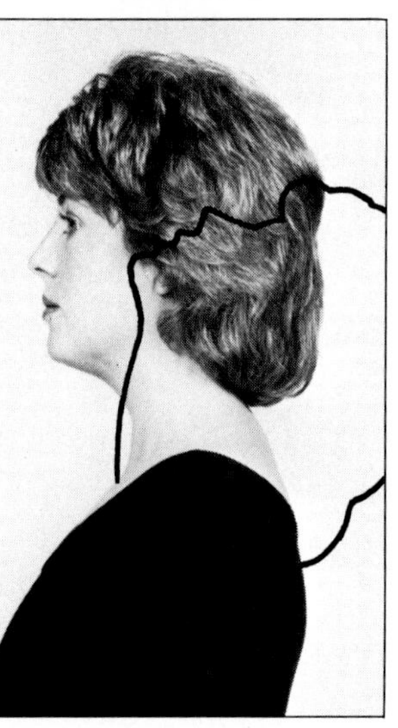

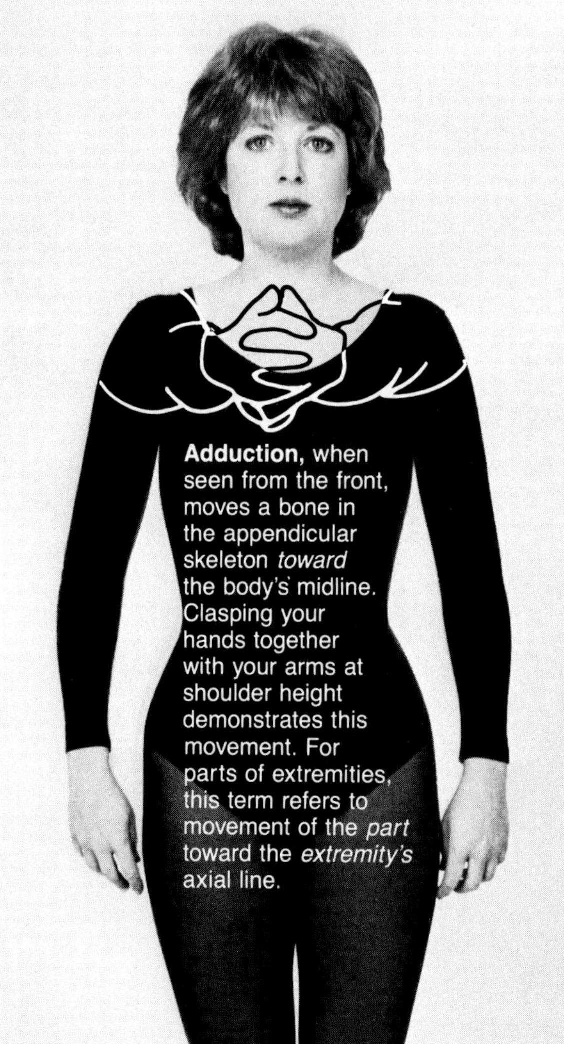

Adduction, when seen from the front, moves a bone in the appendicular skeleton *toward* the body's midline. Clasping your hands together with your arms at shoulder height demonstrates this movement. For parts of extremities, this term refers to movement of the *part* toward the *extremity's* axial line.

Rotation pivots the bone on its axis.

External rotation is motion around a central axis *away* from the midline; for example, moving your head from looking straight ahead to looking to the side.

Internal rotation is motion around a central axis *toward* the midline; for example, moving your head from looking to the side to looking straight ahead.

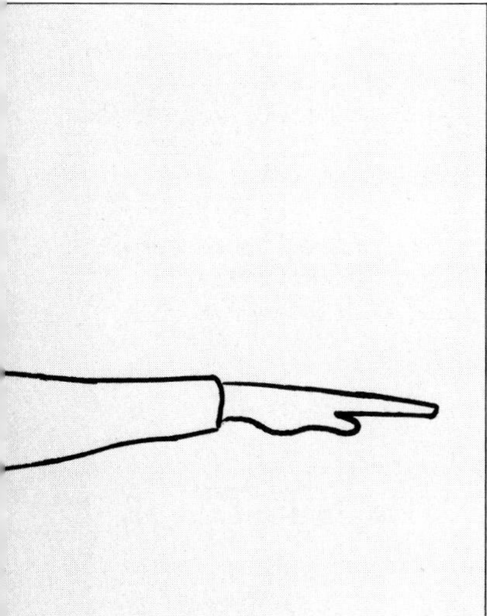

Circumduction combines a number of movements to cause the distal end of a bone to describe a circle. One example is dropping your head to one shoulder, then to your chest, then to the other shoulder, and finally backwards.

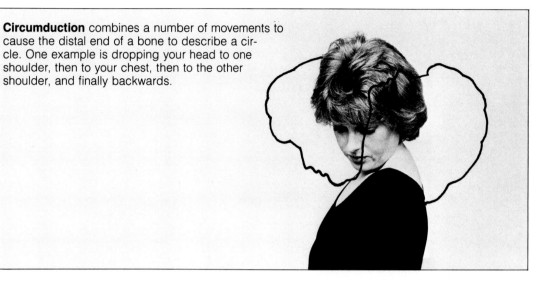

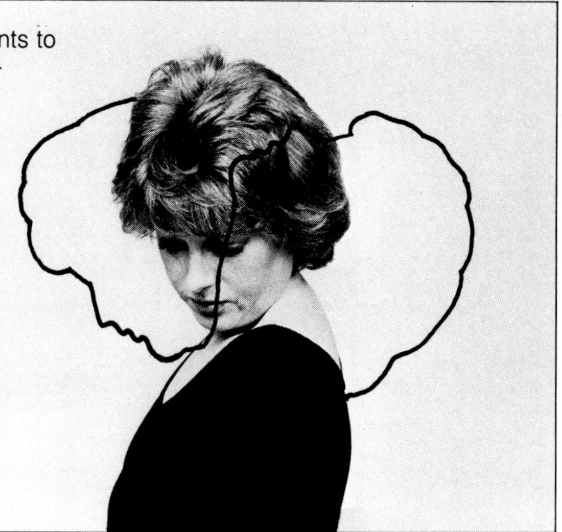

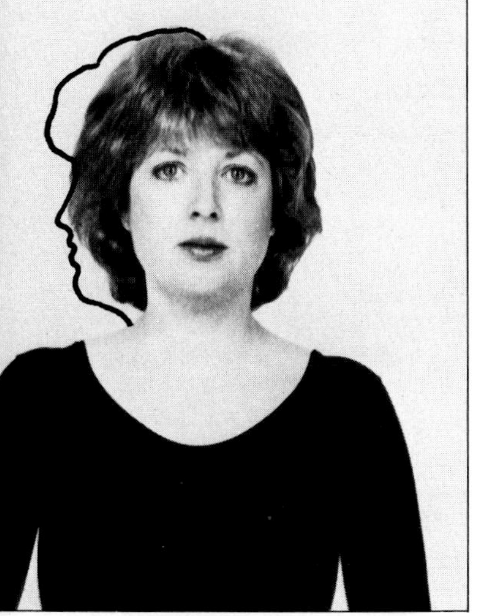

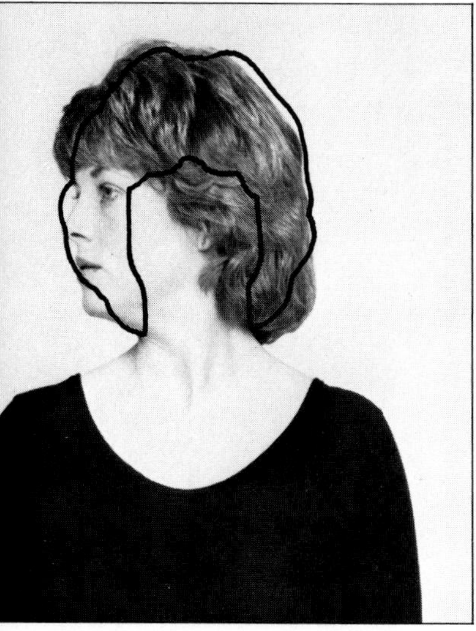

Inversion turns an extremity or part of an extremity *inward* toward the body's midline. Moving the sole of your foot inward is an example of this movement.

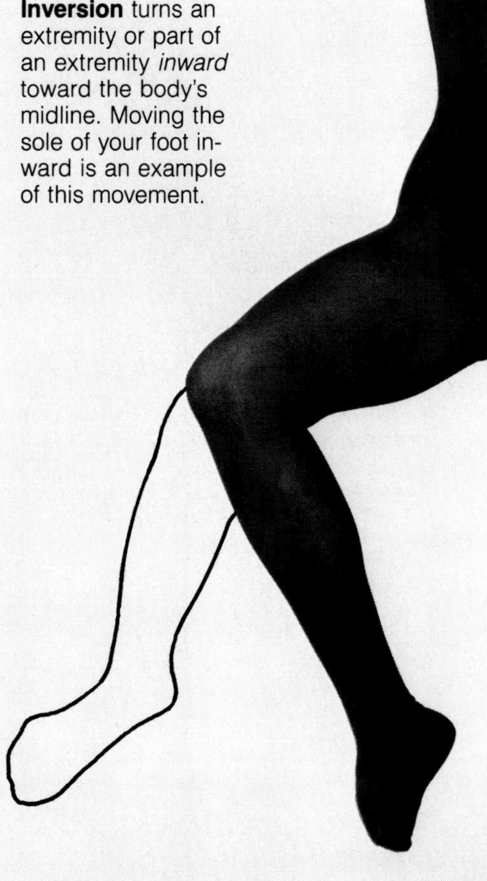

Eversion turns an extremity or part of an extremity *outward* from the body's midline; for example, moving the sole of your foot outward.

Pronation turns the palm, foot, or body's front toward the floor.

Supination turns the palm, foot, or body's front toward the ceiling.

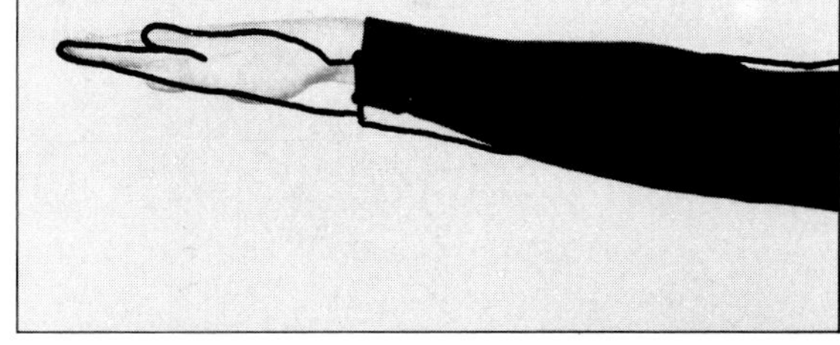

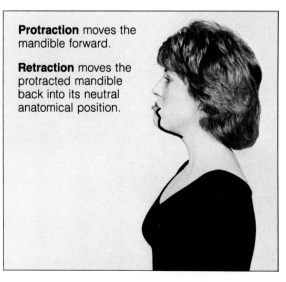

Protraction moves the mandible forward.

Retraction moves the protracted mandible back into its neutral anatomical position.

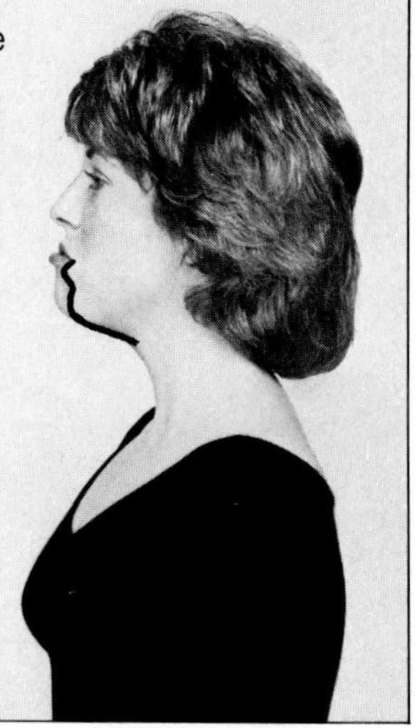

Anatomy and physiology

Bones and joints: A nurses' guide

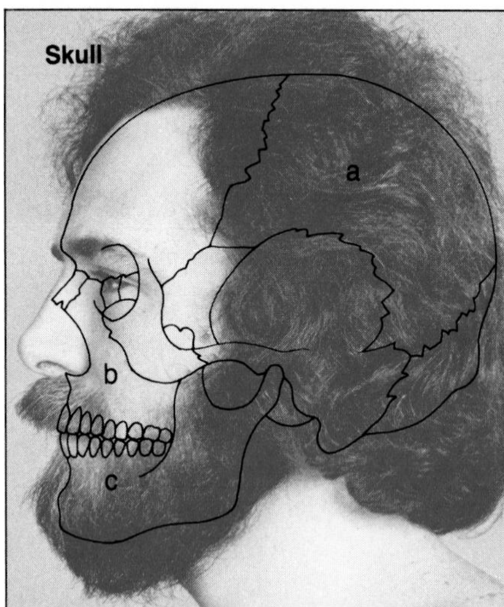

Description

- Twenty-eight bones form the skull, which is divided into the cranium, face, and internal earbones.
- The frontal, occipital, temporal, sphenoid, and two parietal bones form the cranium (a).
- Two maxillae bones (b) form the main portion of the face below the frontal bone.
- The mandible (c), the largest, strongest facial bone, forms the lower jaw.
- The U-shaped hyoid bone (actually located in the neck region) is suspended by ligaments from the styloid processes of the temporal bones. The hyoid bone supports the tongue. It is the body's only nonarticulating bone.

Joint types

- *Sutures.* Parietal bone articulates with frontal bone, occipital bone, and temporal bones. Parietal bones articulate with each other.
- *Condyloid (ellipsoidal).* The mandible articulates with the temporal bone (the only moving joint in the skull). The skull articulates with the first cervical vertebra, the atlas.

Range of motion

- Suture permits no movement.
- Condyloid joints between mandible and temporal bones allow these two bones to separate and join together again, (as in talking or chewing). These joints also allow minimal protraction, retraction, and rotation. Condyloid joint between skull and atlas allows flexion (about 70°); extension (head is straight in neutral position); and hyperextension (about 35°).

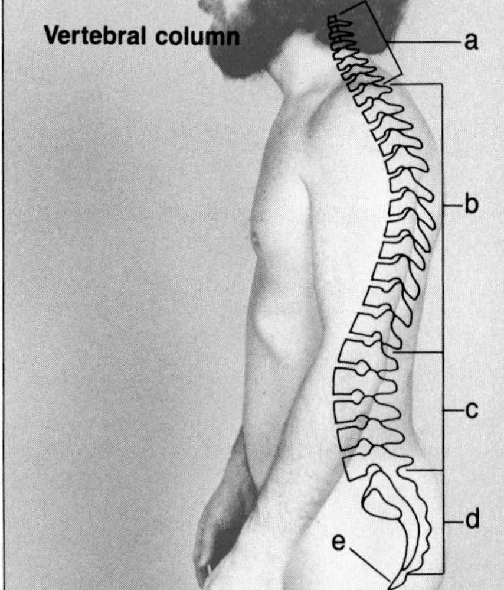

Description

- The vertebral column consists of 26 separate bones connected to form a flexible column. When viewed from the side, the vertebral column has four curves: cervical (a), thoracic (b), lumbar (c), and sacral (d).
- The seventh cervical vertebra's long spinous process can be seen and felt through the skin at shoulder level.
- The thoracic vertebrae possess facets for articulation with ribs.
- The sacrum, the fusion of five lower vertebrae, articulates with the hip bones. The three lowest vertebrae on the spinal column are fused to form the coccyx (e), which articulates with the sacrum.
- The spinal cord passes through the vertebral column from the atlas to the second lumbar vertebra, where it terminates in a cone of nerves with peripheral nerve characteristics.

Joint types

- *Cartilaginous.* Main bodies of vertebrae are cushioned by intervertebral discs.
- *Gliding.* Articular processes of vertebrae connect with each other.
- *Pivot.* The first cervical vertebra, the atlas, articulates with the second cervical vertebra, the axis.

Range of motion

- Gliding joints permit flexion (90°) of entire spinal column; hyperextension (30°); lateral deviation (30°); and rotation (45 °).
- Pivot joint allows rotation of head from side to side (about 90° to each side from midline).

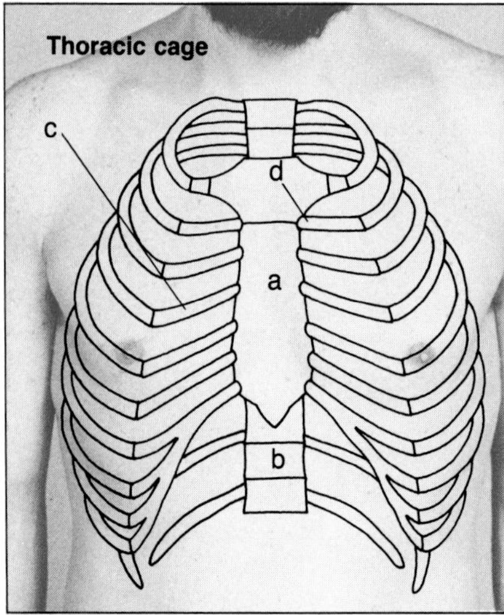

Description

- The thoracic cage includes sternum (a), thoracic vertebrae (b), ribs (c), and costal cartilage (d).
- The sternum has three parts: manubrium (top), gladiolus (body), and xiphoid process (bottom).
- Twelve pairs of ribs form a person's rib cage, each articulating with two vertebrae in his back. Only the top seven pairs articulate with the sternum in front. In the next three pairs, each rib connects with the one above it, in front. The remaining two pairs connect only to the vertebrae.
- A costal cartilage connects each of the top seven rib pairs with the sternum. The cartilage allows thoracic cage expansion and contraction during respiration.

Joint types

- *Gliding.* Ribs articulate with vertebrae.

Range of motion

- *Gliding joints* permit minimal gliding movement between ribs and vertebrae and between sternum and clavicles.

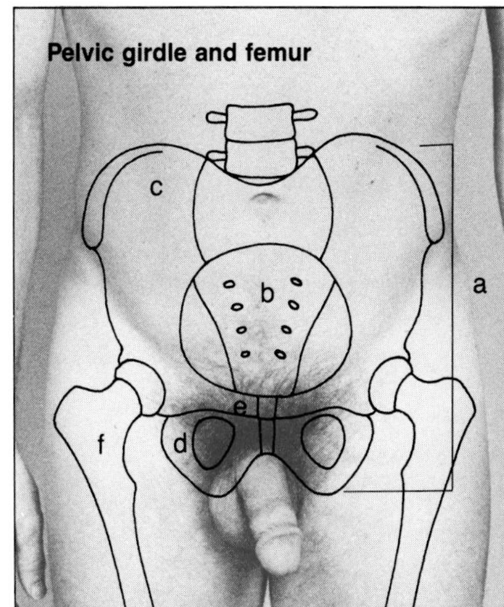

Description
- The pelvic girdle consists of two hip (innominate) bones (a), the sacrum (b), and the coccyx.
- Each hip bone is divided into the ilium (c), ischium (d), and symphysis pubis (e).
- The femur (f), the longest and strongest bone in the body, extends from the hip to the knee.
- The iliofemoral ligament, one of the body's strongest, firmly connects the femur's proximal end to the ilium.

Joint types
- *Cartilaginous.* Pubic portions of the innominate bones fuse to form the symphysis pubis.
- *Gliding.* Iliac portions of the innominate bones fuse with the sacrum.
- *Ball and socket.* The femur's head fits into the acetabulum socket of the innominate bone.

Range of motion
- Ball and socket joint allows flexion (about 120°); extension (leg is straight in neutral position); minimal hyperextension (42°); abduction (about 65°); adduction (about 30°); cross-adduction (about 45°); internal rotation (varies between 45° and 60°); external rotation (about 90°); and circumduction (about 360°). Gliding and cartilaginous joints allow no movement except expansion during childbirth.

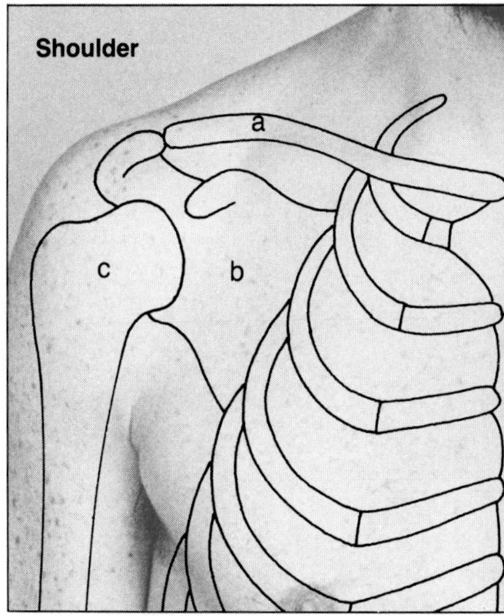

Description
- The clavicle (a) articulates with the sternum proximally, and with the scapula distally.
- The scapula (b) is attached to the thoracic cage by a sheath of strong muscles.
- The humerus (c), composed of a head, body, and condyle, extends from shoulder to elbow.
- The scapula and upper extremity are suspended primarily by two strong ligaments, the trapezoid and the conoid, which extend from the clavicle's underside to the scapula's coracoid process.
- The scapulohumeral articulation is one of the body's most unstable joints.

Joint types
- *Ball and socket.* The humerus' head fits in the scapula's glenoid fossa.
- *Gliding.* The clavicle's distal end articulates with the scapula at the acromioclavicular joint. Sternum articulates with clavicle's proximal end at sternoclavicular joint.

Range of motion
- Movement is possible between scapula and thorax, and between scapula and humerus. However, the acromioclavicular joint and the sternoclavicular joint allow only minimal movement.
- Normal scapulothoracic movement includes: the shoulder shrug; forward rotation (about 180°); backward rotation (about 180°); adduction (between 45° and 90° forward and about 45° backward).
- Ball and socket joint allows abduction (about 180°); adduction (about 75°); cross-adduction (about 45°); flexion (about 180°); extension (shoulder straight in neutral position); hyperextension (about 65°); circumduction (about 360°); internal rotation (about 90°); and external rotation (about 90°).

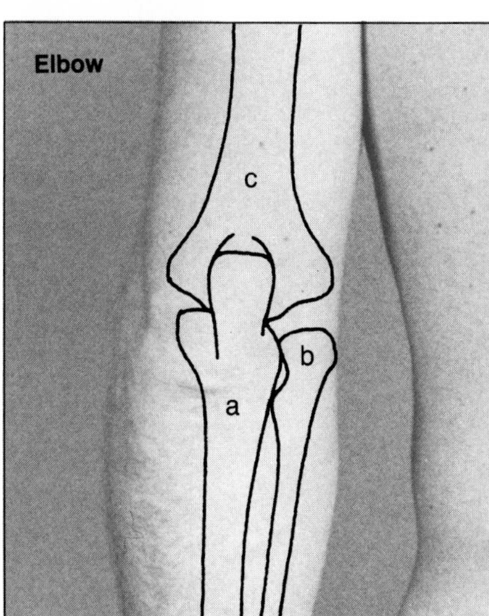

Description
- The elbow includes two joints: the humero/ulnar/radial articulation and the radial/ulnar articulation.
- The ulna (a), the larger of the two lower arm bones, runs from elbow to wrist on the arm's lateral (outer) side.
- The radius (b), the smaller of the two lower arm bones, runs from elbow to wrist on the arm's medial (inner) side.
- The articulation of the humerus (c) and the ulna's proximal surface (called the olecranon) possesses great stability.

Joint types
- *Hinge.* Humerus articulates with ulnar olecranon. Humerus articulates with head of radius.
- *Pivot.* Head of radius articulates with proximal radial notch of ulna.

Range of motion
- Hinge joints allow flexion (about 135°) and extension (elbow is straight in neutral position).
- Pivot joint allows supination (about 90°) and pronation (about 80°).

Anatomy and physiology

Bones and joints: A nurses' guide continued

Wrist

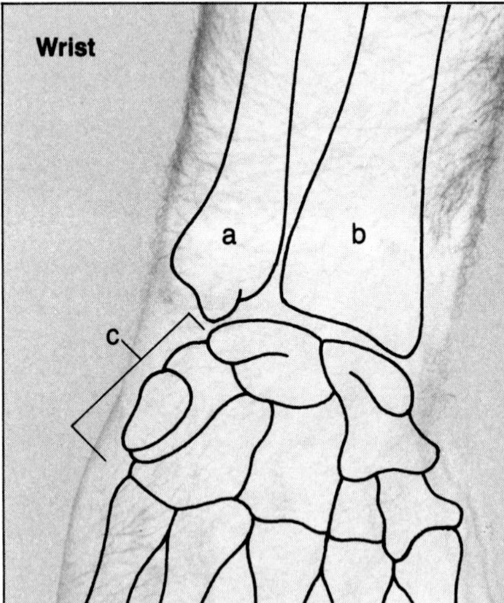

Description
- Distal end of radius (a) articulates with distal end of ulna (b) to make up proximal portion of wrist joint.
- Eight carpal bones (c), firmly bound together by ligaments, make up the wrist proper.
- The radius articulates with the proximal row of carpals (the distal portion of the wrist joint).

Joint types
- *Pivot.* Radius connects with radial notch of ulna.
- *Condyloid.* Scaphoid, lunate, and triquetral carpals articulate with the radius and the ulna.
- *Gliding.* Carpals articulate with each other.

Range of motion
- Pivot joints allow supination (about 150°) and pronation.
- Condyloid joints allow palmar flexion (about 90°); extension (wrist is straight in neutral position); and hyperextension (called dorsiflexion; about 75°).
- Gliding joints allow minimal flexion, extension, adduction, and abduction.

Hand and fingers

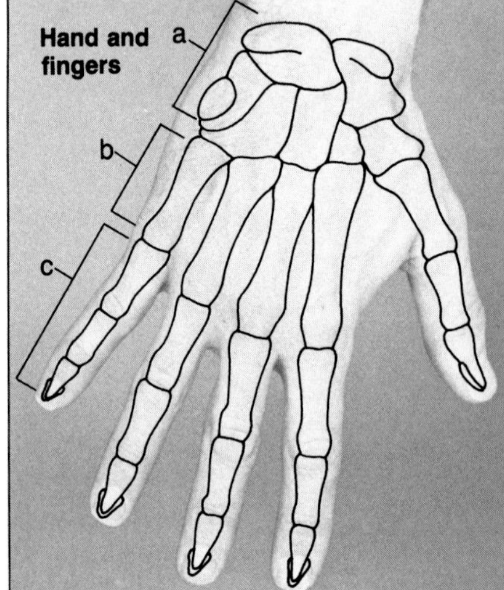

Description
- Hand and fingers include the eight carpals that make up the wrist proper (a), the five metacarpals of the palm (b), and the twelve phalanges of the fingers (c).
- Four of the metacarpal bones articulate with the first phalanx in each finger.
- Each finger contains three phalanges.

Joint types
- *Gliding.* Wrist carpals articulate with each other. Carpals articulate with metacarpals.
- *Condyloid.* Metacarpals articulate with phalanges.
- *Hinge.* Phalanges articulate with each other.

Range of motion
- Gliding joints allow minimal palm and wrist flexion, extension, adduction, and abduction.
- Condyloid joints allow flexion (approximately 95°); extension (wrist is straight in neutral position); hyperextension (about 12°); limited adduction (about 12°); limited abduction (about 12°); and circumduction (minimal circular movement).
- Hinge joints allow flexion (about 90°), and extension (fingers are straight in neutral position).

Thumb

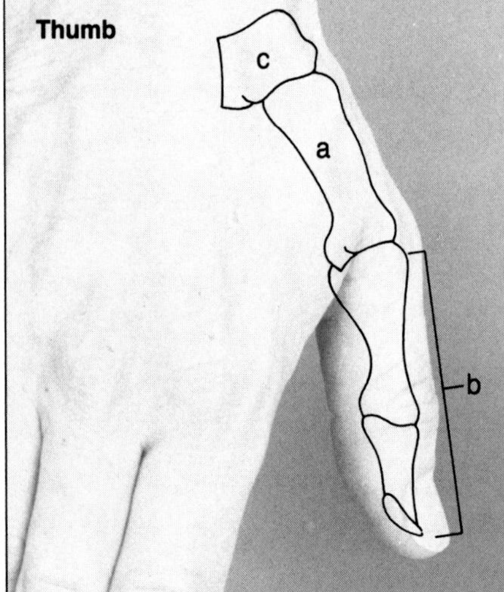

Description
- The thumb is composed of one metacarpal bone (a) and two phalanges (b).

Joint types
- *Saddle.* Proximal end of thumb's metacarpal articulates with wrist's trapezium carpal (c).
- *Condyloid.* Metacarpal articulates with proximal phalanx.
- *Hinge.* Phalanges articulate with each other in distal thumb.

Range of motion
- Saddle joint allows flexion (about 90°); extension (thumb is straight in neutral position); hyperflexion (about 45°); abduction (about 50°); adduction (about 50°); and opposition (thumb moves toward fingers).
- Condyloid joint allows flexion (about 45°); extension (thumb is straight in neutral position); adduction (about 35°); abduction (about 45°); and circumduction (minimal circular motion).
- Hinge joint allows flexion (about 90°), and extension (distal thumb is straight in neutral position).

Knee and fibula

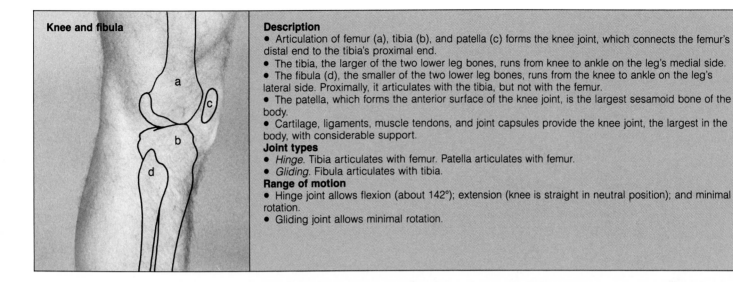

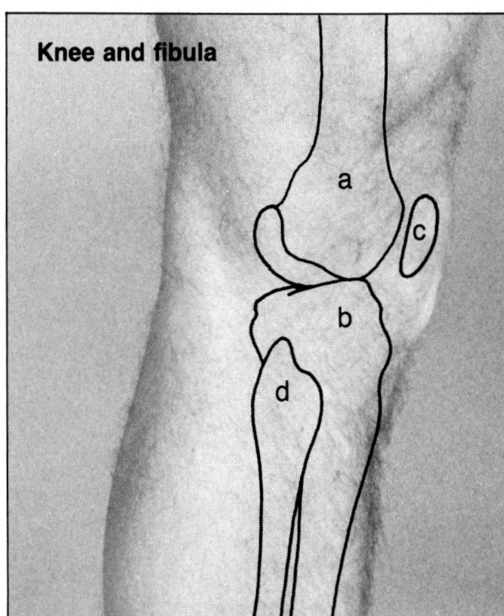

Description
- Articulation of femur (a), tibia (b), and patella (c) forms the knee joint, which connects the femur's distal end to the tibia's proximal end.
- The tibia, the larger of the two lower leg bones, runs from knee to ankle on the leg's medial side.
- The fibula (d), the smaller of the two lower leg bones, runs from the knee to ankle on the leg's lateral side. Proximally, it articulates with the tibia, but not with the femur.
- The patella, which forms the anterior surface of the knee joint, is the largest sesamoid bone of the body.
- Cartilage, ligaments, muscle tendons, and joint capsules provide the knee joint, the largest in the body, with considerable support.

Joint types
- *Hinge.* Tibia articulates with femur. Patella articulates with femur.
- *Gliding.* Fibula articulates with tibia.

Range of motion
- Hinge joint allows flexion (about 142°); extension (knee is straight in neutral position); and minimal rotation.
- Gliding joint allows minimal rotation.

Ankle

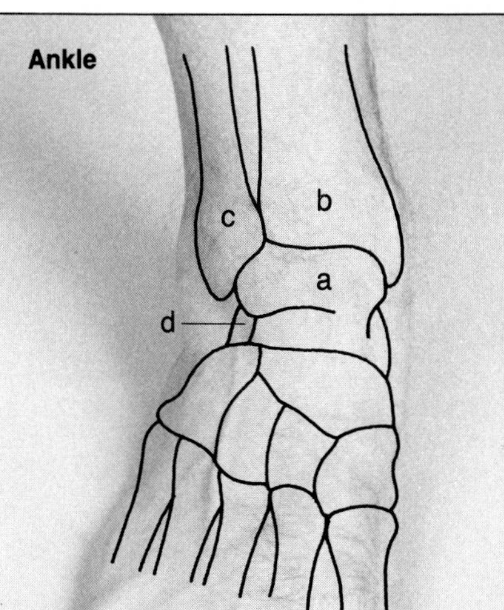

Description
- Articulation of (a) talus (ankle bone) with distal ends of tibia (b) and fibula (c), and with (d) calcaneus (heel bone).

Joint types
- *Hinge.* Talus fits into boxlike socket formed by projections of the tibia and the fibula.
- *Syndesmosis.* Tibia articulates with fibula.
- *Gliding.* Talus articulates with calcaneus bone.

Range of motion
- Hinge joint permits extension (normally, ankle is straight in neutral position); flexion (called dorsiflexion; about 10°); hyperextension (called plantarflexion; about 45°).
- Gliding joint allows inversion (about 20°), and eversion (about 20°).

Foot

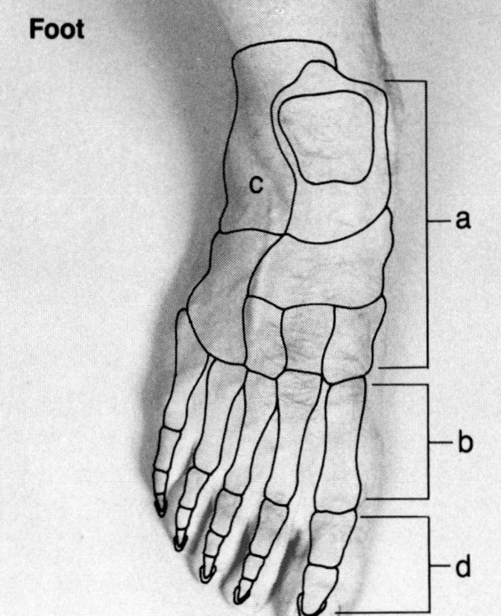

Description
- Foot bones are arranged to form springy, weight-bearing arches lengthwise and crosswise. Ligaments, muscles, and tendons support the arches.
- The innermost five tarsals (a) and three metatarsals (b) form the medial longitudinal arch. The outermost two tarsals and metatarsals form the lateral longitudinal arch. The metatarsals and the distal row of tarsals form the transverse arch.
- The calcaneus bone (c) forms the heel.
- Two phalanges (d) make up the big toe; three phalanges make up each of the small toes.

Joint types
- *Gliding.* Tarsals articulate with each other. Tarsals articulate with metatarsals.
- *Condyloid.* Metatarsals articulate with phalanges.
- *Hinge.* Phalanges articulate with each other.

Range of motion
- Gliding joints permit minimal flexion, extension, adduction, and abduction.
- Condyloid joints permit flexion (about 45°); extension (normally, toe is straight in neutral position); hyperextension (about 90°); adduction (about 20°); and abduction (about 20°).
- Hinge joints allow flexion (about 90°), and extension (normally, toe is straight in neutral position).

Assessment

How familiar are you with orthopedic assessment procedures? Do you know how to perform a complete step-by-step assessment? For example, do you know how to evaluate your patient's muscle power?

Also, do you know what signs and symptoms indicate a fracture? Or, how to detect neurovascular damage associated with fractures? Do you know the difference between a strain, sprain, and dislocation? Or how to identify your patient's musculoskeletal deformity?

In this section, we use easy-to-follow charts, illustrations, and photos to help you assess your patient's orthopedic problem. Remember, performing a quick and accurate assessment helps you provide the care your patient requires.

Learning about fractures

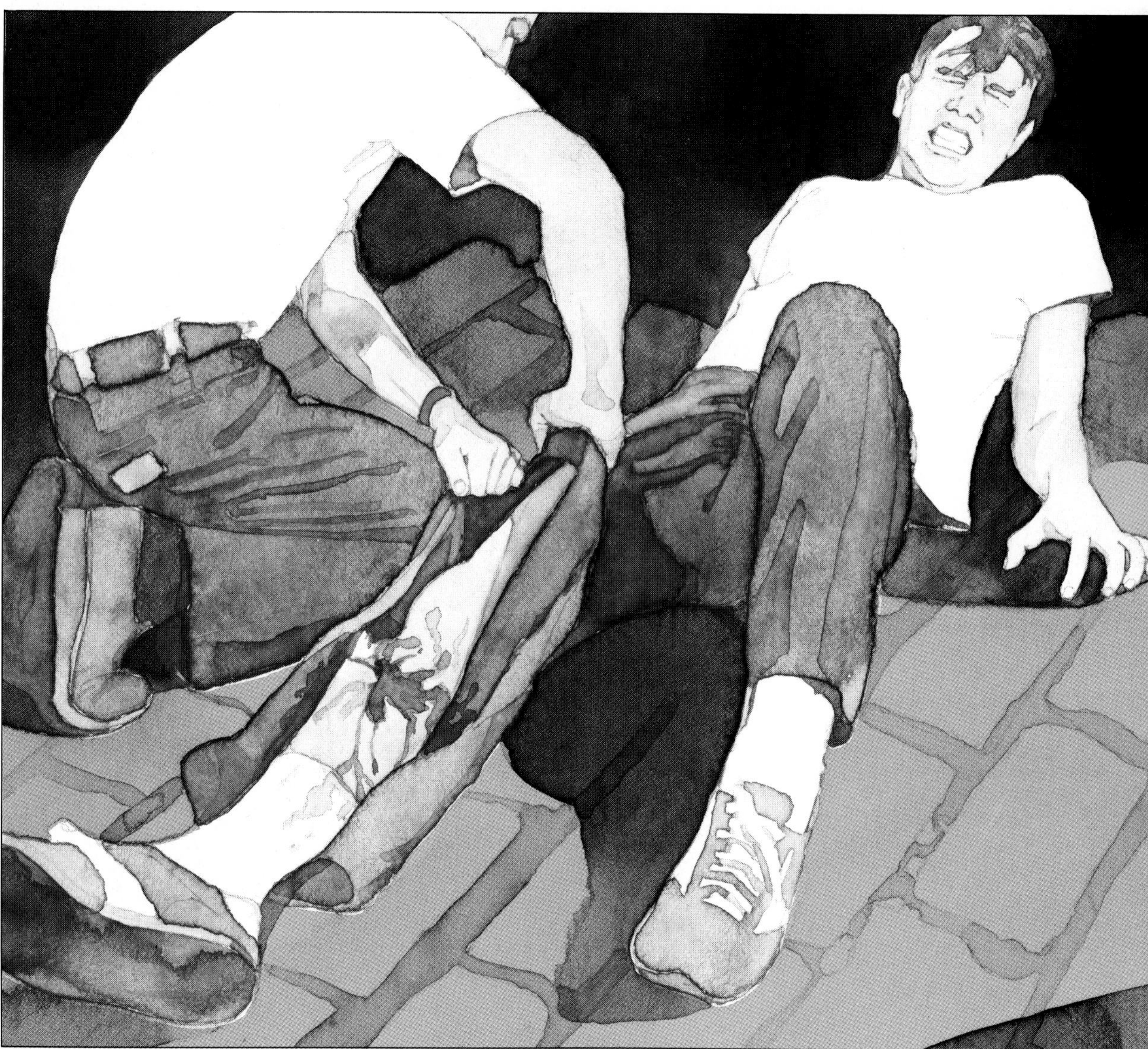

Fractures, though not usually life threatening, are painful disruptions of a bone's normal continuity. Fractures are associated with automobile, home, sports, and on-the-job accidents, as well as with aging's degenerative changes. The specific causes can be categorized as follows:

- *Direct force,* in which the bone absorbs more stress than it can endure from impact with a solid object; for example, when a person is hit with a baseball bat.
- *Twisting force* (torsion), in which severe twisting of a limb breaks the bone at a site different from where the force was actually applied. This type of fracture occurs most often in the legs (for example, in a skiing accident). Twisting force often causes a spiral fracture.
- *Powerful muscle contractions,* in which highly developed muscles contract so violently that muscle tears from bone, sometimes pulling a small piece of bone with it; for example, in a grand mal seizure.
- *Fatigue or stress,* in which the bone breaks after repeated stress. This phenomenon is associated with soldiers, who may break foot bones during prolonged marching.
- *Pathologic decay,* in which bones are weakened by disease (for example, osteoporosis), and become susceptible to fracture from the slightest movement.

Direction of the force causing a fracture determines the direction of the fracture line. See the illustrations at right for terms describing the fracture line's direction in relation to the affected bone's longitudinal axis.

Fractures are divided into two major categories: *closed* (simple; bone does not break through skin) and *open* (compound; one or both broken bone ends protrude through or communicate with a wound at the fracture site). They are also classified according to the direction of the fracture line, the fracture's proximity to a joint, and the condition of the broken bone. Also, fractures affecting specific bones may be named after the doctor who first identified them. (See the chart on the following page.)

Fractures in adults usually sever both the periosteum and cortical tissue, completely splitting the bone. This is called a *complete* fracture. Children frequently experience *incomplete* fractures, which only partially break the bone.

Any of these classification terms can be used in combination to better describe the break's location and severity. For example, an open-complicated-complete-oblique fracture describes an injury in which the bone has broken at an angle and completely snapped, with either one or both broken ends protruding through or communicating with the wound site. Also, the fracture has injured surrounding nerves and blood vessels, causing additional complications.

Are you familiar with some common fracture types? If not, study the following X-rays and descriptions. But, remember, these are only a few examples.

Direction of a fracture line

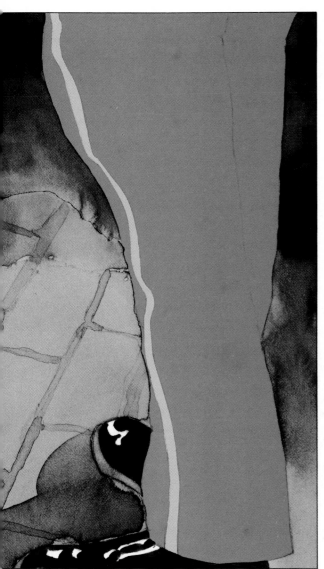

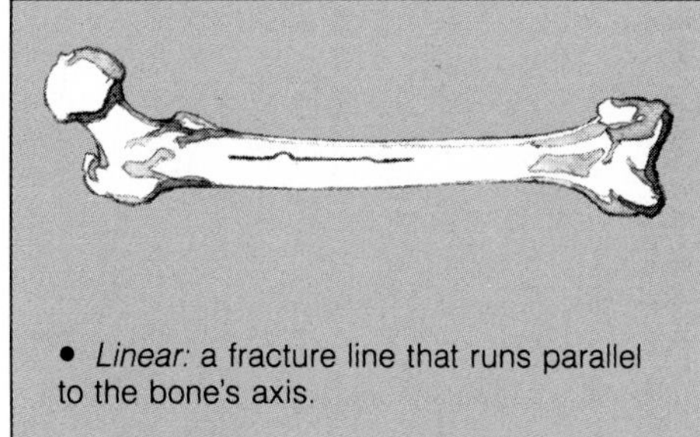

• *Linear:* a fracture line that runs parallel to the bone's axis.

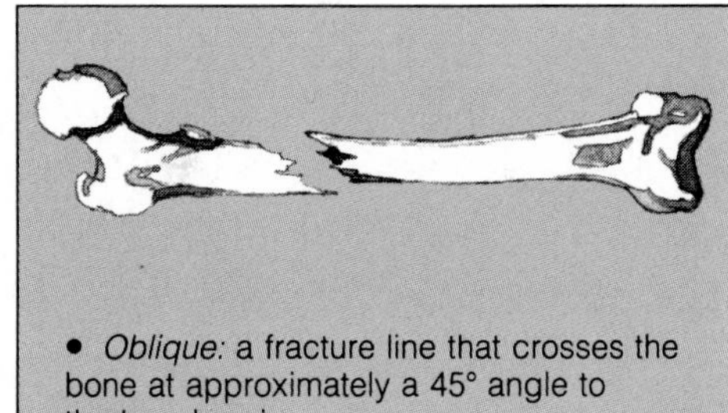

• *Oblique:* a fracture line that crosses the bone at approximately a 45° angle to the bone's axis.

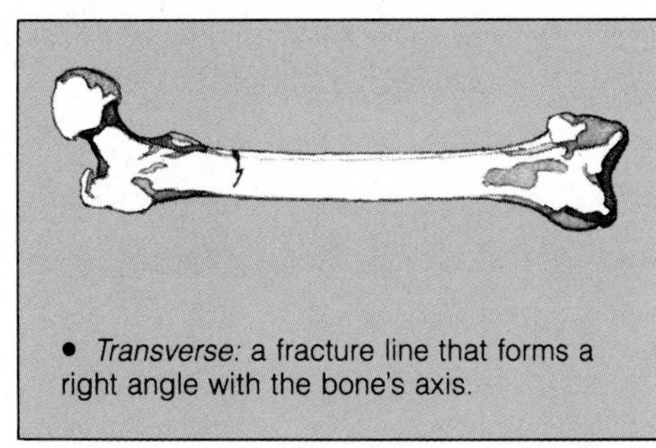

• *Transverse:* a fracture line that forms a right angle with the bone's axis.

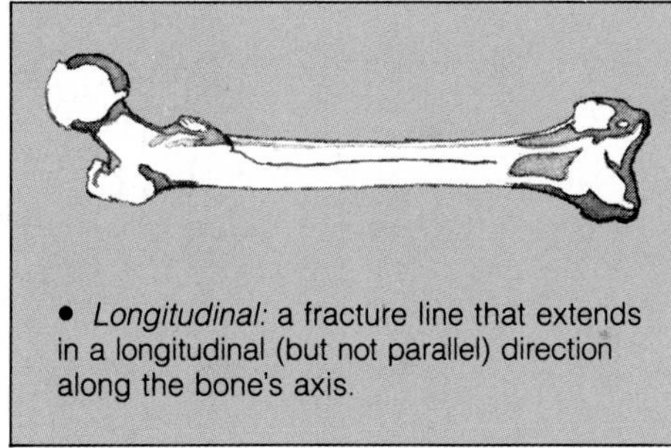

• *Longitudinal:* a fracture line that extends in a longitudinal (but not parallel) direction along the bone's axis.

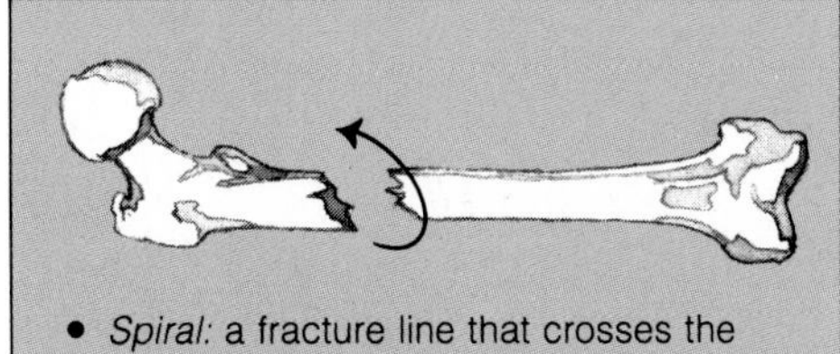

• *Spiral:* a fracture line that crosses the bone at an oblique angle, creating a spiral pattern. This kind of break usually occurs in a long bone.

MINI-ASSESSMENT

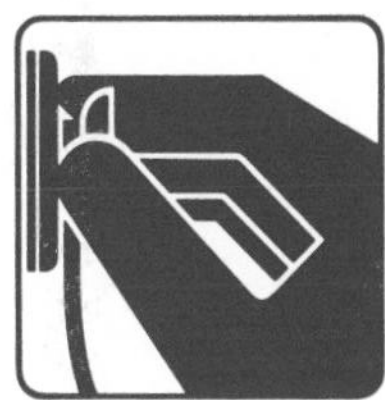

Identifying fracture signs and symptoms

Specific fracture signs and symptoms vary, depending on the fracture type and its location. Of course, if a patient's bones are protruding from an open, bleeding wound, you'll know he has a fracture. But a *closed* fracture can be much more difficult to assess visually.

Look for these physical signs and symptoms that generally accompany a fracture:

- deformity or shortening of the injured area
- localized discoloration and edema
- pain in injured area (especially at time of injury occurrence)
- patient's tendency to guard the injured area by holding it in a protected position
- tenderness of injured area several hours to several days after the injury occurs
- presence of crepitation (crackling sound) during skin palpation
- decrease or complete loss of muscle power at injured area
- presence of grating sound when testing for range of motion during standard assessment.

If the grating sound is detected, call the doctor immediately. Avoid moving the limb any further. Doing so can cause additional injury and pain. *Note:* Never deliberately test range of motion if you suspect a fracture.

Assessment

Nurses' guide to fractures

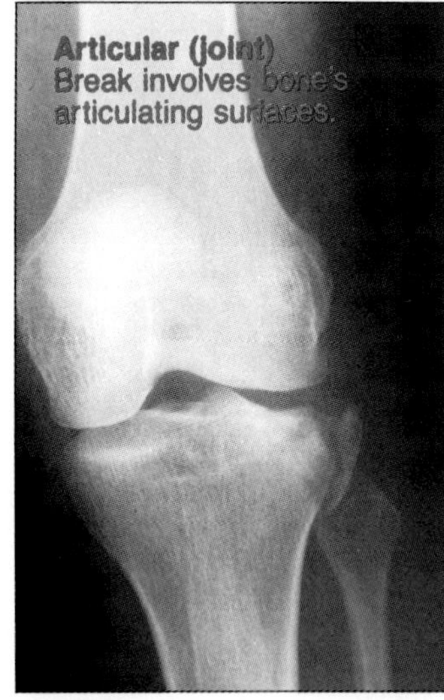
Articular (joint)
Break involves bone's articulating surfaces.

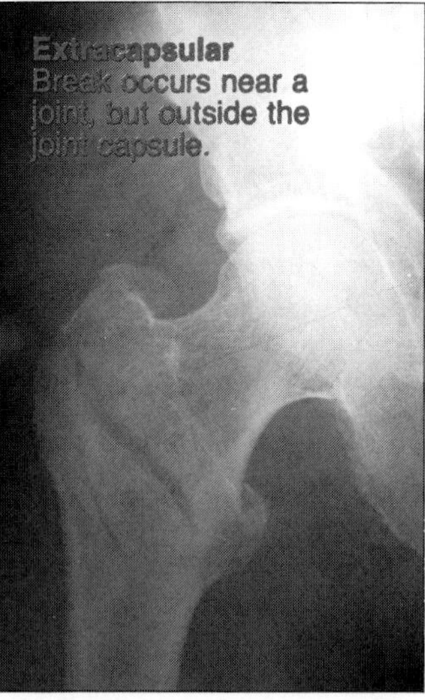
Extracapsular
Break occurs near a joint, but outside the joint capsule.

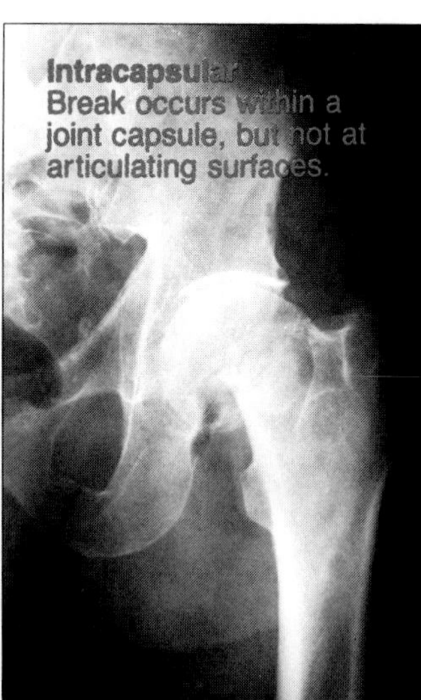
Intracapsular
Break occurs within a joint capsule, but not at articulating surfaces.

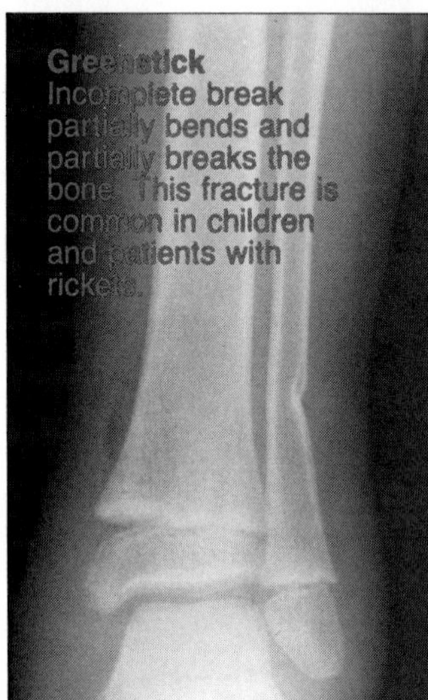
Greenstick
Incomplete break partially bends and partially breaks the bone. This fracture is common in children and patients with rickets.

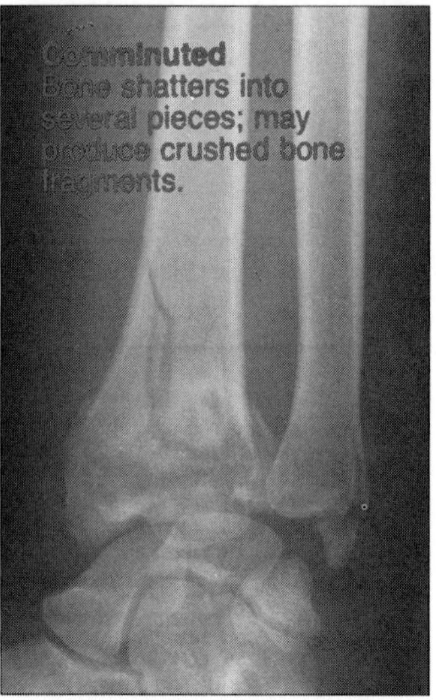
Comminuted
Bone shatters into several pieces; may produce crushed bone fragments.

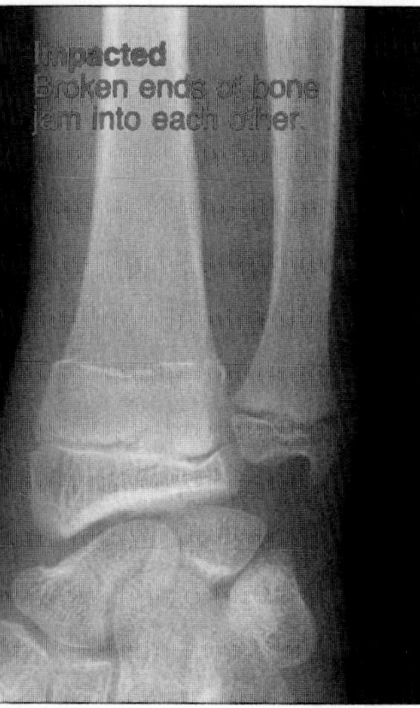
Impacted
Broken ends of bone jam into each other.

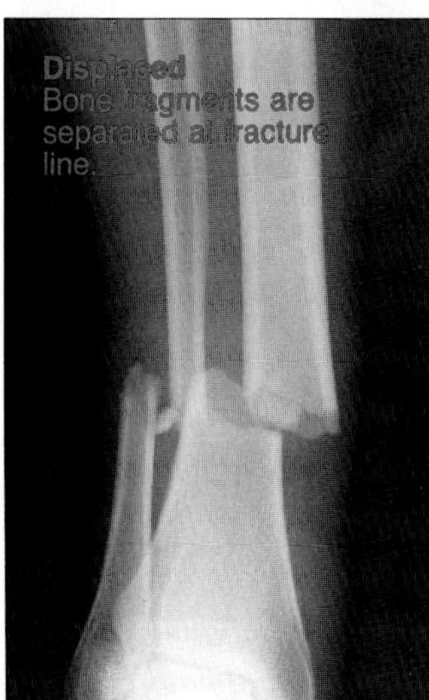
Displaced
Bone fragments are separated at fracture line.

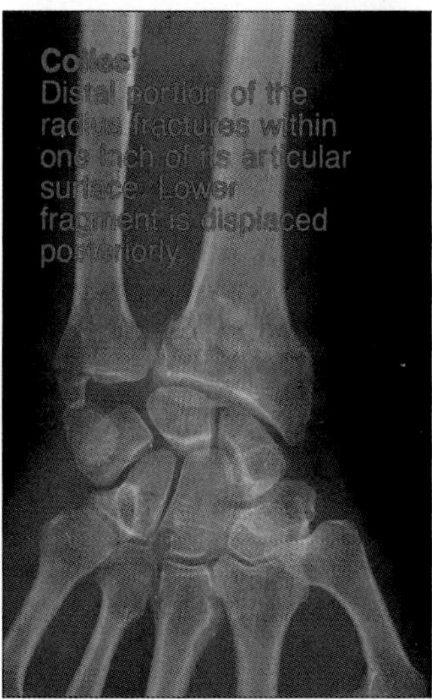
Colles'
Distal portion of the radius fractures within one inch of its articular surface. Lower fragment is displaced posteriorly.

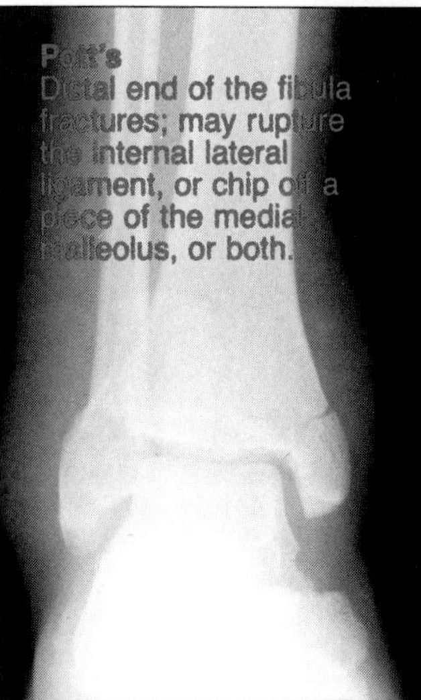
Pott's
Distal end of the fibula fractures; may rupture the internal lateral ligament, or chip off a piece of the medial malleolus, or both.

Coping with hemorrhage from a long-bone fracture

Has your patient fractured a long bone, such as his femur? Such a fracture may cause traumatic hemorrhage, even if the break is closed. How does the hemorrhage occur? Ruptured blood vessels surrounding the bone ooze blood into the injury site. Within 24 to 48 hours, as much as 1 to 2 liters (2 to 4 units) of blood may accumulate in the patient's thigh. This blood loss may eventually cause hypovolemic shock.

Observe your patient for the following signs and symptoms of shock: low or erratic blood pressure; weak, rapid pulse; tachypnea; cold, clammy skin; pallor; restlessness; nausea and vomiting; and lab tests showing decreased hemoglobin and hematocrit. These signs and symptoms, plus increasing ecchymosis of his injury, may indicate internal hemorrhage.

To provide care, take these steps:

- Notify the doctor immediately.
- Administer oxygen.
- Keep the affected limb immobilized.
- Keep the patient warm.
- Check vital signs frequently.
- Measure and record the circumference of the affected extremity at and below the injury site. An increase in size indicates blood accumulation.
- Monitor your patient's fluid balance. To do so, measure intake and output hourly for 24-hour periods.

Of course, a long-bone fracture can be open instead of closed. If the bone's not protruding, stop bleeding by applying pressure on the wound, using a sterile dressing. However, if your patient's bone protrudes through his wound, or if the bleeding can't be controlled by direct pressure, apply pressure either above or below the bleeding site. If the blood's spurting from an artery, apply pressure above the bleeding site, at a pressure point. If the blood's flowing steadily from a vein, apply pressure directly below the bleeding site.

Understanding compartment syndrome

In addition to the direct damage caused by a fracture, a patient with a fractured arm or leg may experience a complication called *compartment syndrome.* Compartment syndrome is a form of vascular impairment that can lead to permanent deformity of the affected limb.

But, a fracture isn't the only cause of compartment syndrome. This syndrome can occur with any musculoskeletal injury. Constriction or occlusion from tight dressings, sutures, casts, poor positioning, swelling, a severed artery, or bleeding into a tissue can all contribute to the syndrome.

The *compartment* referred to is a muscle group enveloped by a tough, inelastic fascial tissue (see illustration). The entry and exit points from the compartment are only large enough to accommodate major arteries, nerves, and tendons. So, tissue swelling from an injury rapidly begins to compress the arteries and nerves, causing muscle ischemia. Or, ischemia can occur when an artery is severed, interrupting blood supply to a compartment.

The initial ischemia induces histamine release, which leads to capillary dilation and increased edema. Increased compression from edema occludes the compartment's larger arteries, causing further muscle ischemia. The increased ischemia, in turn, leads to further histamine release. As you can see, a viscious cycle rapidly compounds the initial ischemia.

If the condition's left untreated, irreversible damage will occur to the patient's muscles and nerves within 6 hours. Within 24 to 48 hours, contracture, paralysis, and sensation loss will completely disrupt function in his limb and leave it permanently deformed. One common example of deformity resulting from compartment syndrome is Volkmann's contracture of the hand (shown at right), in which the patient's wrist and fingers contract in a clawing position. This may occur following a supracondylar fracture of the elbow.

To detect compartment syndrome, frequently perform the neurovascular assessment given on page 24. Signs and symptoms of this condition include:

- increasing pain in limb
- pallor or cyanosis distal to the injury site
- absent pulse distal to the injury site
- decreased active and passive muscle movement distal to injury site; passive muscle stretching causes pain
- edema of limb distal to injury site
- sensory changes (late symptom) such as numbness or tingling.

To help prevent the effects of compartment syndrome, take the following steps:

- Report any complaints of pain to the doctor immediately.
- Elevate a swollen extremity above the patient's heart level. If elevation doesn't relieve the swelling, notify the doctor.
- Then, remove any obvious constriction, such as a dressing or wrap. Or, make sure your patient's cast is cut enough to relieve any pressure. If these measures don't relieve the signs and symptoms within 4 to 6 hours, the doctor may surgically relieve the compression.

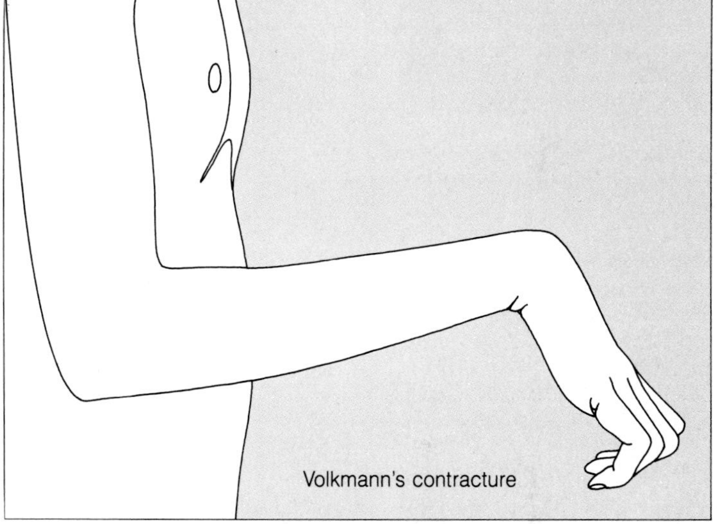

Volkmann's contracture

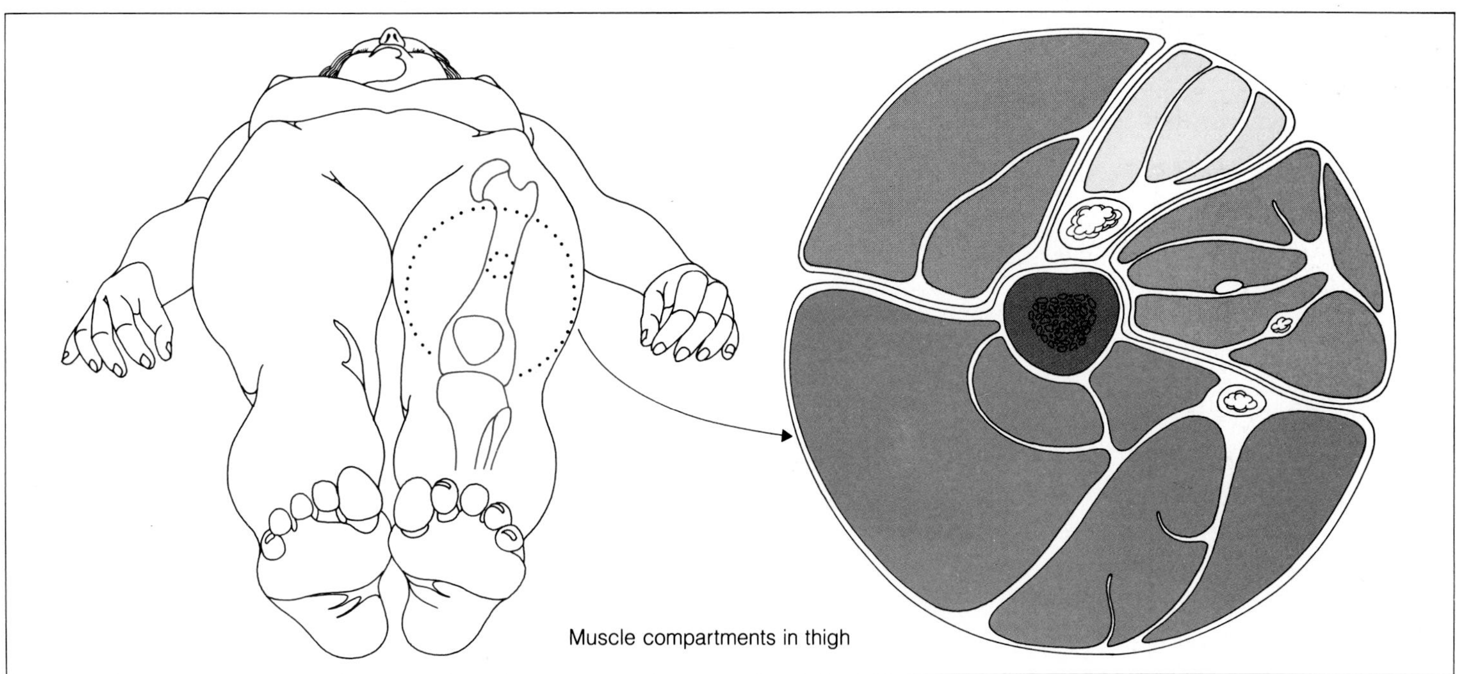

Muscle compartments in thigh

Assessment

Detecting neurovascular impairment

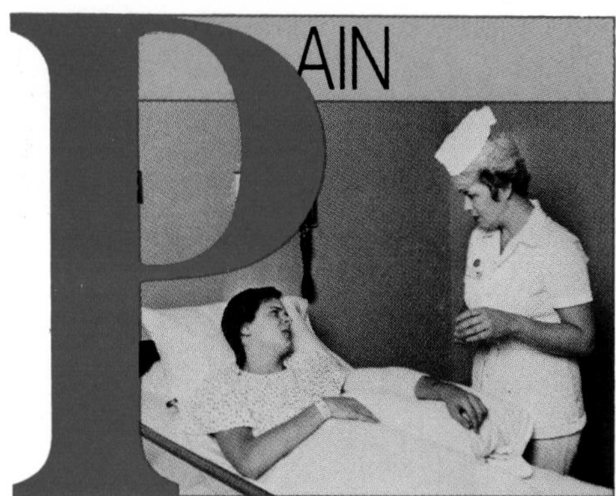

If you're caring for a patient with a fracture, keep in mind that he may be suffering associated nerve and vascular damage. To evaluate his neurologic and circulatory status, assess him for the following signs and symptoms (also known as the *5 Ps*). For specific information about hemorrhage associated with long-bone fractures, see page 22.

• *Pain.* Determine the pain's location and whether it seems to be getting worse or better. Remember, pain worsens with increased edema from secondary nerve compression, lack of blood supply, and soft tissue damage.

Note: Most unconscious patients react to painful stimuli. Evaluate your unconscious patient by palpating injured areas and noting any response such as twitching, jerking, or grimacing.

If your patient's received any analgesics, observe him for signs of pain relief. Check his medication record to determine any pattern in his pain relief. For example, if his pain hasn't diminished since he first began receiving medication, he may need a different drug.

• *Pulse.* Assess his peripheral pulses, especially those distal to the injury site. Always compare bilateral pulses at the same time to detect any discrepancies between them. *Remember:* Many patients have a congenital unilateral or bilateral lack of the *dorsalis pedis* pulse. Check your patient's medical history, or ask if he's ever been told that he lacks pulses in his feet.

• *Paresthesia.* Lightly touch, prick with a pin, or pinch the involved area, both distally and proximally to the injury site. Note any increase or decrease in sensation; lack of sensation; numbness; or tingling. Check the same area on his affected side. Compare your findings.

Presence of paresthesia indicates local, cerebral, or spinal injury.

Note: If your patient's unconscious, note whether he moves, twitches, grimaces, or otherwise responds to stimuli. Compare your findings with his previous assessments. Report any differences to the doctor for interpretation.

• *Pallor or patchy cyanosis.* Carefully check the skin color and temperature of your patient's injured extremity. Note where pallor or cyanosis occur with respect to his injury. Above the injury site, these signs indicate venous impairment. Below the injury site, these signs indicate arterial impairment.

Compress a nail bed in his injured limb momentarily and observe how quickly the blood returns (capillaries usually refill in 3 to 5 seconds). Also, check his unaffected side and compare your findings.

• *Paralysis.* For an arm or leg, assess mobility in the first intact joint distal to the fracture. Or, if the patient's arm or leg is already in a cast, check his fingers or toes for mobility. Be sure to check his unaffected side as well. For a spinal injury, check mobility in all his extremities.

Presence of paralysis may indicate peripheral nerve injury, spinal cord injury, or brain injury.

Document your assessment accurately. If your findings indicate any problems, notify the doctor immediately. Then, provide the care described at right.

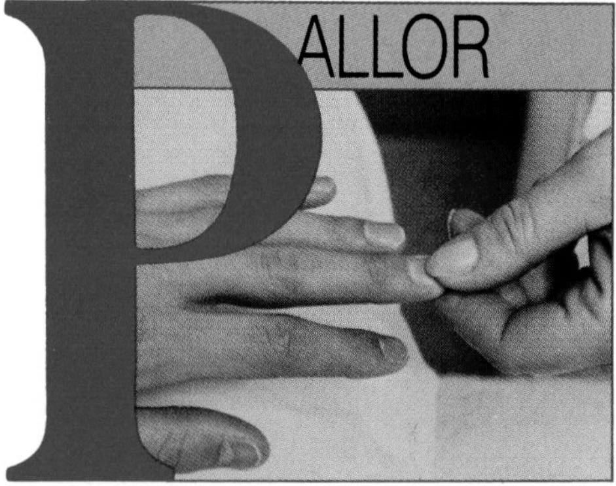

Caring for a patient with suspected neurovascular impairment

Your neurovascular assessment indicates that your patient's suffering impairment. Provide the following immediate care.

• First, raise his injured extremity above his heart level. Doing so will decrease edema and increase vascular return.

• Then, determine your patient's vital signs, including temperature, pulse rate, respirations, and consciousness level.

• Now, check any dressings, bandages, or traction equipment to make sure they're not too tight. Also, check the patient's position to minimize pressure points.

• If your patient's already in a cast, check the cast for tightness. You should be able to fit one finger between the cast and his skin. If the cast is constricting your patient's circulation, notify the doctor. Obtain a cast cutter and spreader for the doctor's use.

• Warm a cool extremity by covering it.

• Administer analgesic medication, as ordered. Request additional medication if the patient still has pain.

• If you've noted paresthesia or paralysis, check whether spinal X-rays have been taken. If not, obtain an order from the doctor for X-rays.

• Document all nursing care on the appropriate forms.

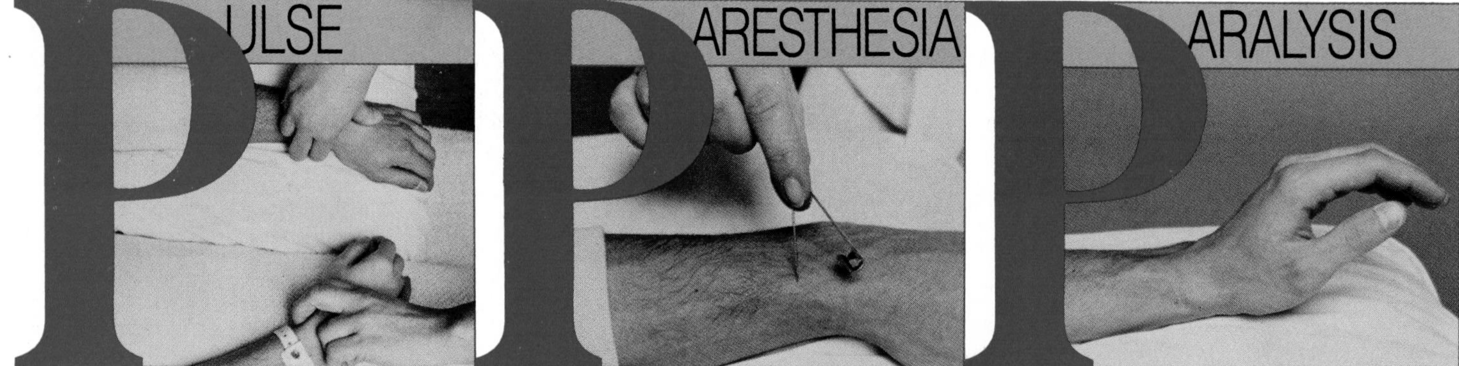

Testing your patient for nerve damage

Bone fractures and dislocations may damage nearby nerves, causing temporary or permanent numbness or paralysis. Always perform the neurovascular assessment we've outlined on the opposite page for any patient with a fracture.

But, for a quick assessment of specific nerve damage, instruct your patient to perform the following active range-of-motion tests. Of course, which tests you choose will depend on your patient's injury site.

Humerus fracture
Your patient should be able to hyperextend her thumb. If she can't, she may have radial nerve damage.

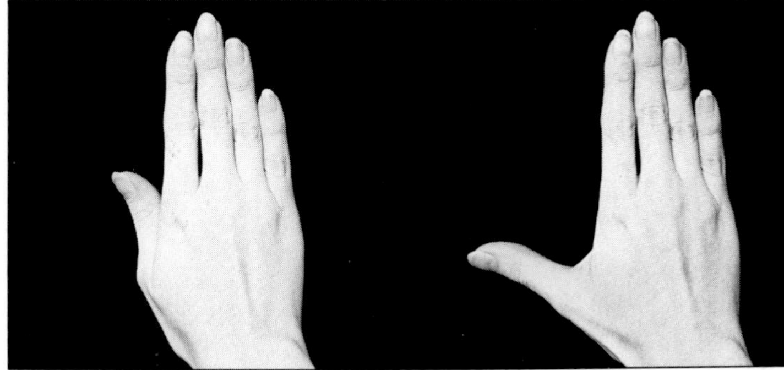

Ulna fracture
Your patient should be able to abduct all her fingers. If she can't, she may have ulnar nerve damage.

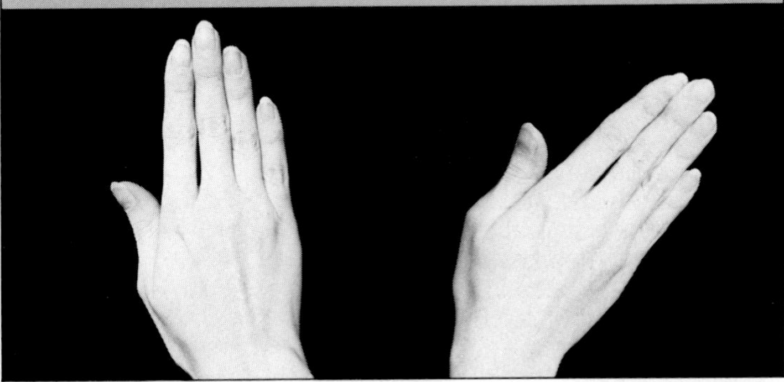

Radius fracture
Your patient should be able to oppose her thumb to her little finger. If she can't, she may have median nerve damage.

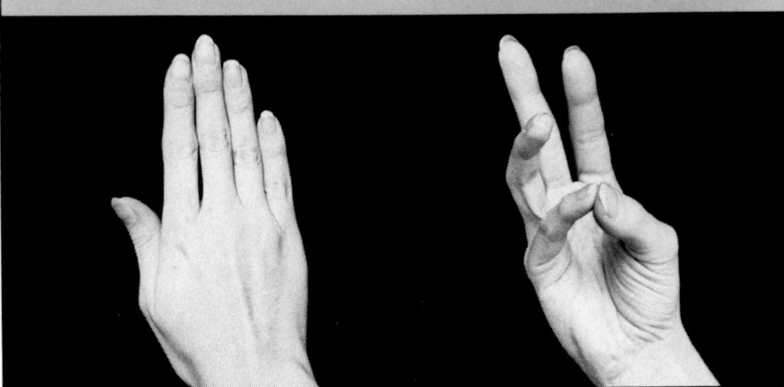

Tibia fracture
Your patient should be able to plantarflex her ankle. If she can't, she may have tibial nerve damage.

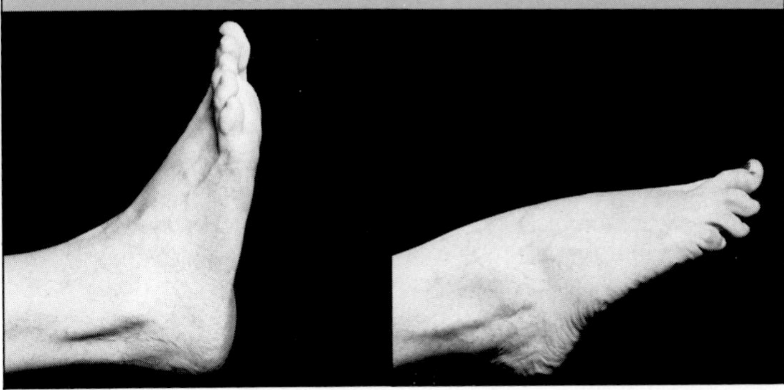

Radius fracture
Your patient should be able to hyperextend her thumb. If she can't, she may have radial nerve damage.

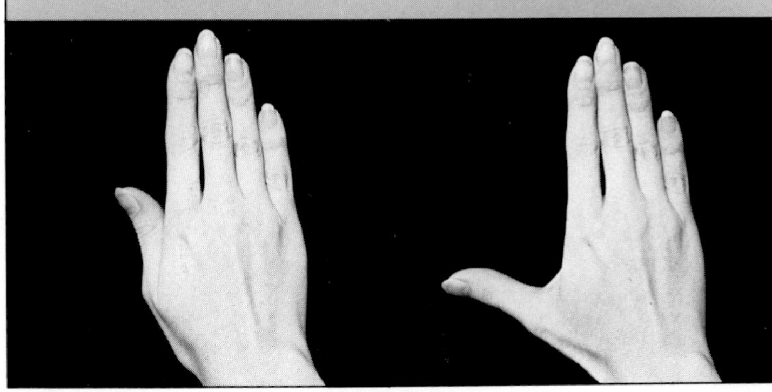

Fibula fracture
Your patient should be able to dorsiflex her ankle. If she can't, she may have peroneal nerve damage.

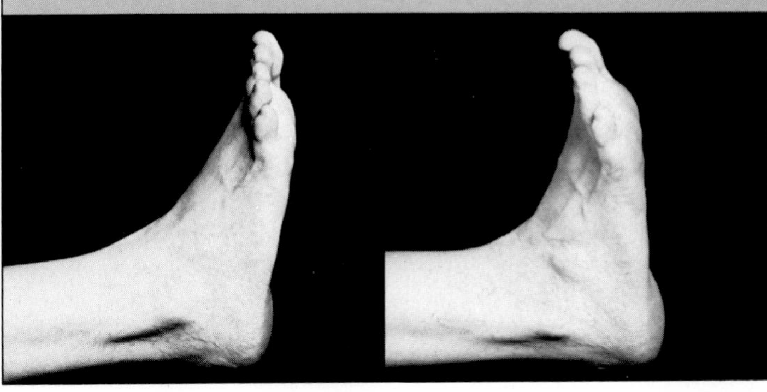

Assessment

Preparing your patient for an orthopedic X-ray

Barbara Bowen, a 25-year-old computer programmer, has been transported to your hospital's emergency department (ED) after falling off a ladder. She tells you she has severe pain in her right leg. The doctor has ordered X-rays to determine whether she has a fracture.

You must quickly assess your patient to determine whether she can be transported to the radiology department for X-rays. If she shows signs and symptoms such as bleeding, hypotension, or chest pain, obtain an order for a portable X-ray machine for use in the ED.

Suppose you've decided that Ms. Bowen can be moved to the radiology department safely. Although you won't accompany her there, you must prepare her for the X-ray procedure. Adequate preparation will help alleviate any fears she may have. In preparing her, follow these guidelines:

- First, since your patient's in pain, obtain an order for an analgesic. Administer the medication before she goes to the X-ray department. Be sure to notify the X-ray room staff that she's received an analgesic.
- Then, explain the X-ray procedure to your patient. Tell her that the technician will take X-rays from several different angles. Make sure she realizes that the technician will probably move her right leg, which may increase her pain temporarily. Explain that only by moving her injured limb can her bone damage be thoroughly assessed.
- Explain that X-rays of other body parts, besides the obviously affected one, may be taken to rule out possible injuries. For example, the doctor will order X-rays of Ms. Bowen's vertebral column because she might have sustained vertebral fractures during her fall.
- Describe the X-ray room setting to your patient. The large and probably unfamiliar equipment could make her apprehensive. Warn your patient that the X-ray table will feel cold and hard and that she'll have to remain motionless during the procedure. Mention that she'll hear a thudding sound as each picture is taken.
- Assure your patient that she'll receive only a small amount of radiation.

Nursing tip: When she enters the X-ray room, she may be puzzled if the staff is wearing radiation shields and she's not. So, explain ahead of time that these staff members shield themselves because they're exposed to many X-rays daily.

Note: Any time you prepare a female patient for an X-ray, find out the date of her last menstrual period. If she's had her last period more than a month ago (or if she suspects she's pregnant), specify a shield for her pelvic area on the X-ray requisition form. Inform her of this special precaution. To make sure she actually gets a shield, tell her to verbally request one from the X-ray technician.

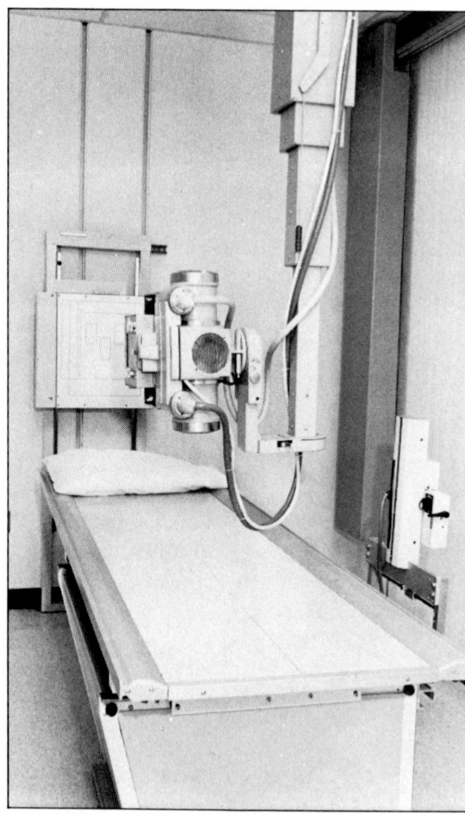

- Ask your patient to remove watches, rings, or any other metal objects she's wearing. Explain that the metal distorts the X-ray picture. Make sure all your patient's valuables (jewelry, purse, wallet, etc.) are placed in a safe or given to a waiting family member. Remember to document the disposition of any valuables.
- After you've thoroughly explained the X-ray procedure, ask your patient to disrobe. Clean all extraneous material, such as mud, grass, or broken glass, from her skin. Then, assist her in putting on a hospital gown or pajamas.

Remember: Never use a gown with metal snaps.

- Now, fill out your patient's X-ray requisition form thoroughly and accurately. Be sure to write legibly. Correctly identify your patient, the specific X-rays ordered, and the reason for each desired X-ray. Note your patient's age, hospital number, and whether she's been X-rayed previously. List any special instructions.

Including accurate and complete information contributes to correct evaluation of the X-rays. By avoiding the necessity for further X-rays, you can minimize your patient's expenses, her exposure to radiation, and any discomfort associated with the procedure.

- All patients should be accompanied to the radiology department by a hospital staff member. Give the X-ray requisition form to whomever will accompany your patient. If your patient's being transported on a stretcher or a bed, make sure the side rails are raised and safety straps are in place before she leaves the ED.

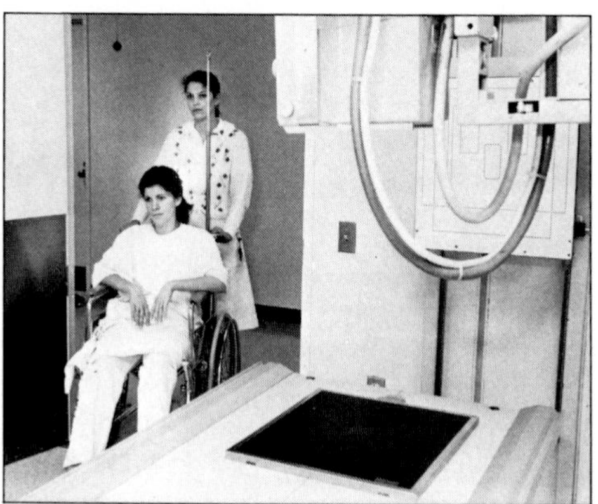

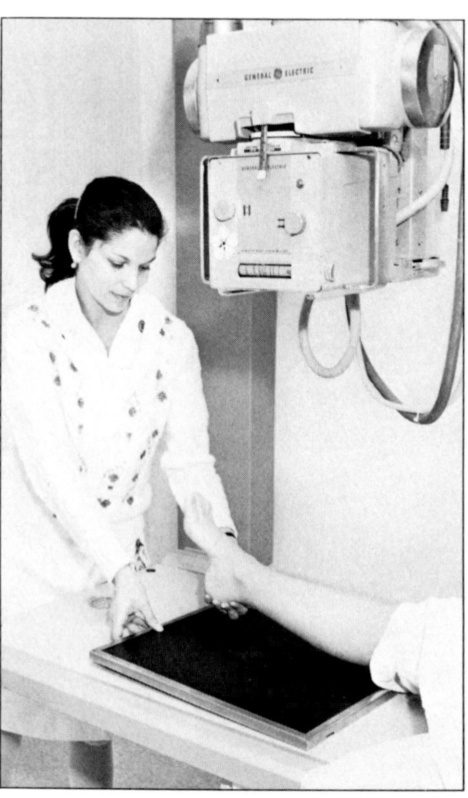

How a bone heals

X-ray films confirm that your patient has a fracture. You know that his injured bone will require immobilization in order to heal. But, do you understand the healing process itself?

Bone healing consists of five basic steps: hematoma formation; cellular proliferation; callus formation; ossification; and consolidation and remodeling. Although the process occurs in the order listed, keep in mind that the five phases overlap, with no clear division between them.

Also, remember that the time spans we give for each phase are only approximations. Several factors affect the length and outcome of the healing process: the patient's general physical condition, including his health and age; the fracture type and its severity; proper bone fragment immobilization; and adequate care, such as good nutrition, during the healing period. Another factor in healing time is bone type; for example, dense bone will heal more slowly than cancellous (spongy) bone.

Hematoma formation

Immediately after a fracture occurs, a hematoma forms, as blood escaping from damaged tissues accumulates around bone fragments at the fracture site. Within 24 hours, a fibrin mesh develops from the hematoma. This mesh will provide a framework for the growth of granulation (wound repair) tissue.

Cellular proliferation

After the fibrin network's been established, connective tissue cells (fibroblasts) and capillaries infiltrate and reinforce it. White blood cells surround and contain the network.

You remember that bone is covered with a special connective tissue called periosteum. Injury or trauma to this tissue stimulates osteoblast (bone-forming cell) production. The osteoblasts infiltrate and fortify the fibrin network. In doing so, they lift the periosteum away from the bone, allowing granulation tissue, the cell-reinforced fibrin network, to form between bone and periosteum.

Within a few days, a collar of granulation tissue and periosteum surrounds each bone fragment.

Callus formation

Six to ten days after the injury, fibroblasts begin forming provisional callus from the granulation tissue. They do so by developing into either cartilage or bone. Fibroblasts underneath the periosteum, close to capillaries, usually form bone. Internal fibroblasts, distant from capillaries, usually form cartilage. *Note:* Cartilage also forms where motion occurs; for example, at the bone fragment ends. Consequently, excessive motion during healing will promote cartilage rather than bone formation, resulting in a weaker bone.

Provisional callus is a loosely woven mesh of bone and cartilage, much wider then the bone's normal diameter. It extends beyond the bone fracture line for some distance, bridging the gap between bone fragments, and acting as a splint. It usually reaches its maximum size within 14 to 21 days.

Ossification

From the third to the tenth weeks after injury, newly formed blood vessels begin depositing calcium salts in the affected area, ossifying the bony callus. Cartilage callus, however, requires additional changes to become bone.

After ossification, the bone fragments are firmly bound together, and the healing process is essentially complete.

Consolidation and remodeling

While calcium salts continue to be deposited, excess callus and bone resorption begins. Muscle and weight-bearing stresses determine this remodeling process, so that the bone will be strongest where it usually absorbs the most stress. This last stage in healing may continue for as long as a year. When it's complete, the bone should be as strong as it was before the injury.

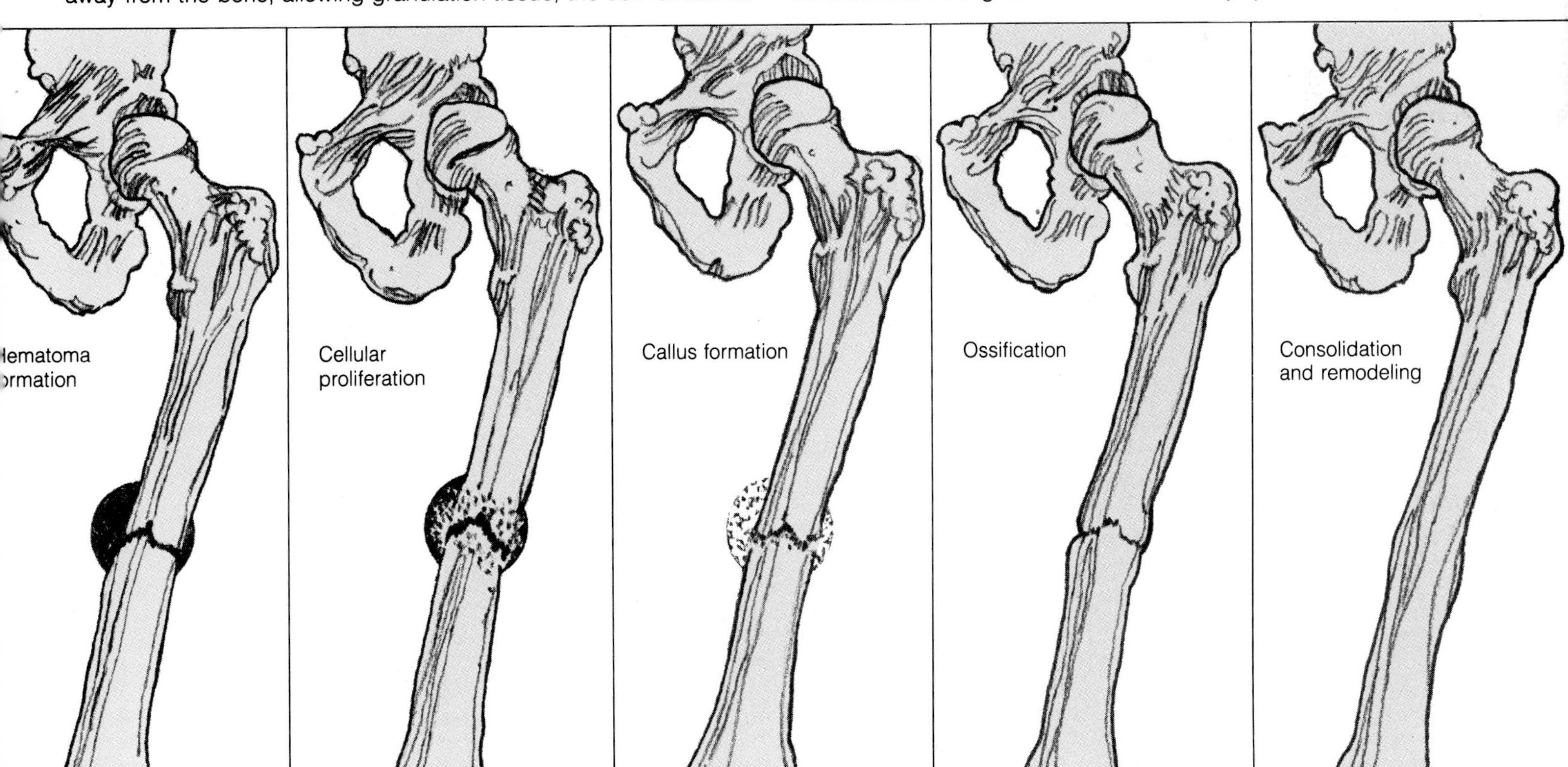

Assessment

Identifying common musculoskeletal injuries

Dislocation (subluxation)

Description
Displacement of a bone end from a joint. Associated ligaments may be torn or stretched.
Causes
Trauma; disease; congenital condition
Signs and symptoms
- Burning pain at joint
- Deformity of joint
- Stiffness and loss of joint function
- Moderate or severe edema around joint

Nursing considerations
- Notify doctor of patient's condition immediately.
- To lessen swelling, elevate the affected extremity immediately. Keep it elevated after dislocation is reduced, because manipulation increases swelling.
- Don't splint until the dislocation's been reduced. Deformity caused by dislocation automatically immobilizes joint.
- Assess affected extremity frequently for signs of neurovascular problems, such as pain, absent pulse, paresthesia, peripheral cyanosis, pallor, and paralysis (see page 24). Be sure to check bilateral pulses distal to the point of dislocation.
- Because condition causes severe pain, give pain medication (as ordered). Doctor may order additional analgesics or muscle relaxants during reduction of dislocation.
- Doctor may order traction or immobilization with a splint, wrap, or cast until dislocation's completely healed.
- After immobilization device has been removed, encourage gradually increasing levels of exercise.
- Some dislocations reduce themselves without therapeutic intervention. The patient then has a sprain (from torn or stretched ligaments), rather than a dislocation.

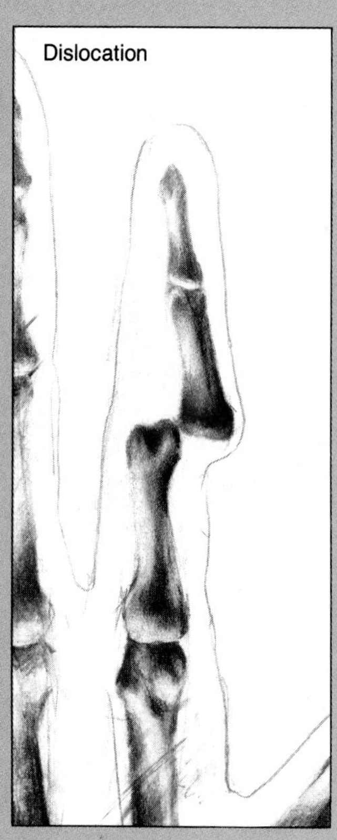
Dislocation

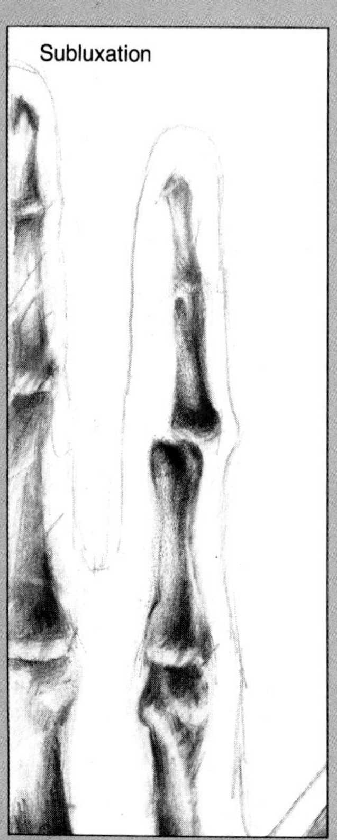
Subluxation

Sprain

Description
Incomplete tearing of joint capsule or ligaments surrounding a joint, which doesn't disrupt ligament continuity or cause joint instability
Cause
Sudden twisting of joint beyond its normal range of motion
Signs and symptoms
- Pain at joint
- Edema around joint
- Discoloration around joint
- Decreased joint function

Nursing considerations
- To reduce swelling, apply cold treatment, such as an ice bag or a cold pack, for the first 48 hours.
- Then, after swelling's controlled, apply warm treatment such as warm compresses or a heating pad.
- Immobilize the sprain to prevent further ligament damage, as ordered. The doctor may order the extremity wrapped, taped, or placed in a cast for several weeks.

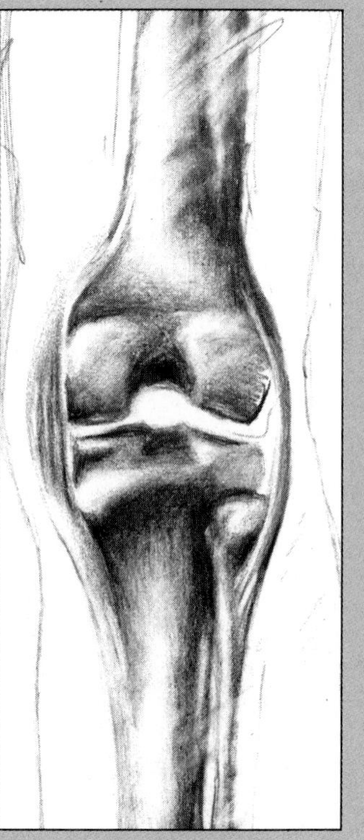

Torn ligament

Description
Partial or complete tearing of ligaments around joint, which usually causes joint instability
Cause
Trauma
Signs and symptoms
- Joint feels unstable
- Rapid swelling after injury
- Pain at joint

Nursing considerations
- Apply a splint immediately.
- Assess affected extremity frequently for neurovascular damage.
- For mild condition, doctor may order rest and cold treatment of swelling.
- For moderate condition, doctor may order aspiration of excessive joint fluid and wrapping or taping of extremity to compress swelling and support joint.
- For a severe condition, indicated by gross instability, prepare the patient for surgery, as ordered.
- Range-of-motion exercises help restore joint strength.

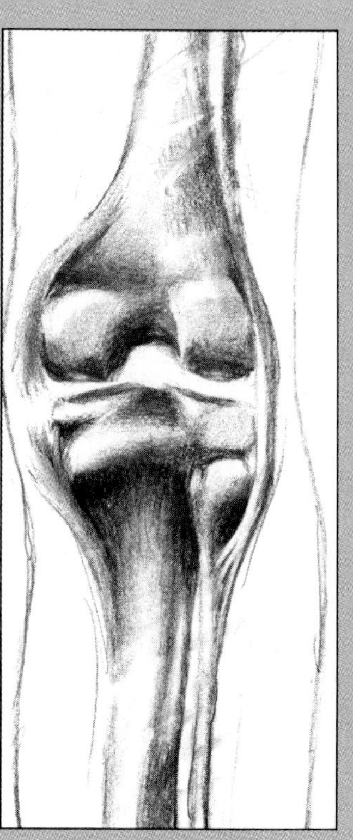

Strain

Description
Injury to a tendon/muscle unit close to a joint. May be acute or chronic.
Causes
Overstretching tendons or overusing muscles
Signs and symptoms
- Acute strain produces sudden, severe pain at the time of injury, which then subsides to local tenderness. Swelling occurs rapidly.
- Chronic strain produces gradual onset of stiffness, soreness, and tenderness.

Nursing considerations
- For acute strain, apply ice packs for the first 48 hours to control swelling.
- Then, after swelling's controlled, apply warm treatment, such as warm compresses or a heating pad.
- Doctor may order rest for affected area for 4 to 6 weeks.
- For both acute and chronic strains, permit only minimal movement of affected area.

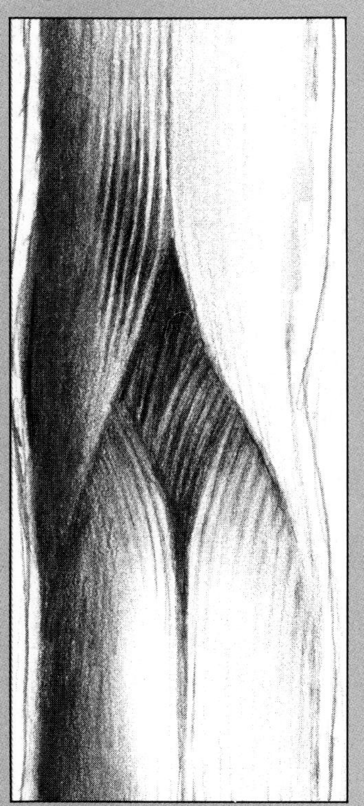

Lacerated tendon

Description
Partial or complete tear across tendon
Causes
Laceration or other trauma
Signs and symptoms
- Local edema and tenderness; inability to move the injured part

Nursing considerations
- Check any lacerations, particularly on flexor side of wrist or arm, for underlying tendon injury. But, never *probe* an open wound, or you may further damage a lacerated tendon.
- Check active range of motion in affected extremity.
- To reduce swelling, provide cold treatment, such as ice bags or cold packs.
- For mild to moderate lacerated tendon, doctor may order rest and splinting or wrapping.
- Prepare patient for surgery (as ordered), if laceration is severe.

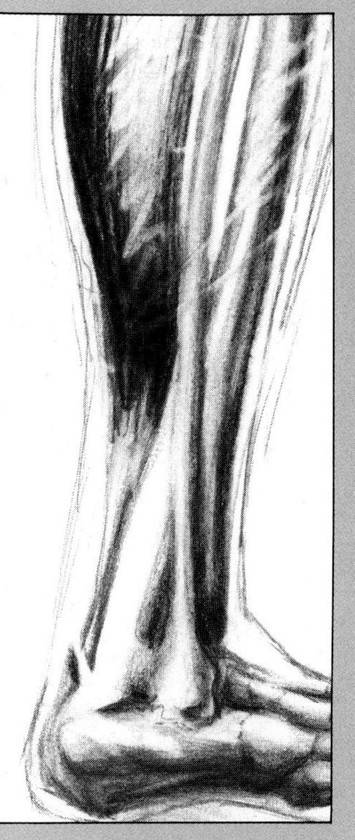

Pulled tendon

Description
Tearing away of tendon from bone. A small piece of bone may be torn away with the tendon.
Cause
Trauma
Signs and symptoms
- Local edema and tenderness

Nursing considerations
- Check patient's active range of motion in affected extremity.
- Elevate extremity and apply ice bag or cold packs to reduce swelling.
- Doctor will order rest for affected area until it's healed.

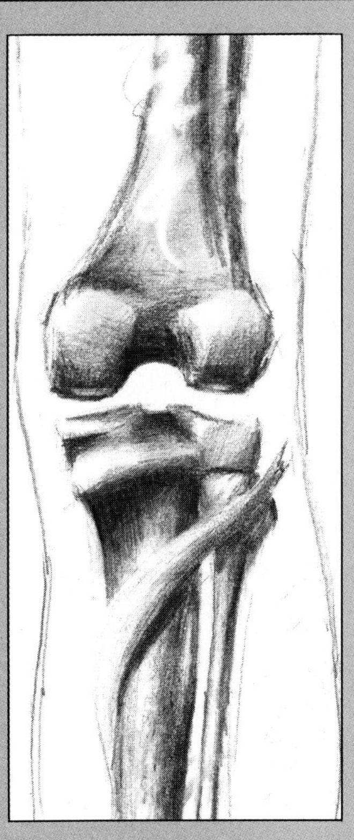

Contusion

Description
Injury to soft tissue or muscle tissue, without accompanying break in skin
Cause
Trauma
Signs and symptoms
- Initially, local tenderness and minor swelling. After 48 hours, local ecchymosis (bruise mark).

Nursing considerations
- Apply cold treatment, such as ice bags or cold packs, to reduce swelling and ecchymosis.
- Check size of discoloration, and measure width of extremity frequently to determine whether trauma is localized, or whether contusion indicates serious hemorrhage.

Nursing tip: Mark point of measurement with pen; compare with future measurements.
- Suspect further damage (dislocation or fracture) beneath ecchymosed areas.
- If no underlying problem exists, contusion will resolve spontaneously.

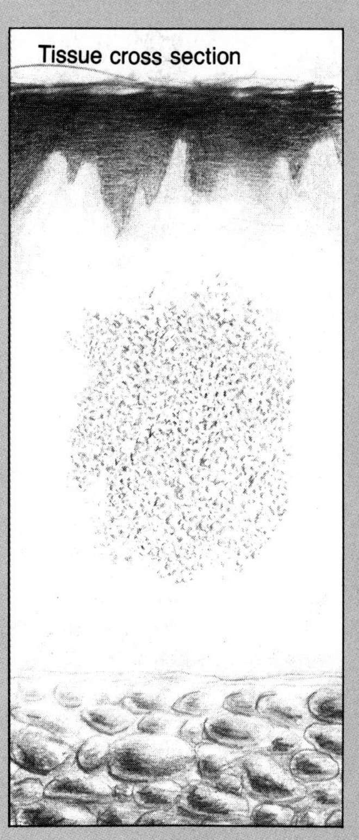

Assessment

Identifying common deformities

Body part	Deformity	Possible causes	Signs and symptoms
SPINE 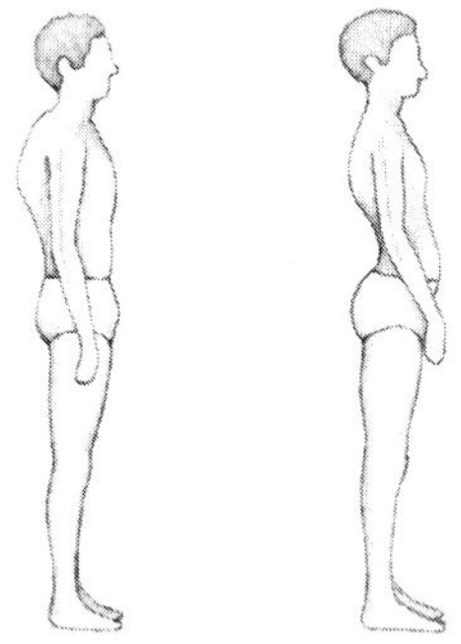	**Kyphosis** Abnormally increased convexity in the spine's thoracic curve, as viewed from the side	Tuberculosis of the spine; chronic arthritis; osteoporosis; thoracic vertebrae compression fractures	• Obviously rounded back • Poor posture • Possible decreased respiratory function
	Lordosis Anterior concavity in the spine's lumbar and cervical curves, as viewed from the side	Spondylolisthesis in lower lumbar region	• Swayback appearance, accompanied by forward protrusion of abdomen and backward protrusion of buttocks
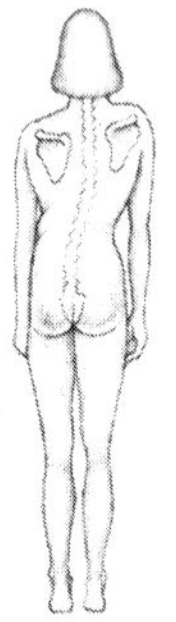	**Scoliosis** Lateral *C*-shaped or *S*-shaped curvature of the spine; may be thoracic, lumbar, or thoracolumbar	Poor posture from muscle weakness or asymmetric muscle paralysis; vertebral body deformity; congenital condition; rib or spinal cord tumor	• Lateral spinal curve, either confined to a localized region or involving the entire spine • One shoulder lower than the other; hip on same side prominent • Protrusion of ribs toward the patient's back on the curve's convex side and toward the patient's front on the curve's concave side
SHOULDER 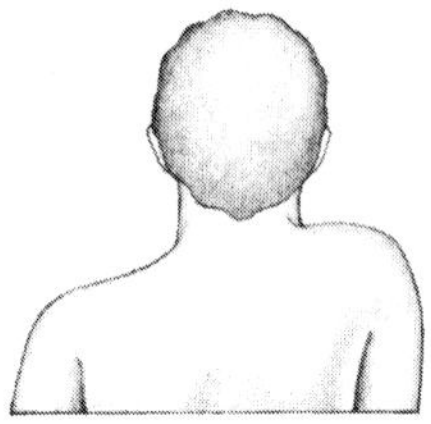	**Sprengel's deformity** Larger portion of scapula is present in cervical region, instead of in the thoracic region, where it's normally located	Congenital failure of scapula to descend into adult position	• Elevated and asymmetric shoulder • Restricted shoulder abduction • With bilateral deformity, shortened neck • Possible cervicothoracic scoliosis and torticollis
WRIST AND HAND 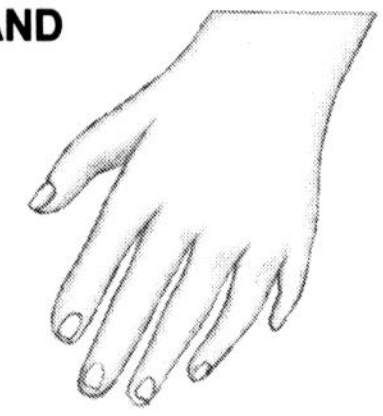	**Polydactyly** Extra digits formed by abnormal soft tissue masses on hand; masses may include bone	Congenital condition	• Extra digits on hand; tissue amount and location vary • Possible abnormal hand function
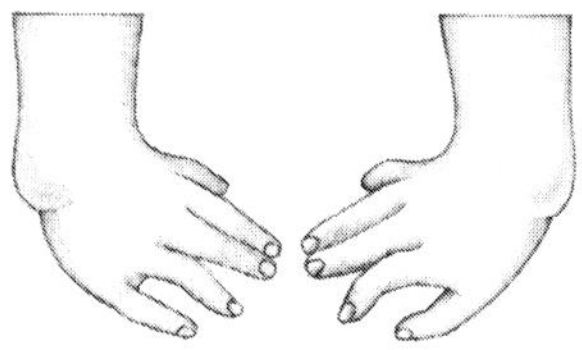	**Talipomanus (clubhand)** Twisting of hand out of normal position or shape into strong flexion and adduction	Congenital condition (absence of either the radius or the ulna)	• Marked deviation of hand in direction of radius; patient still has use of hand • Extremely short forearm

Body part	Deformity	Possible causes	Signs and symptoms
HIP 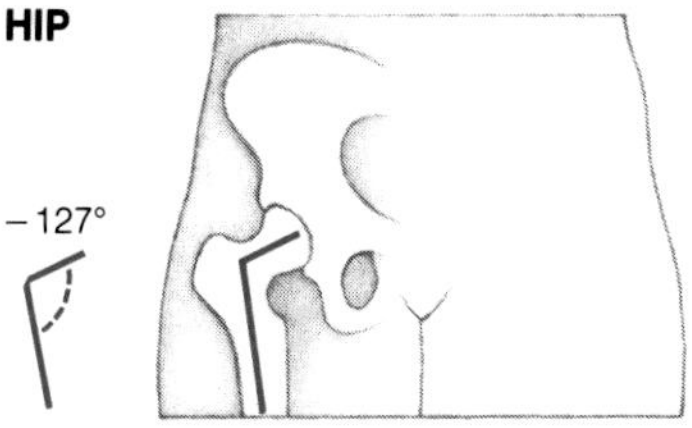 −127°	**Coxa vara (gluteus medius limp)** Hip angulated toward body's midline	Congenital condition (diminished angle between axis of femoral shaft and femoral neck)	• Increased hip adduction • Decreased distance from iliac crest to greater trochanter • Ability to cross thighs at higher than normal level • Swaying gait
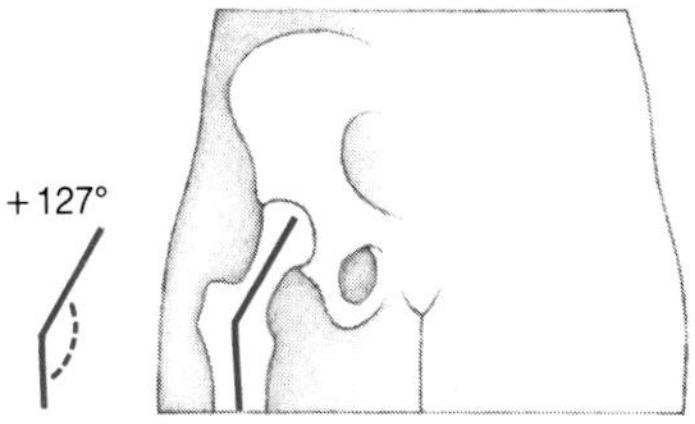 +127°	**Coxa valga** Hip angulated away from body's midline	Congenital condition (increased angle between axis of femoral shaft and femoral neck)	• Not usually indicated by any limp or external deformity, although normal hip mechanics may be distorted
KNEE 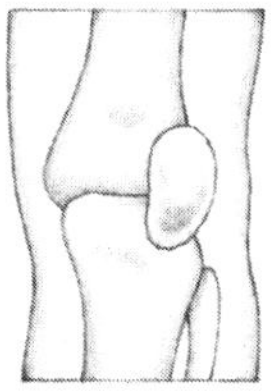	**Recurrent patella dislocation** Repeated patella displacement leading to patellofemoral arthritis	Traumatic injury; weakened ligaments; contracture and abnormal attachments of area; knock-knee condition with external tibia deformity; displaced patella (unusually high and laterally positioned)	• Unstable knee joint causing knee to give way • Knee edema • Possible severe pain • Pain, which may diminish with frequent episodes
FOOT AND ANKLE 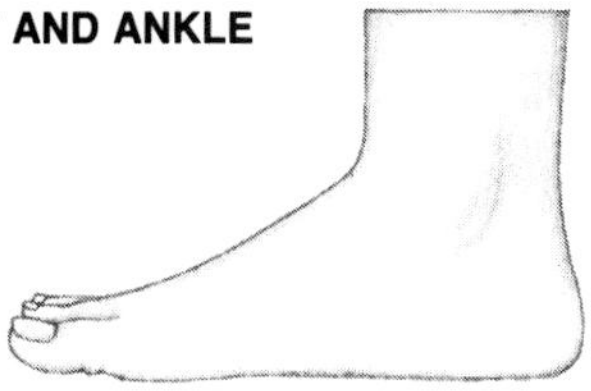	**Pes planus (pronated foot, flatfoot)** Laxity of ligaments supporting foot's longitudinal arch, flattening the arch	Congenital condition; or may be from muscular imbalance, postural alterations, arthritic changes, or ligament or bone injuries	• Convex medial border of foot • May be permanent or may occur only when patient stands, putting weight on his foot
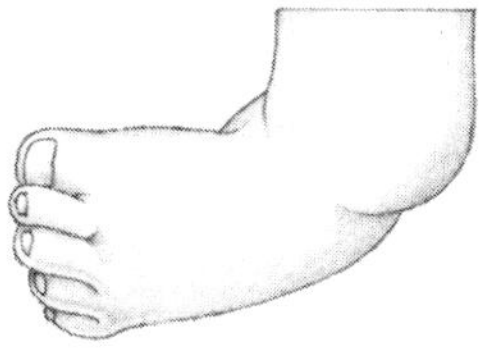	**Talipes (clubfoot)** Combination of deformities such as foot inversion, forefoot adduction, and equinus	Congenital condition	• Foot permanently twisted out of shape or position. Foot may assume variety of positions. • Shortened Achilles tendon • Decreased leg muscle size • Thickened joint capsule and ligaments on affected ankle's medial side • Fatigue • Marked muscle atrophy
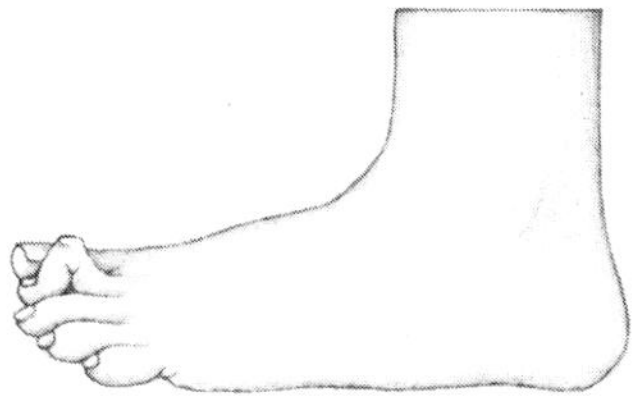	**Hammertoe** Flexion contracture of proximal interphalangeal joint; with flexion, neutral extension, or slight hyperextension contracture of distal interphalangeal joint; most often affects the second toe, although it may affect more than one toe	Congenital condition; may also be produced by improperly fitted shoes that force involved toe into flexed position	• Involved toes point downward • Possible painful calluses over proximal interphalangeal joint

Assessment

Learning about inflammatory conditions

Name and description	Possible causes	Signs and symptoms
Osteoarthritis		
Progressive joint disorder, most commonly diagnosed in patients over age 40, which is characterized by articular cartilage degeneration and bony outgrowths at joint margins	Genetic predisposition; factors affecting onset are age, sex, heredity, and obesity.	• Early stages: stiffness, pain, and swelling of one or more joints; moderate joint movement relieves stiffness, but continual movement produces discomfort; symptoms worsen in cold, wet weather. • Later stages: joint limitation with considerable disability; pain may occur with or without joint movement; malalignment and crepitation may be present. • May resemble or accompany rheumatoid arthritis
Rheumatoid arthritis		
Chronic inflammatory disease, characterized by synovial membrane damage, which results in joint destruction, ankylosis, and deformity	Precipitating factors include infection, allergic reaction, metabolic disorders, and stress	• Fatigue, weakness, and sweating with no accompanying fever • Symmetric inflammation and swelling at interphalangeal joints in hands and feet, or at wrists and knees • Stretched and shiny skin over joint • Limited joint movement from swelling; joints may become semiflexed. • Pain on joint motion • Cold, clammy extremities • Subcutaneous nodules at bony prominences of joint; nodules are firm, nontender, and unattached to overlying tissues. • In very late stages, signs and symptoms also include lymph node and spleen enlargement, weight loss, malnutrition.
Bursitis		
Inflammation of bursa (lubricating sacs surrounding joint capsule), causing friction on joint movement	Trauma, overuse of joint, infection, gout, rheumatoid arthritis, metabolic disease, abnormal tissue growth	• Pain, tenderness, and possible edema; specific signs and symptoms vary depending on inflammation site. • Joints most commonly involved include knee, elbow, shoulder, hip, and heel.
Neuropathic joint disease (also known as Charcot's joints)		
Chronic, progressive degeneration of one or more joints	Neurologic disorders, such as tabes dorsalis, diabetic neuropathy, syringomyelia, myelomeningocele, spinal cord compression, peripheral nerve section, leprosy, and congenital lack of pain in joints in extremities	• Noticeable absence of pain in a swollen and unstable joint • Synovial fluid effusion into joint cavity • Possible compression fractures and loose bone fragments in joint cavity
Synovitis		
Synovial membrane inflammation. Two types exist: *toxic* form occurs commonly in toddlers; *traumatic* form results from traumatic injury.	Toxic synovitis: streptococcal infection, excessive joint use, or undetected traumatic injury Traumatic synovitis: twisting or jarring injury to weight-bearing joint, which causes synovial membrane irritation and synovial fluid effusion into joint cavity; viral infection may be a precipitating factor.	• Limited, and possibly painful, joint movement • Painful limp, accompanied by muscle spasms • In toxic synovitis, possible low-grade fever • Can be distinguished from pyogenic septic joint or tubercular joint conditions by synovial fluid studies

Documenting your patient's orthopedic history

Clarence Michie, a 41-year-old insurance underwriter, was injured in an automobile accident 4 days ago. He came to the emergency department today, and was admitted to the orthopedic service with neck pain, an ecchymosed area on his left shoulder, and a right knee contusion.

Before assessing your patient physically, obtain his musculoskeletal history. Understanding Mr. Michie's medical and family history, and the details of his current injuries, will help you better respond to his needs.

Use the following questions as a guide in obtaining his history. *Remember:* Mention each body part as you ask your patient about specific problems. Doing so may help him remember past problems. Also, encourage him to be as specific as possible.

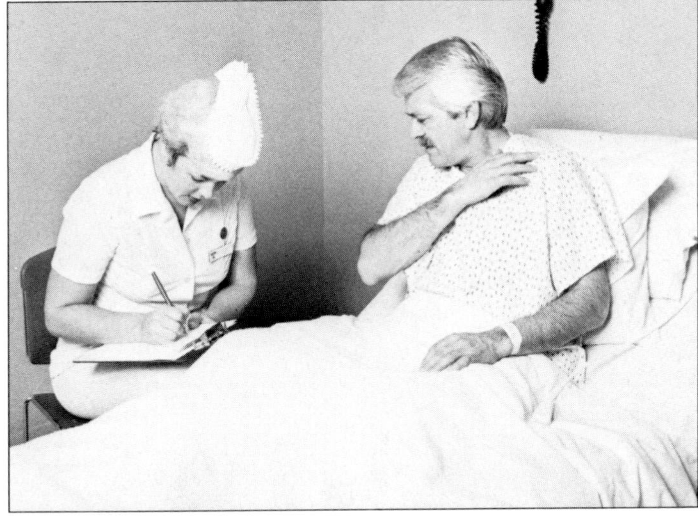

- When did your injuries occur? How did you receive them? Did you notice any immediate signs and symptoms? How often do your symptoms occur? Do they occur at a particular time of day? What treatment have you received for your injuries? What effect has it had on your symptoms? Does anything seem to relieve or aggravate them?
- Name any other past or present major bone or muscle injuries, such as fractures, dislocations, or lacerations. How were they treated? Did they heal successfully?
- Have you ever damaged any tendons? Have you pulled or strained muscles? Injured ligaments? Torn cartilage? When? What caused the injuries? How were these injuries treated? Did you suffer any long-term damage?
- How active are you? Do you exercise regularly, or participate in any athletic activities, such as running? What sports have you played in the past? Have you ever suffered any sports-associated injuries? If so, when? How was the injury treated? Was there any long-term damage?
- Were you born with any physical deformities? What kind? Has your condition been treated? Have any other deformities developed?
- Have you ever experienced muscle weakness in your arms or legs? When?
- Have you ever suffered any temporary or permanent muscle paralysis? When? In what area of your body?
- Have you ever noted any numbness or tingling? In what part of your body?
- Do you have any problem walking or keeping your balance? Do you associate this problem with any particular activity, such as climbing stairs or standing on a stool or ladder? How long have you had this condition?
- Have you ever suffered any muscular pain? If so, where? Do you have it now? Is it continuous or intermittent? Is it aggravated by using a joint? Does it prohibit or limit joint movement?
- Have you noted any swelling, tenderness, discoloration, or pain in any of your joints? Or, have you ever been aware of any stiffness, or inability to use a particular joint? If so, which joints were affected?
- Have you ever been diagnosed as having arthritis? When? In what area of your body?
- Have you had surgery for any bone, muscle, ligament, tendon, or nerve problems? When? Was your recovery complete, or was there any long-term damage?
- Does any family member have a bone or muscle problem; for example, osteoporosis, flatfoot, clubfoot, or muscular dystrophy?

When you've completed a successful interview, you'll have the following information about your patient's musculoskeletal condition:

- details of his present injuries including location of any signs and symptoms, their frequency and intensity, times of day they're most noticeable, and factors which seem to exacerbate or relieve them
- details of any previous injuries which might have a bearing on your patient's present condition
- any treatment of previous injuries and the treatment outcome
- existence of any deformity
- existence of any paresthesia or paralysis
- existence of any muscle problems
- existence of any joint problems.

Document all your findings accurately on the appropriate forms.

Preparing for an orthopedic assessment

You've documented Clarence Michie's orthopedic history. Now, you must thoroughly assess his musculoskeletal system. A musculoskeletal examination includes general observation, inspection, palpation, range-of-motion evaluation, and muscle power assessment.

Always conduct your assessment in a quiet, private setting that's well lighted. Make sure you allot sufficient time for the assessment, as each joint must be examined extensively.

Nursing tip: If your patient's receiving pain medication, schedule your assessment approximately 2 hours after his medication has been administered. This way, he'll still be receiving some pain relief, but not enough to mask his signs and symptoms.

When inspecting and palpating your patient's joints, use the checklist on page 34 as a guide. Be sure to check each joint for all the conditions listed.

Always remember to compare bilateral body parts. *Important:* If your patient's been injured, examine his uninjured side first. Otherwise, his muscles may tense bilaterally in response to discomfort, inhibiting range of motion on his uninjured side.

When you conduct range-of-motion tests, perform the movements listed for each joint in the chart on pages 16 to 19. Encourage your patient to actively perform the range-of-motion tests. But, don't let him strain to do so. Also, whenever you must use passive range of motion because of your patient's condition (for example, his muscles are weak, or he's comatose), stop the movement at the first signs of discomfort or joint resistance.

In performing your assessment, use the following photostory as a guideline. But, always consider your patient's individual condition. Examine his body parts in a way that will cause him the least discomfort. For example, if he has a leg injury, try to reduce the time he'll spend standing.

Assessment

Joint signs and symptoms

When assessing your patient, check each joint for the following signs and symptoms.

Joints
- Pain or tenderness
- Full range of motion
- Abnormal mobility
- Temperature (warmth)
- Redness
- Pain on motion
- Crepitation
- Discoloration
- Synovial fluid effusion
- Swelling or deformity
- Instability
- Ankylosis (joint immobility)
- Thickened synovial membrane
- Bony enlargement
- Congenital defects

Condition of tissues surrounding joint
- Spasm
- Muscle atrophy
- Subcutaneous nodules
- Skin changes
- Swelling
- Contractures

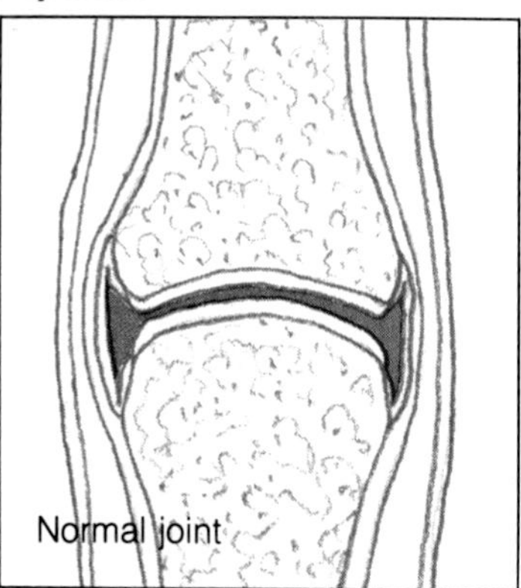

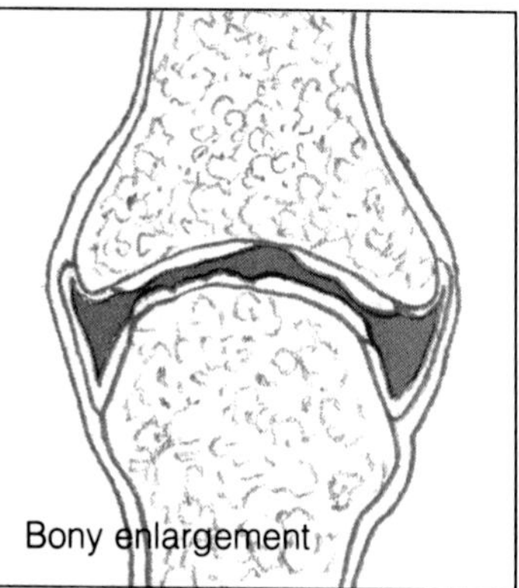

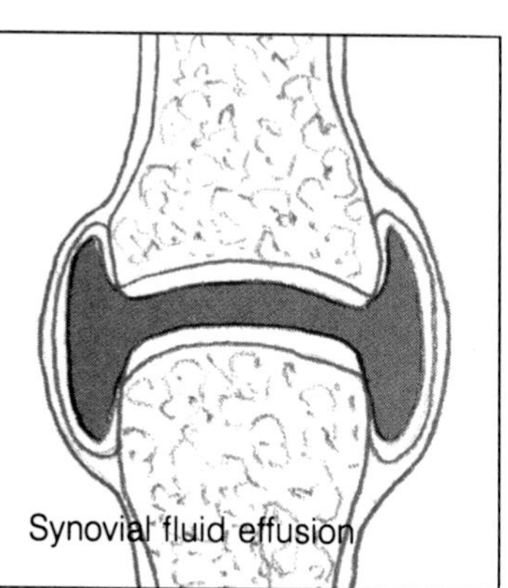

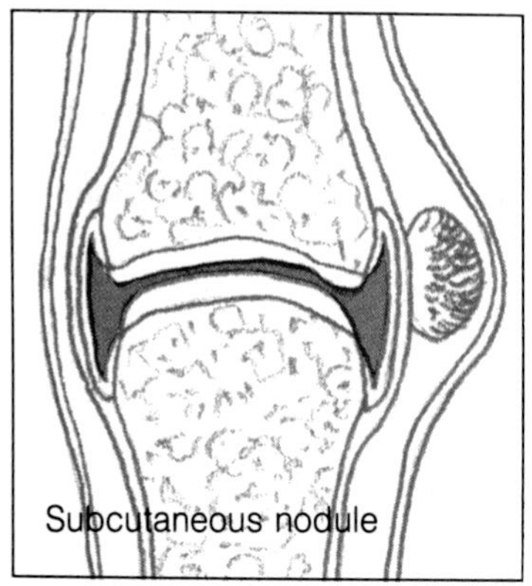

Performing an orthopedic assessment

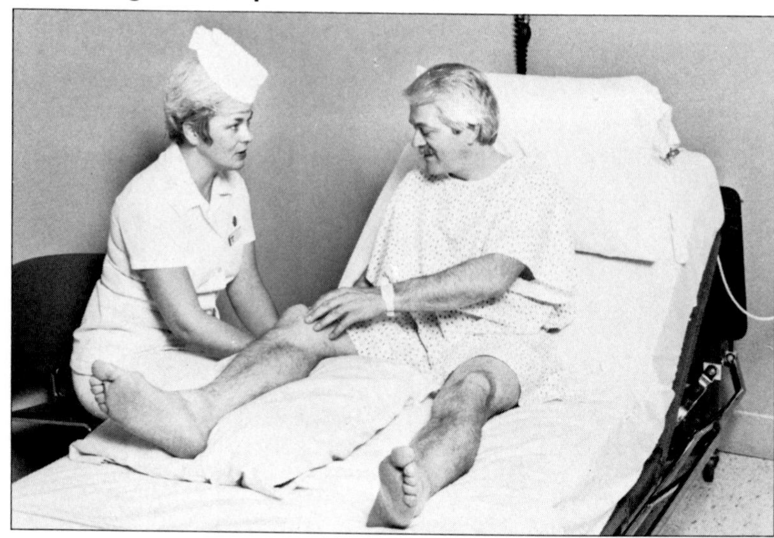

1 *Are you ready to begin Mr. Michie's assessment?* First, obtain a tape measure for measuring body parts. Then, wash your hands.

Next, spend a few minutes explaining the assessment procedure to Mr. Michie. To help relax him, discuss the procedure in a reassuring, conversational way. *Note:* You'll obtain a more accurate assessment if your patient's muscles are relaxed.

Also, take this opportunity to observe his facial expressions, skin color, level of consciousness, and body posture, including placement of his arms and legs.

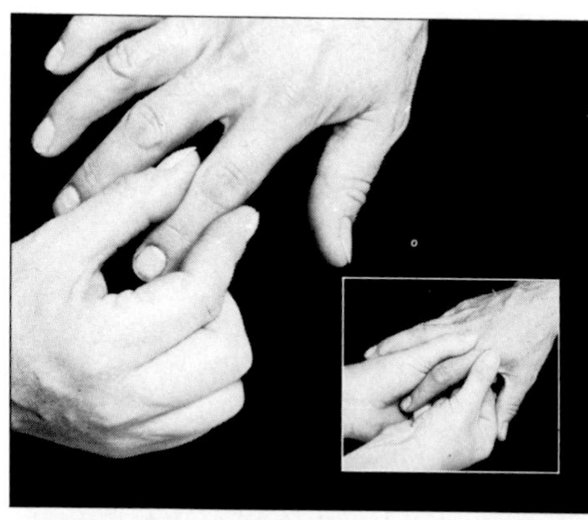

2 Now, you're ready to perform inspection, palpation, and range-of-motion testing. Begin by inspecting your patient's right hand and fingers. Then, using your thumb and forefinger, palpate the medial and lateral aspects of each interphalangeal joint, as the nurse is doing here.

(Inset) Then, palpate each metacarpophalangeal joint.

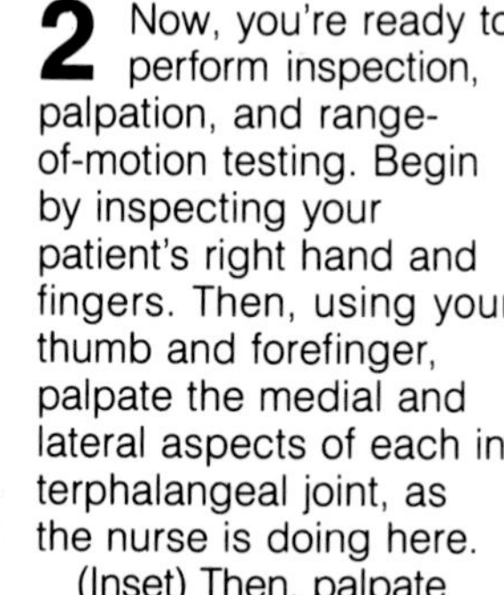

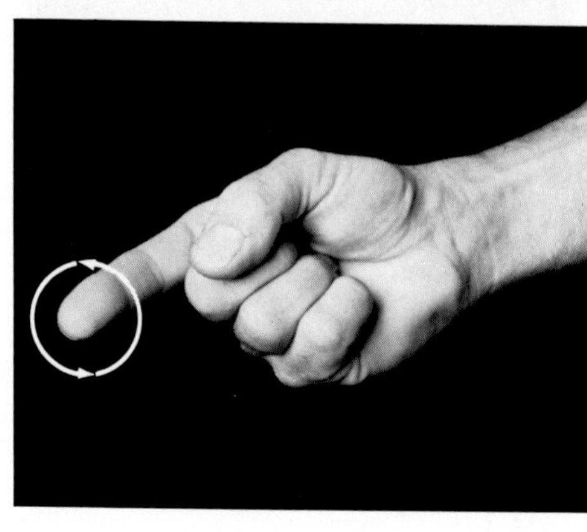

3 Test your patient's metacarpophalangeal joints, and his proximal and distal interphalangeal joints, for full range of motion.

Then, inspect, palpate, and test range of motion for Mr. Michie's left hand and fingers as you did for his right hand and fingers.

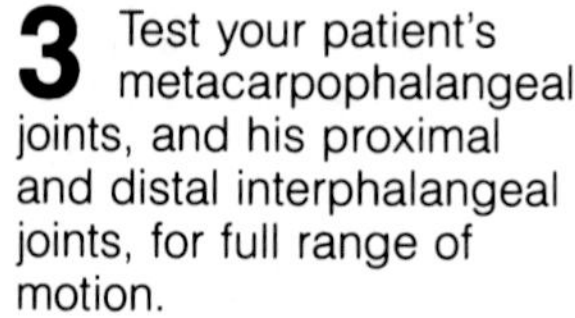

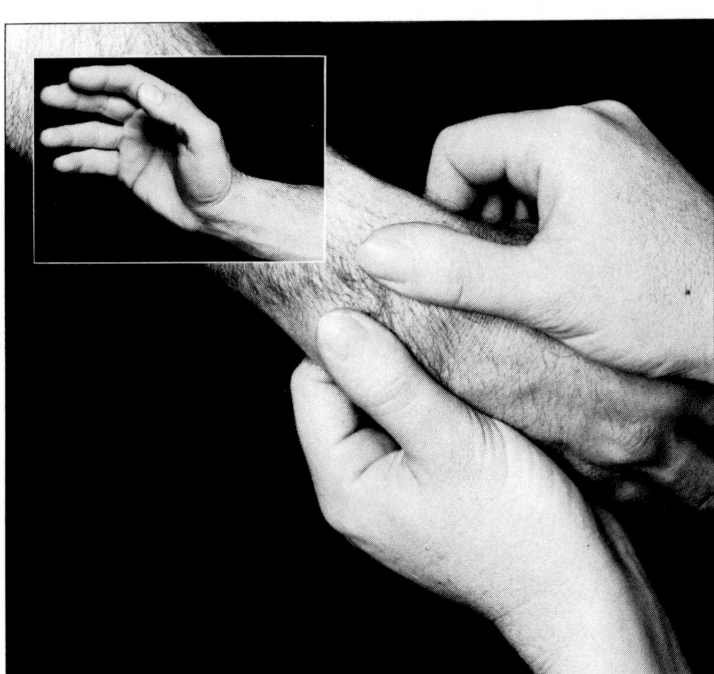

4 Next, palpate each wrist joint, as shown here, placing your thumbs on his wrist's upper surface and your fingers underneath his wrist. Palpate the distal ends of his radius and ulna, and the group of carpal bones.

(Inset) Evaluate each wrist for range of motion.

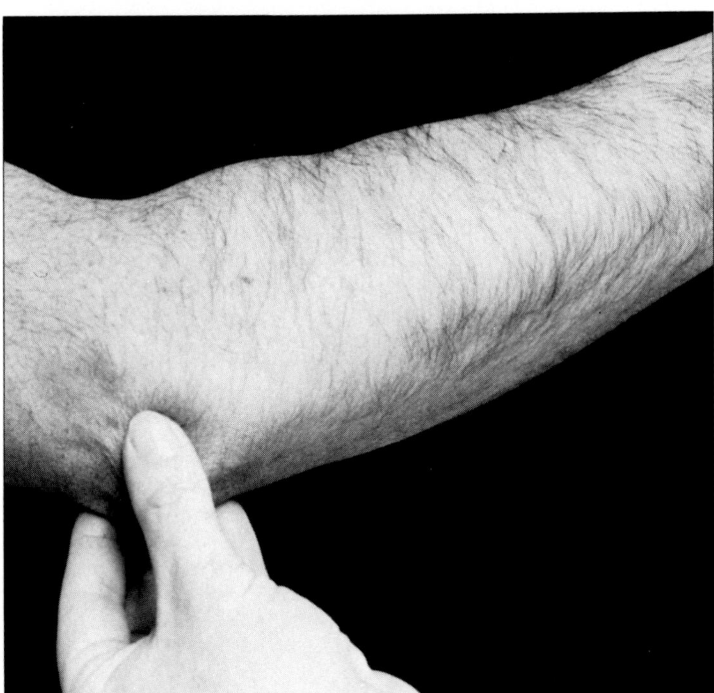

5 Then, inspect and palpate each elbow, examining the olecranon, the humerus' bony prominences (medial and lateral epicondyles), and the humeroulnar joint space, as shown here. Also, test each elbow's range of motion.

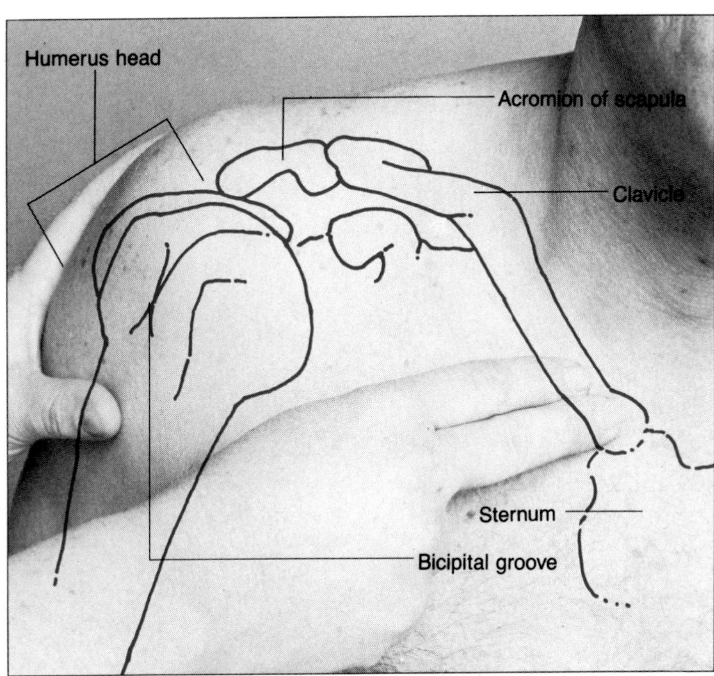

6 Now, ask Mr. Michie to disrobe to his waist. Then, examine his shoulders and scapulae.

First, examine his uninjured right shoulder. Palpate the length of his clavicle, including the sternoclavicular and acromioclavicular joints. Also, palpate the acromion of his scapula and the anterior surface of the humerus' head. (You won't be able to palpate the portion of the humerus' head which rests in the glenoid fossa.) Locate his bicipital groove, between the greater and lesser tubercles on the humerus' anterior surface. Conduct range-of-motion exercises, observing his scapulohumeral and scapulothoracic movement.

Then, cautiously follow the same procedure on your patient's injured left shoulder. Check for crepitation, grating sounds, pain, and tenderness, in addition to the other signs, symptoms, and tissue conditions listed in the chart at left. Gently conduct range-of-motion exercises.

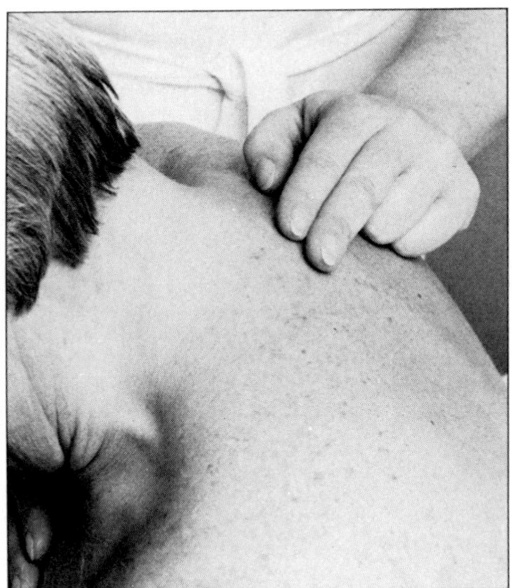

7 Next, carefully inspect your patient's neck.

To assess his complaint of tenderness, palpate his vertebrae, as shown here. Make sure all seven cervical vertebrae are palpable and in proper alignment.

Assessment

Performing an orthopedic assessment continued

8 Now, test range of motion in your patient's head and neck. *Caution:* Conduct range-of-motion tests only if you're certain your patient's cervical vertebrae are intact. Otherwise, you could damage his spinal cord.

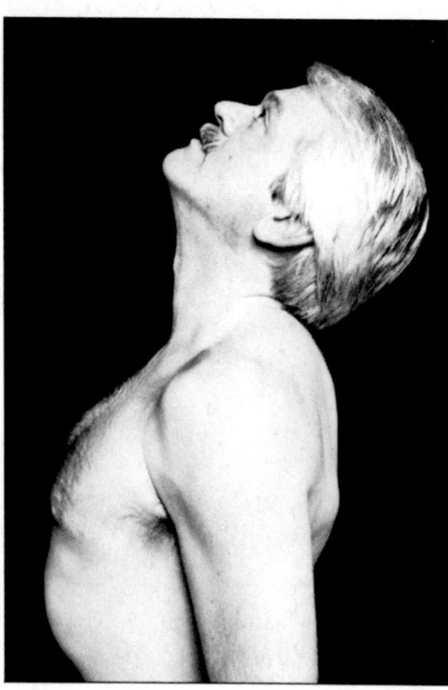

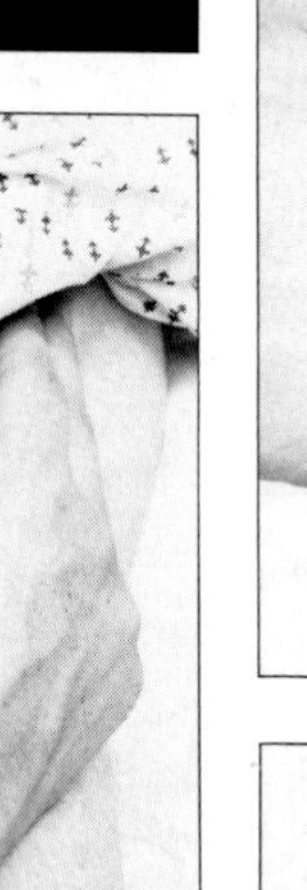

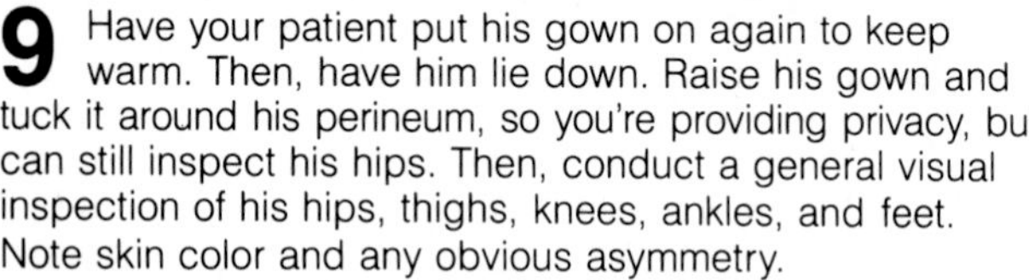

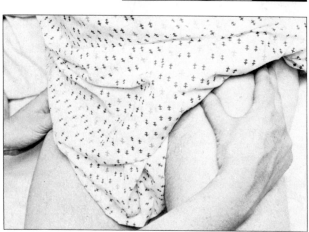

9 Have your patient put his gown on again to keep warm. Then, have him lie down. Raise his gown and tuck it around his perineum, so you're providing privacy, but can still inspect his hips. Then, conduct a general visual inspection of his hips, thighs, knees, ankles, and feet. Note skin color and any obvious asymmetry.

10 Now, inspect his left foot. Observe his toes and nailbeds for any obvious cyanosis or discoloration. Note any deformities, nodules, swelling, calluses, or corns.

To test for tenderness in his metatarsophalangeal joints, compress the sides of his forefoot, as shown here.

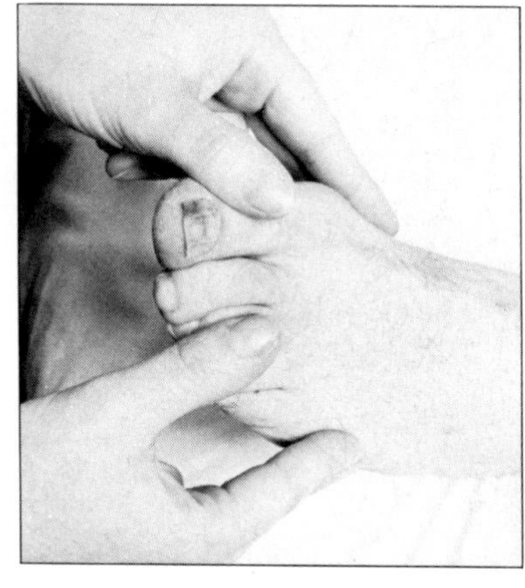

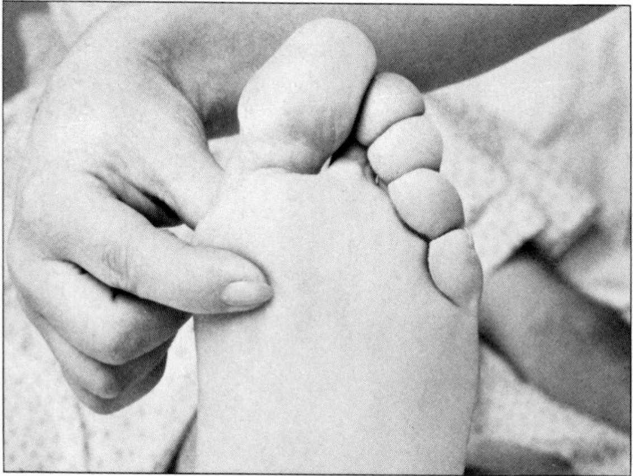

11 To detect a plantar wart, palpate his metatarsophalangeal joints. Do so by compressing each joint between your thumb and forefinger.

Also, evaluate range of motion in his toe joints. Repeat this assessment on Mr. Michie's right foot.

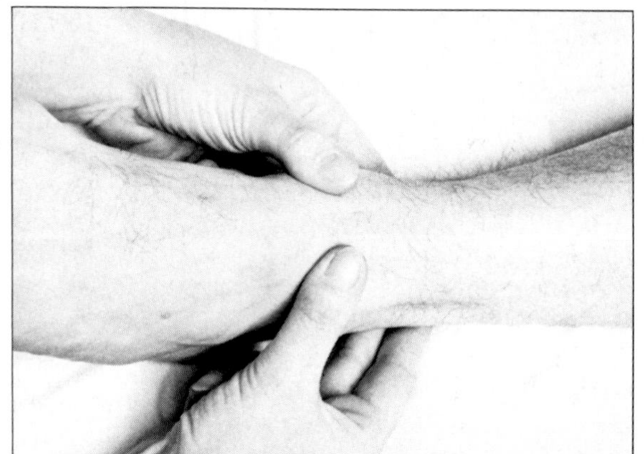

12 Next, palpate his ankle joint's anterior surface, as the nurse is doing here. Also, palpate his ankle's bony prominences (the lateral and medial malleoli). Then, palpate along his Achilles tendon for subcutaneous nodules. Examine both his ankles for full range of motion.

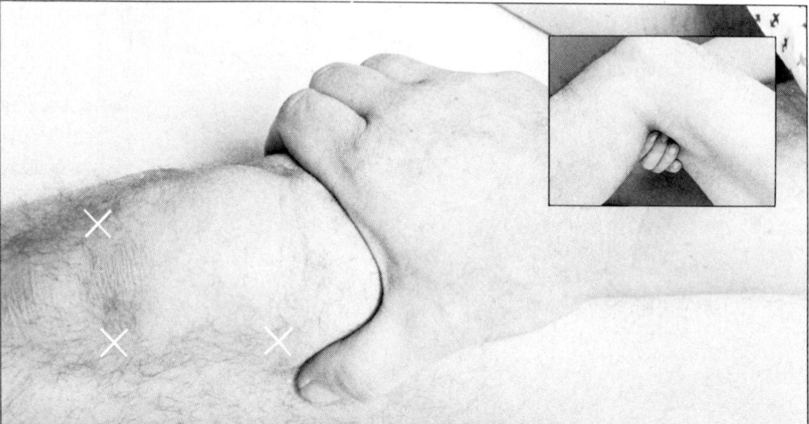

13 Continue your inspection by examining your patient's uninjured knee. Note any atrophy of his quadriceps muscle. Palpate the suprapatellar pouch on each side of the quadriceps, using your thumb and fingers.

Next, compress his suprapatellar pouch with one hand, as you palpate on either side of his patella (position indicated by Xs). Then, palpate over his tibiofemoral joint space (position indicated by Xs).

(Inset) Finally, palpate his popliteal space for swelling, cysts, or nodules. Now, test his joint for range of motion.

Next, examine his injured right knee in the same way. Note any contusion, bogginess, pain, fluid, tenderness, grating, edema, or synovial thickening.

Note: Knee pain may be referred pain from a hip problem.

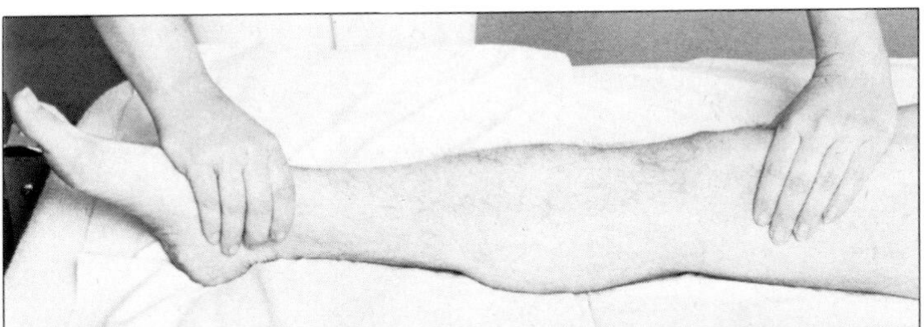

14 Because your patient has a knee injury, you must test his right knee joint for instability. To do so, perform these two special tests. First, have him extend his right leg. Then, fix his femur in place with one hand. With your other hand, grasp his ankle and try to abduct or adduct his leg at his knee. If his joint is stable, it will undergo only minimal motion on this test.

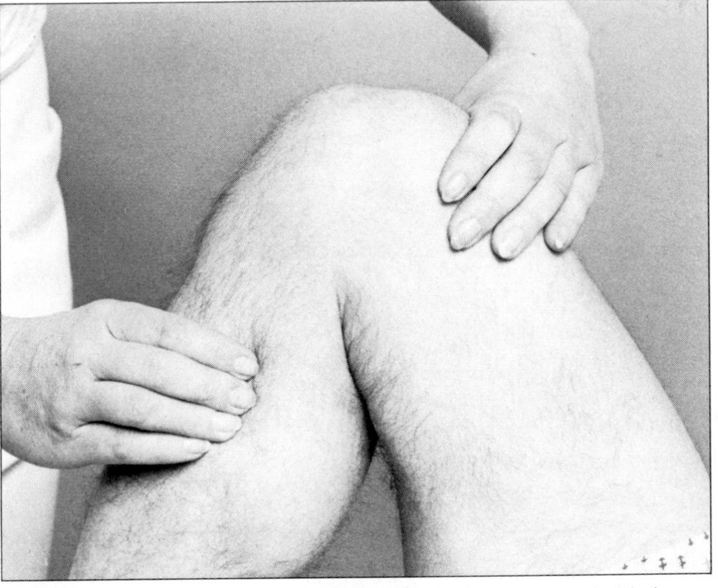

15 Now, perform this second test. First, flex your patient's knee at a 90° angle. Then, stabilize his foot by tucking it under his opposite leg. Hold his upper leg with one hand as you grasp his lower leg below his knee and try to push it backward and forward. Little or no movement should occur in his knee.

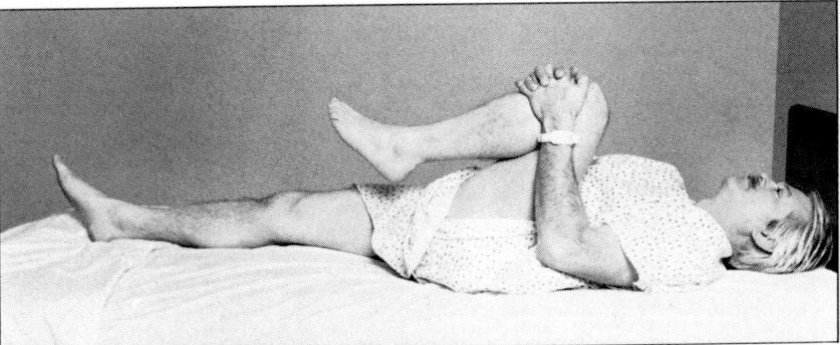

16 Next, inspect and palpate Mr. Michie's left iliac crest and his femur's bony prominence (greater trochanter). To test flexion in his hip, have him pull his knee toward his chest, as shown here. *Note:* If his opposite thigh flexes at the same time, he probably has a flexion deformity in the opposite hip.

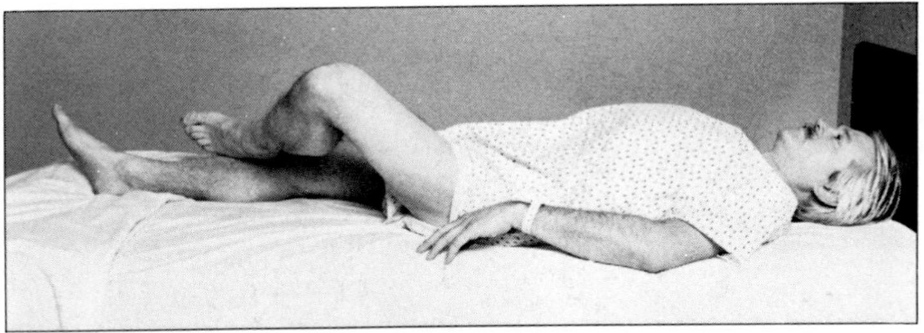

17 To test for arthritis, place his left foot on his opposite patella. Then, have him move his knee down toward his side. Doing so will rotate his leg externally in his hip.

Now, rotate his hip internally by moving his knee back into its original position. Any pain or limitation of motion may indicate arthritis or inflammatory disorder.

Finally, return his leg to its resting position. As you do so, cup your hand over his knee to detect any crepitation.

Examine his opposite hip in the same way.

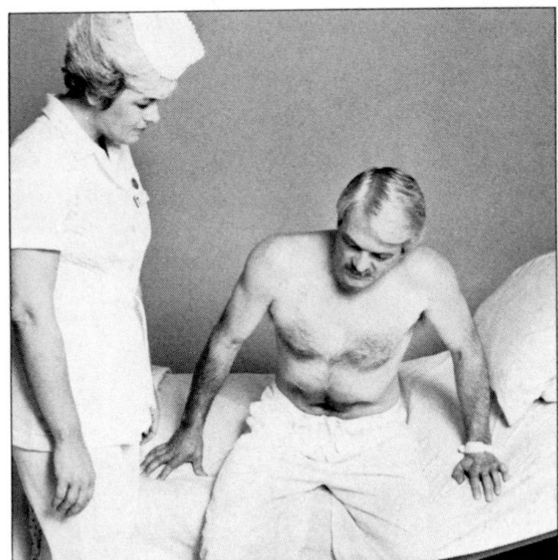

18 Next, give your patient a pair of pajama bottoms to put on. Then, to complete his hip range-of-motion evaluation, have him stand. As he does so, observe how easily he moves from a sitting to a standing position. Note any signs of pain in his right knee. Now, test both hips for other joint movements, such as abduction and adduction.

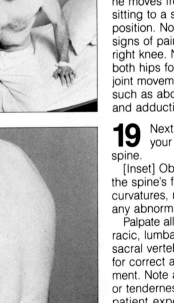

19 Next, inspect your patient's spine.

[Inset] Observe the spine's four curvatures, noting any abnormalities.

Palpate all thoracic, lumbar, and sacral vertebrae for correct alignment. Note any pain or tenderness your patient experiences during palpation.

Assessment

Performing an orthopedic assessment continued

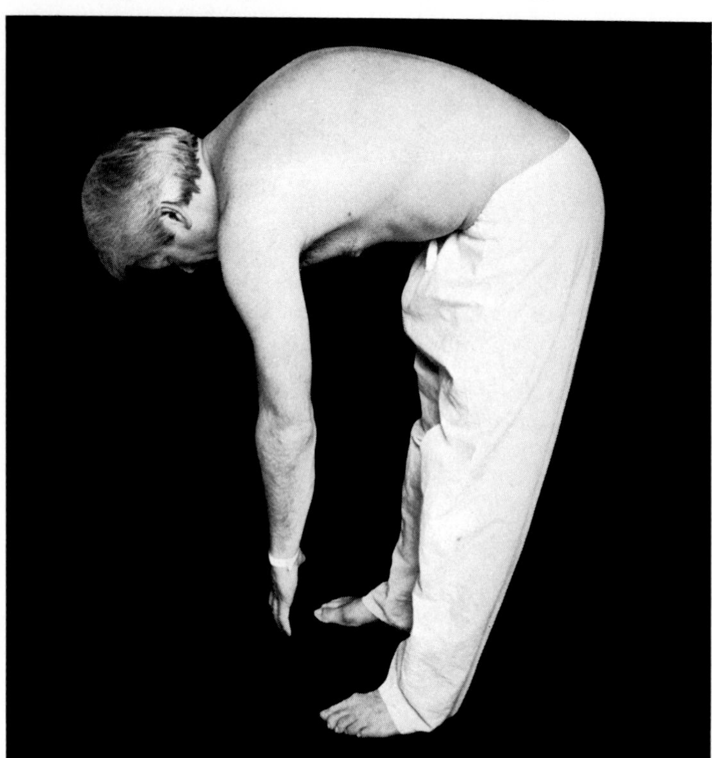

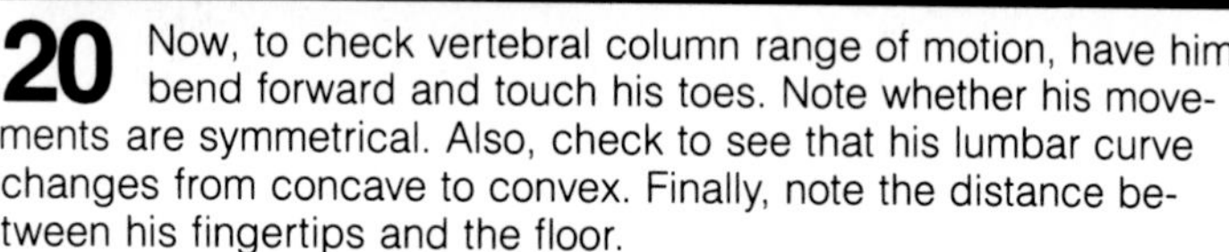

20 Now, to check vertebral column range of motion, have him bend forward and touch his toes. Note whether his movements are symmetrical. Also, check to see that his lumbar curve changes from concave to convex. Finally, note the distance between his fingertips and the floor.

Continue testing vertebral column range of motion by having Mr. Michie bend from his waist, first to each side and then backward. Be prepared to stabilize him by holding his waist, if necessary. Also, have him rotate his shoulders to the right and to the left.

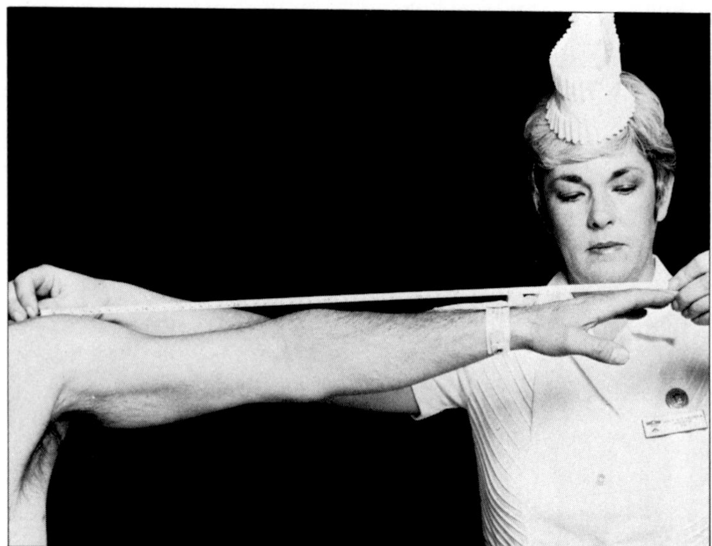

21 Next, measure your patient's extremities. Compare the lengths of symmetrical body parts.

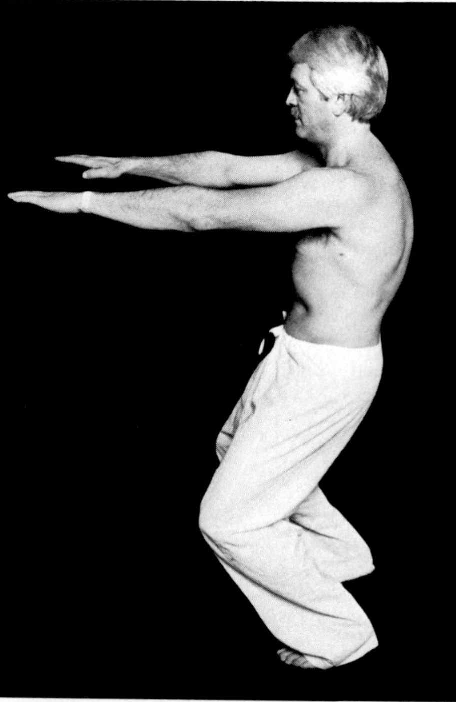

22 Now, ask Mr. Michie to stoop with his arms extended in front of him. As he does so, observe his coordination and movement. Then, have him perform a series of familiar movements, such as sitting down, lying back, sitting up again, rising to a standing position, and bending. As he executes these movements, note his posture, and any signs of discomfort, muscle weakness, and joint stiffness.

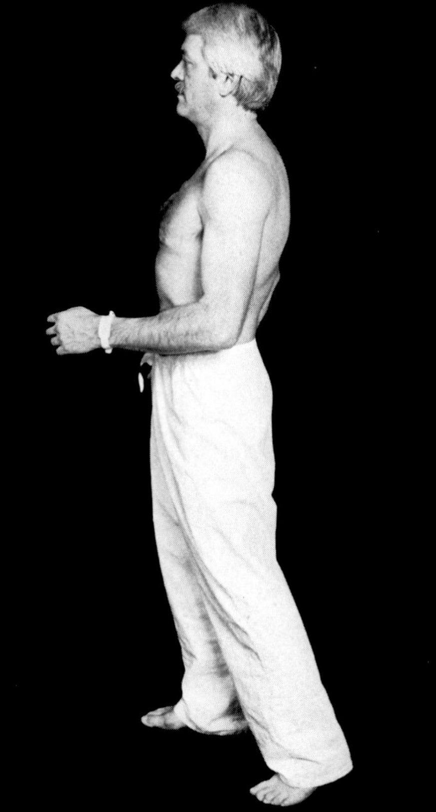

23 Ask Mr. Michie to walk across the room. As you assess his gait, note his stance (position of his foot on the floor) and swing (movement of his leg swinging forward). Note the associated joint movements of his arms and legs. Is his gait smooth, coordinated, and rhythmic? Or does he limp or stumble?

Observe his gait (if possible) both with and without any ambulation aids he uses, such as crutches, braces, or a walker. Listen to his walk for any flopping (indicates foot drop), dragging or scraping (indicates spasticity), or stomping (indicates ataxia). Again, note any signs of pain or stiffness.

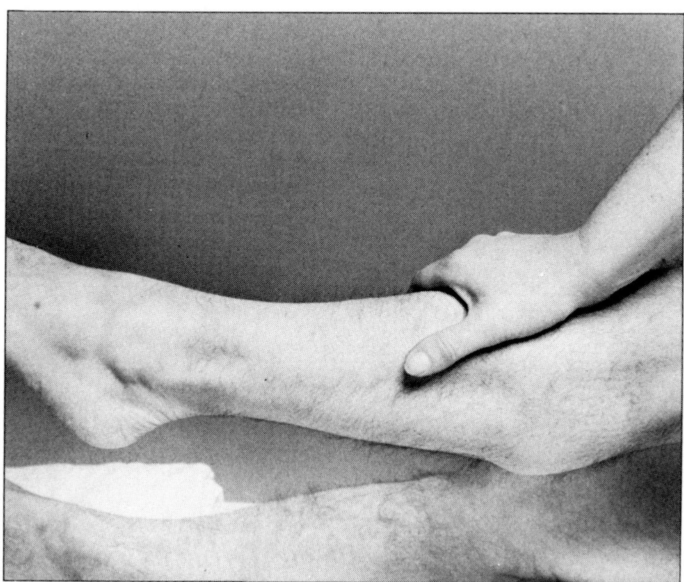

24 For the last step in your assessment, test your patient's muscle power. To do this, help your patient put on his gown, remove his pajama bottoms, and lie down. Then, follow the guidelines at right. Evaluate his range of motion both with your assistance and without your assistance. Then, measure his ability to move his muscles when you apply resistance, as the nurse is doing here.

Important: Never tire a weak muscle by assessing it to the point where motion ceases.

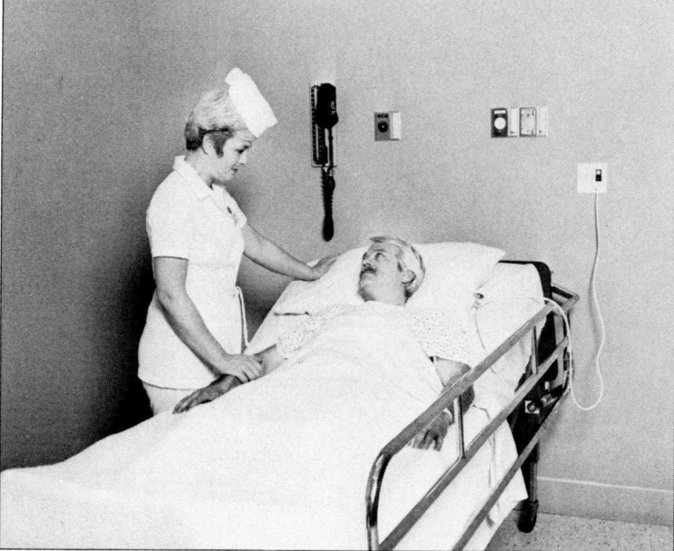

25 After you've finished evaluating his muscle power, adjust his gown. Then, assist him to a comfortable position. Remember to document all your findings on the appropriate assessment forms. Report any new findings to the doctor. Be sure to immediately report any signs or symptoms of a deteriorating condition.

Note: If your patient's scheduled to receive pain medication, administer it when you've completed the assessment.

Assessing muscle power

How strong are your patient's muscles? By range-of-motion testing, you can estimate his muscle power and rate it on a scale of 0 to 5, as shown below.

Usually, you'll assess your patient's muscle function in this order: neck, shoulder, elbow, hand, fingers, hip, knee, foot, and toes. However, if your patient's injured, begin by assessing muscle movement at joints distal to the affected area. Then, work toward the affected area. For example, if he injured his forearm, assess his finger joints first, and then his wrist joints. After that, proceed with the assessment in the usual order.

When assessing your patient's muscle strength, consider these factors: Is his strength appropriate for his size, age, and physical condition? Is his muscle strength equal symmetrically? Carefully document all your findings, including the muscle strength rating, on your hospital's assessment form.

Muscle assessment scale

The following scale for muscle testing divides muscle strength into six categories, ranging from 0 (no muscle movement) to 5 (normal muscle strength).

Note: Your hospital may use a different scale to assess muscle strength. Whatever scale is employed, make sure all staff members who assess the patient use the same one.

Scale value	Description
0	Patient can't use muscle being tested to move the joint. You can't feel muscle contraction or change in muscle tone when he attempts to perform movement.
1	Patient can't use muscle to move the joint. But you can feel muscle contractions and a change in muscle tone when he attempts to perform movement.
2	Patient can use muscle being tested to move joint through a normal range of motion, with your help. However, he can't do it without your help.
3	Patient can move joint through a normal range of motion without help. However, he can't do it when you apply minimal additional resistance.
4	Patient can move the joint through a normal range of motion with minimal resistance applied. However, he can't overcome the amount of resistance you'd expect a person of his size to overcome. Or, if you're testing an injured extremity, he can't overcome the amount of resistance that his unaffected extremity can overcome.
5	Patient can move the joint through its normal range of motion, overcoming the amount of resistance you'd expect, or the amount that his unaffected extremity can overcome.

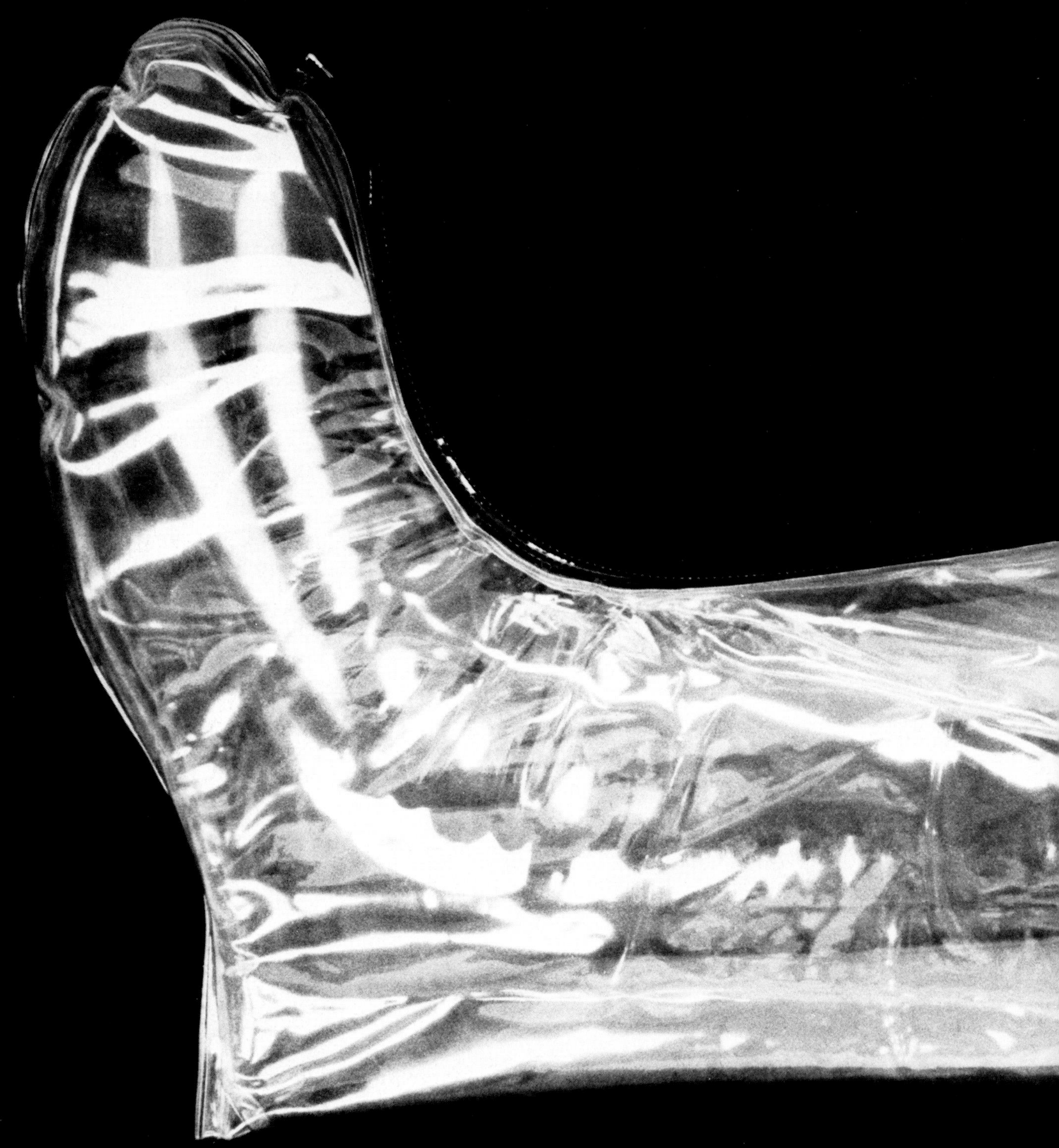

Dealing with Immobilization Devices

Wraps, splints, and slings

Casts

Traction

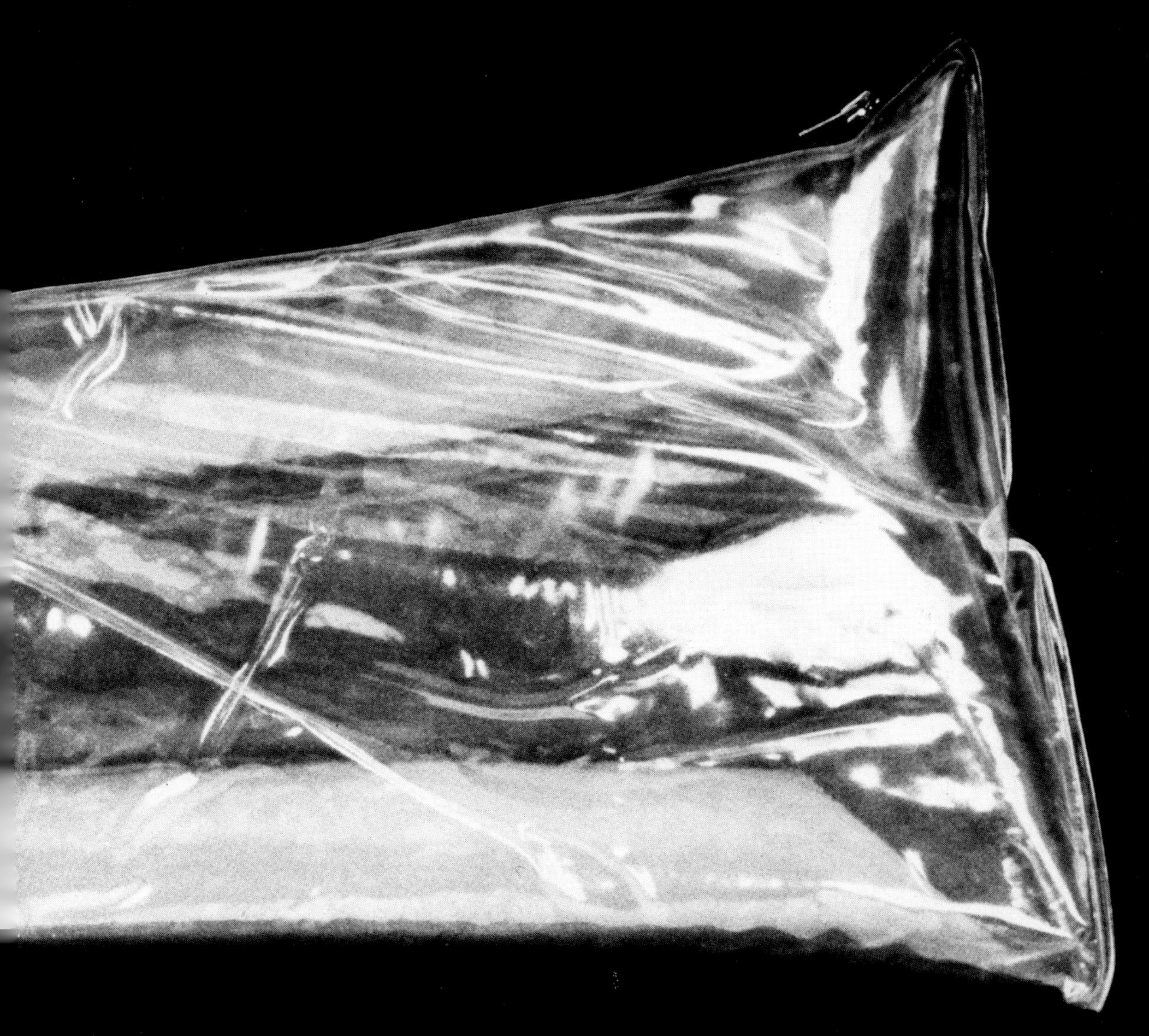

Wraps, splints, and slings

When your patient experiences a musculoskeletal injury, immobilization is a major consideration in proper healing. Why? If the injury site's kept stationary, repair tissue has a chance to form and mature.

In the next few pages, we'll introduce you to several types of immobilization devices. We'll show you:

- how to wrap an injury without causing nerve or circulatory damage.
- how to perform an at-the-scene assessment.
- how to apply a Hare traction splint.
- how to care for a patient with a long-term immobilizer splint.

For a thorough review of immobilization alternatives to casts and traction, read the text, photostories, and charts on the following pages.

Learning about roller bandages

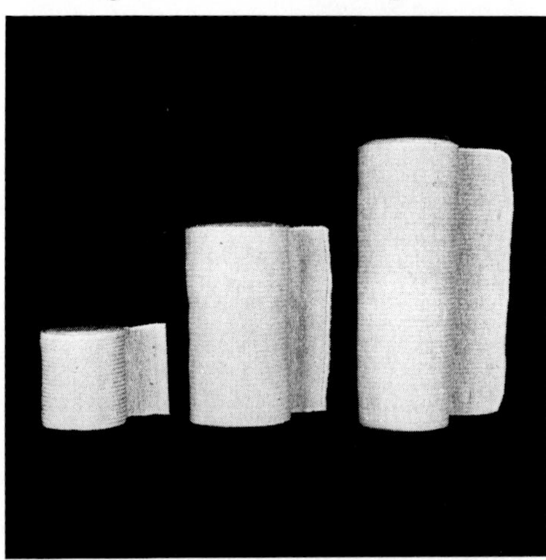

Roller bandages provide one of the simplest forms of immobilization support. Use them to support and protect an injured part or to secure an improvised splint. Roller bandages used for orthopedic injuries are usually made from elastic webbing, although gauze, flannel, muslin, or rubber bandages are also available.

Bandage sizes range from 1″ wide to 8″ (2.5 to 20.3 cm) wide. Use the size that's most appropriate for the injured part. Also, use new bandage rolls whenever possible. The greater the elasticity, the more uniform the bandage pressure will be.

Before applying the bandage, make sure the patient's skin is clean, dry, and free of drainage. Assess and document the condition of the patient's skin. Also, take this opportunity to check for presence of bilateral pulses. If a wound is present, apply a dressing over it before wrapping the injured area.

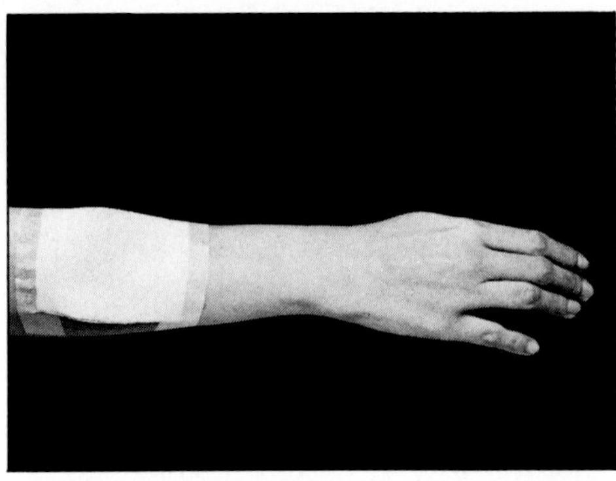

When applying the roller bandage, begin by wrapping the distal end of the injured

Types of turns used in bandaging

- *Circular turn.* Turn encircles previous turn, completely covering it. Use this turn for anchoring a bandage.

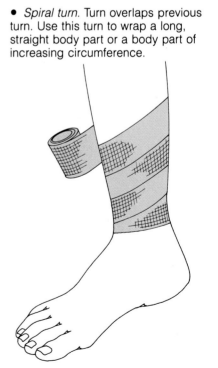

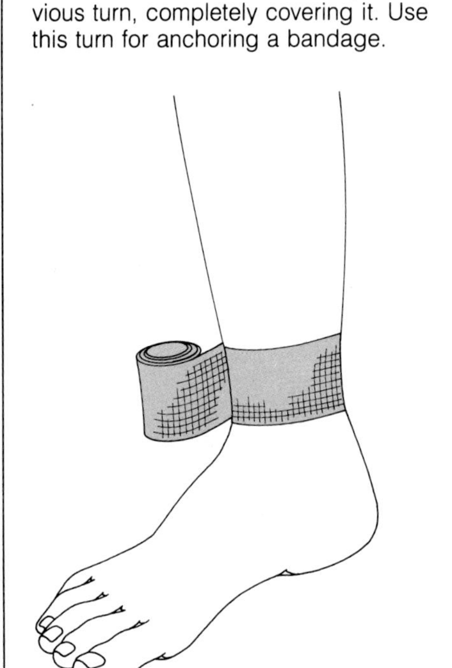

- *Spiral turn.* Turn overlaps previous turn. Use this turn to wrap a long, straight body part or a body part of increasing circumference.

limb. Always wrap from smaller to larger circumferences of the injured limb, for closer shaping of the bandage to the body part. Also, if possible, wrap in the direction of venous blood return to the patient's heart, to prevent blood pooling.

Apply gentle compression as you wind the bandage proximally. Keep the unrolled portion of the bandage close to the surface being wrapped, to create and maintain even pressure. Also, overlap each turn completely to cover the patient's skin. Otherwise, his skin may be pinched between turns of the bandage. Make sure the bandage has no wrinkles, which could cause pressure areas.

Remember: Don't wind the bandage too tightly. Excessive pressure could cause neurovascular impairment. For this reason, any patient wearing a roller bandage requires periodic neurovascular assessment.

Bandage the limb in the position in which you want it maintained. Remind the patient not to bend the limb, because pressure distribution of the bandage will change with joint movement.

Note: Any ordered range-of-motion exercises involving the bandaged area should

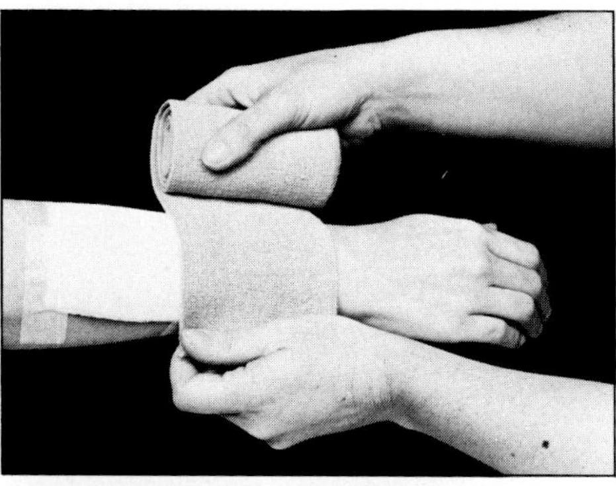

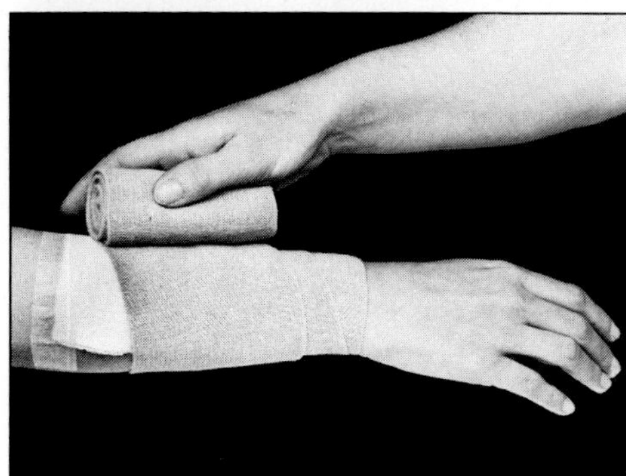

be performed only when the bandage has been removed.

Be sure to cover the limb well above and below the affected area. But, leave the fingers or toes exposed so you can perform

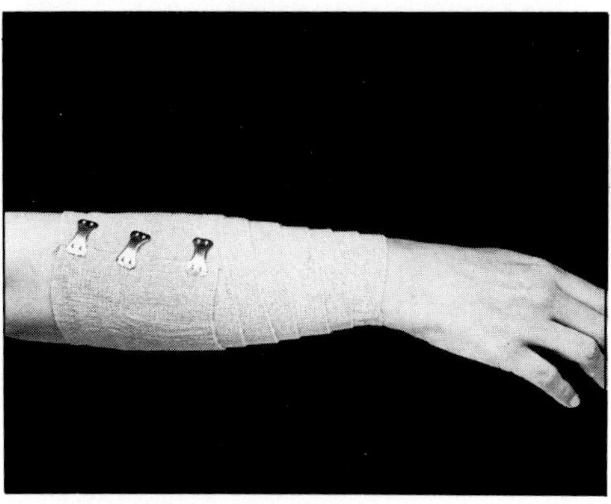

neurovascular checks readily and so your patient can exercise his digits.

See the photostory on the following pages for step-by-step instructions for correctly applying a roller bandage to an injured limb. Also, the chart below shows bandage turns you'll use in wrapping. For skin care of a wrapped limb, see page 55.

- *Spiral-reverse turn.* Turn reverses direction of bandage, halfway through a spiral wrap. Use this turn to accommodate either increasing or decreasing body part circumference.

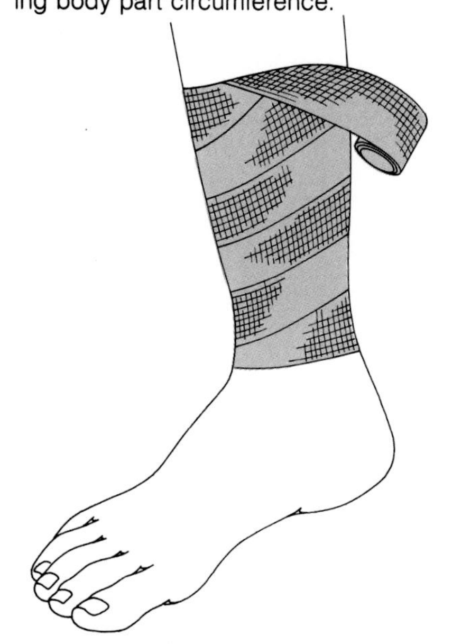

- *Figure-eight turn.* Alternating ascending and descending turns form a figure eight. Use this turn around joints.

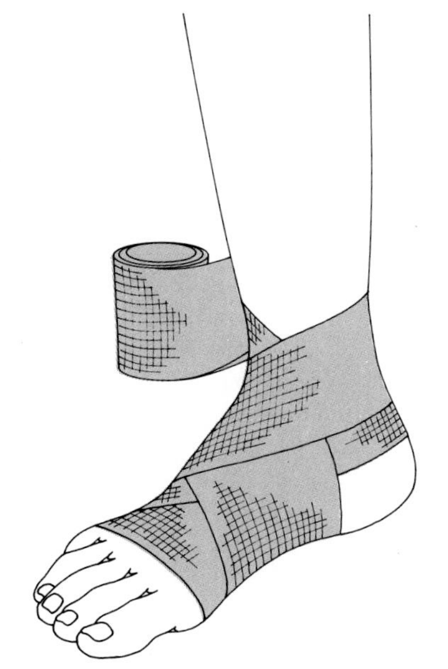

- *Recurrent turn.* Bandage includes a combination of several turn types, such as circular, spiral, spiral reverse, and figure eight. Use this turn for stump or scalp bandaging.

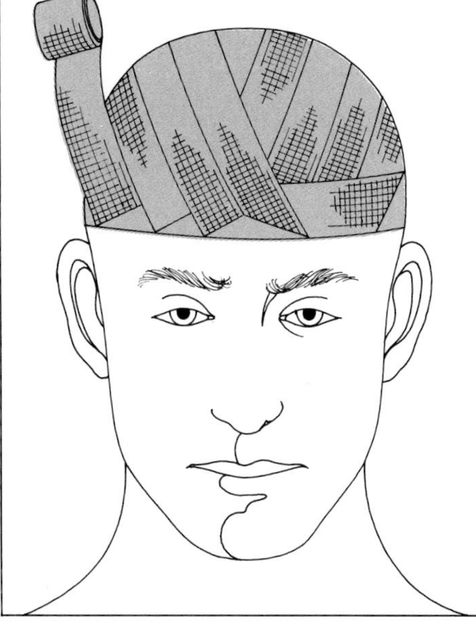

Wraps, splints, and slings

How to wrap an injured limb

1 *The doctor's ordered you to wrap your patient's sprained wrist. As you apply the elastic bandage, instruct your patient in its application. She may have to reapply the bandage at home.*

First, obtain an appropriate size elastic roller bandage, usually 1" to 2" (2.5 to 5.1 cm) wide. Then, wash your hands. To apply the bandage, hold the roll in your working hand with its loose end in your opposite hand.

Apply the outside surface of the loose end to your patient's hand, just proximal to the metacarpophalangeal joints.

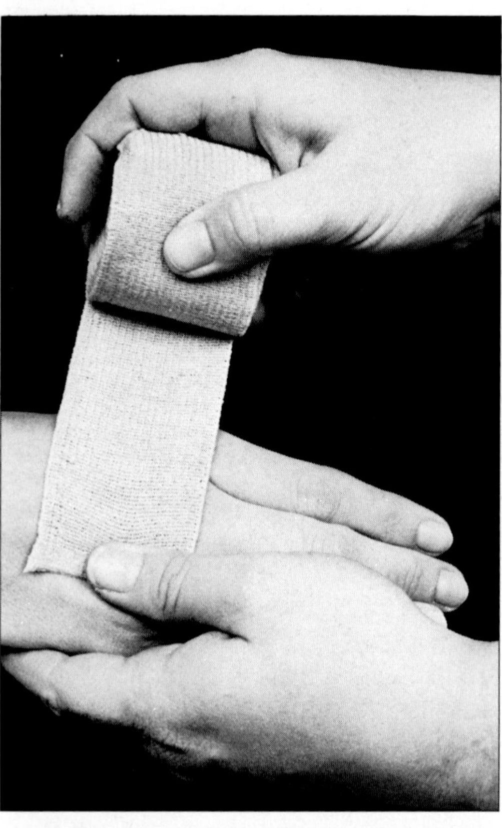

2 With your working hand, pass the roll around her hand. Make two or three circular turns to secure the bandage.

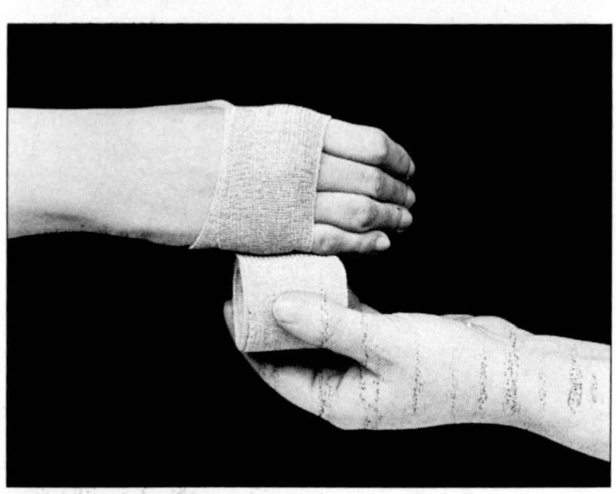

3 Now, angle the bandage, as shown, to begin making a figure-eight turn.

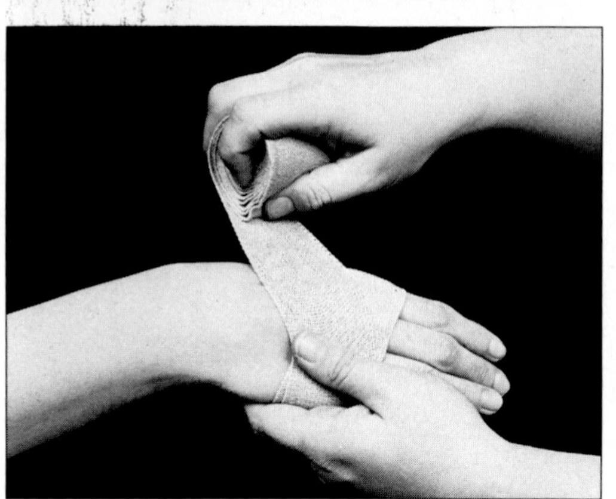

4 Make a figure-eight turn around her wrist, as shown here, until the wrist's completely covered.

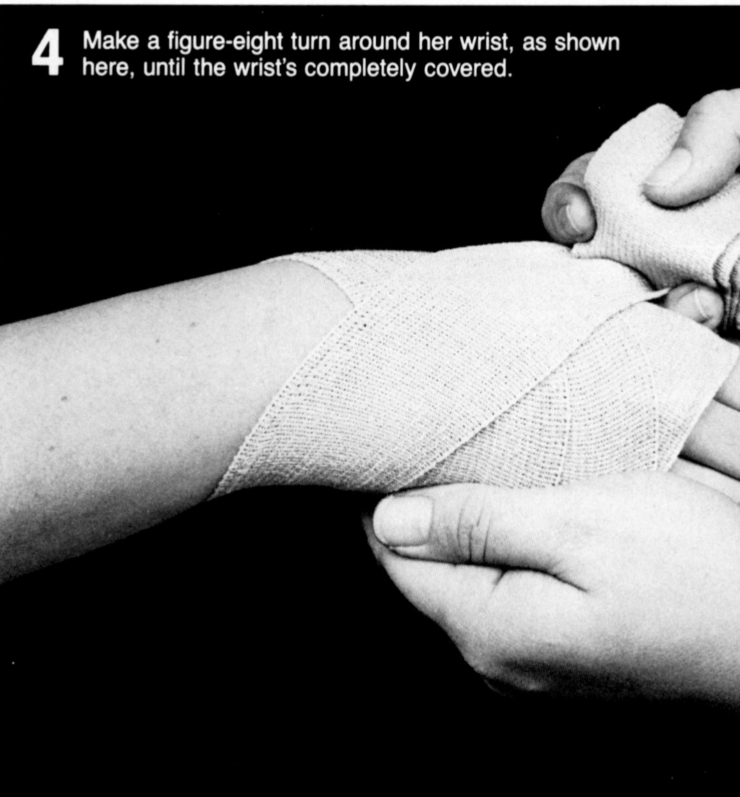

5 After you've wrapped her wrist, continue applying the bandage evenly, using spiral turns. Stretch the bandage gently as you do so.

Be sure to end the wrap away from bony prominences and other areas where the patient will be receiving pressure. Secure the end of the bandage with a clip or pin.

Instruct your patient to check the bandage frequently for tightness by inserting her fingers between the bandage and her skin. Also, instruct your patient to keep her limb elevated as much as possible. Follow the guidelines for patient care (including neurovascular checks and skin care) given on pages 24 and 55.

Finally, document the wrapping on the appropriate forms. Describe the wrist's appearance before wrapping, mentioning signs and symptoms such as ecchymosis and swelling.

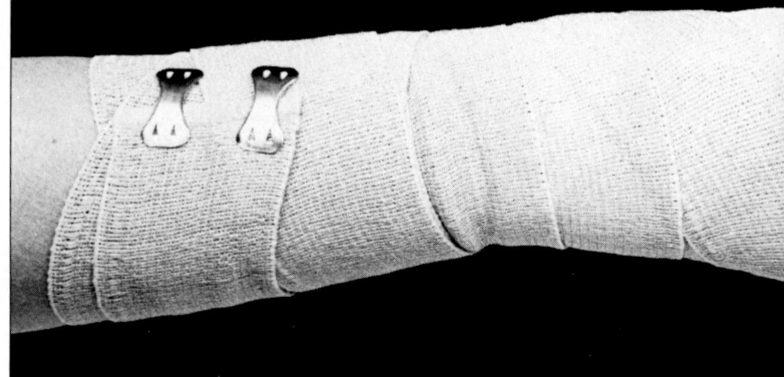

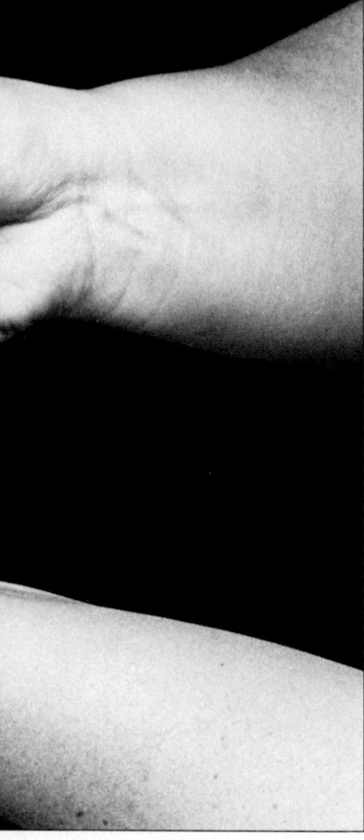

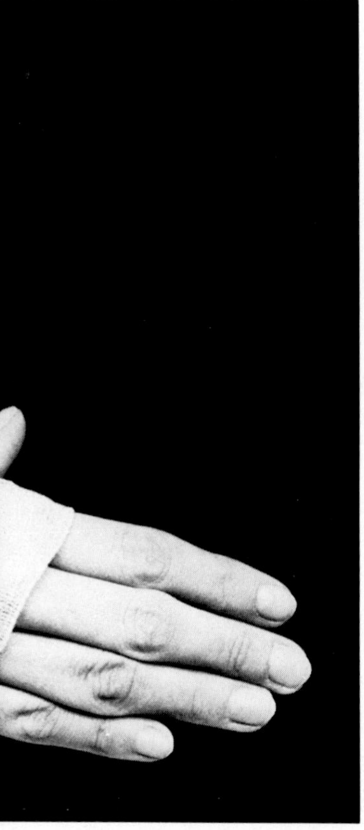

Learning about splints

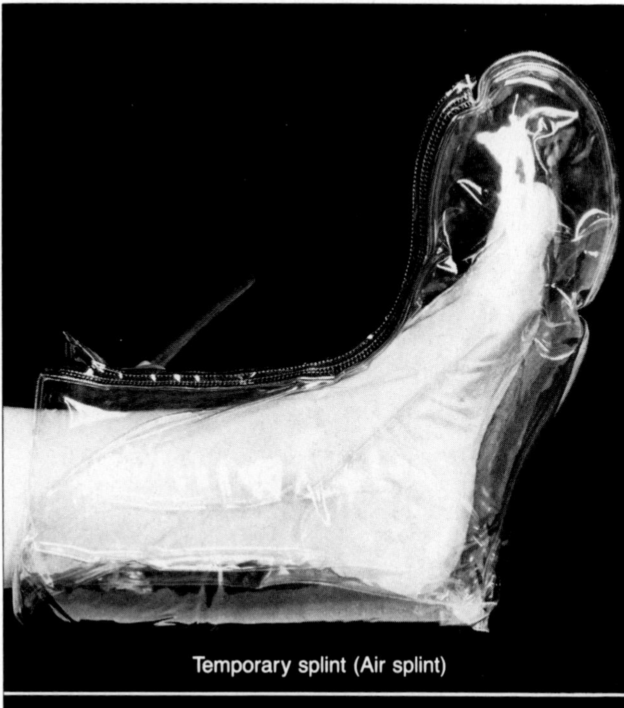

Temporary splint (Air splint)

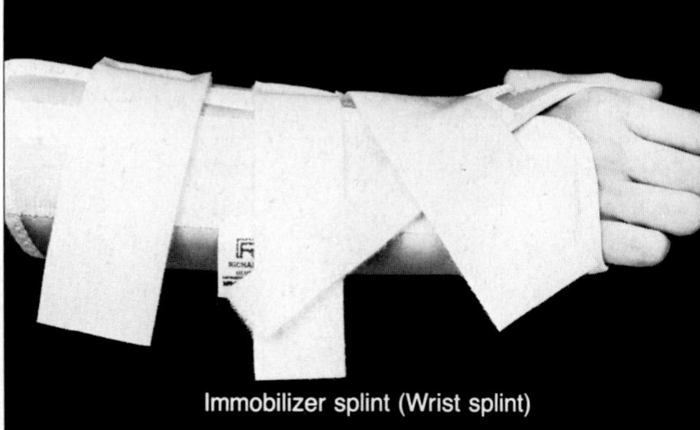

Immobilizer splint (Wrist splint)

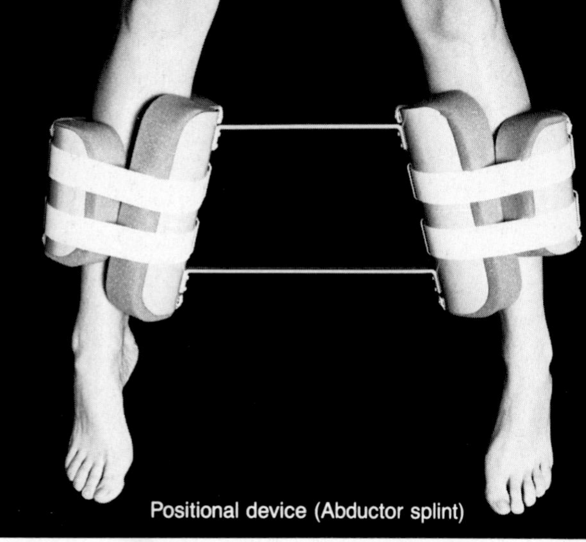

Positional device (Abductor splint)

As you know, a splint is a rigid or flexible device used to immobilize and protect an injured body part. Splints come in a wide range of designs and materials, including cloth, wood, metal, and plastic. Here we'll discuss three types.

• *Temporary splints* prevent further motion and tissue destruction immediately after an injury such as a fracture or a sprain. These include the air splint, the Hare traction splint, and improvised splints made out of rolled magazines, pillows, or even tree limbs. Because you'll usually apply such a splint in an emergency situation, you must carefully assess your patient's physical condition before doing so. See the photostories on pages 46 to 52 for assessment and application guidelines.

• *Immobilizer splints* provide long-term immobilization for such injuries as sprains and dislocations (as well as some fractures) that don't require complete, continuous immobilization in a cast or traction. These splints are also used following surgery.

In recent years, lightweight immobilizers with Velcro® closures have replaced cumbersome metal-and-leather buckled devices. The lighter-weight immobilizers permit quick adjustment as edema increases or subsides. They also provide ready access to the skin for skin care, dressing changes and neurovascular checks. And, as necessary, they can be easily removed for physical therapy.

Immobilizers for almost any body part, including the jaw, shoulder, knee, wrist, cervical vertebrae, and clavicle, are available (see the chart on pages 53 and 54).

• Certain *supportive and positional devices* may also be considered splints. They usually provide immobilization in a specific anatomical position. They maintain a body part in good alignment while a patient's on bed rest, and allow the patient to be turned without changing the healing limb's position. They can be removed for skin care, dressing changes, neurovascular checks, and physical therapy.

These immobilizers include abductor splints or pillows, which maintain the patient's legs in an abducted position after hip surgery. They also include casts that are split into anterior and posterior components, and some molded plastic splints. For more specific information on positioning devices, see the traction, surgery, and positioning aids sections.

Wraps, splints, and slings

Before splint application

James Renner, a 60-year-old maintenance man at the school where you work, has fallen from a stepladder. When you arrive at the scene, you see that his left lower leg is oddly positioned. He tells you he can move his leg, but it's very painful. You conclude that he has a fracture. You'll have to apply a splint so he can be moved safely to a hospital emergency department.

But first, assess him for any other trauma-associated problems such as shock, hemorrhage, or cardiopulmonary collapse. If a life-threatening problem exists, take steps to control it, such as providing proper body positioning, applying direct pressure to a hemorrhage site, or initiating cardiopulmonary resuscitation (CPR).

Then, assess the condition of his affected body part as instructed in steps 1 to 4 of the following photostory. Next, quickly examine his body for additional musculoskeletal injuries as instructed in steps 5 to 11. Check each part for malalignment, pain, ecchymosis, crepitation, grating, swelling, or limited range of motion.

Finally, splint the injured part as shown on pages 49 to 52.

Performing an emergency assessment

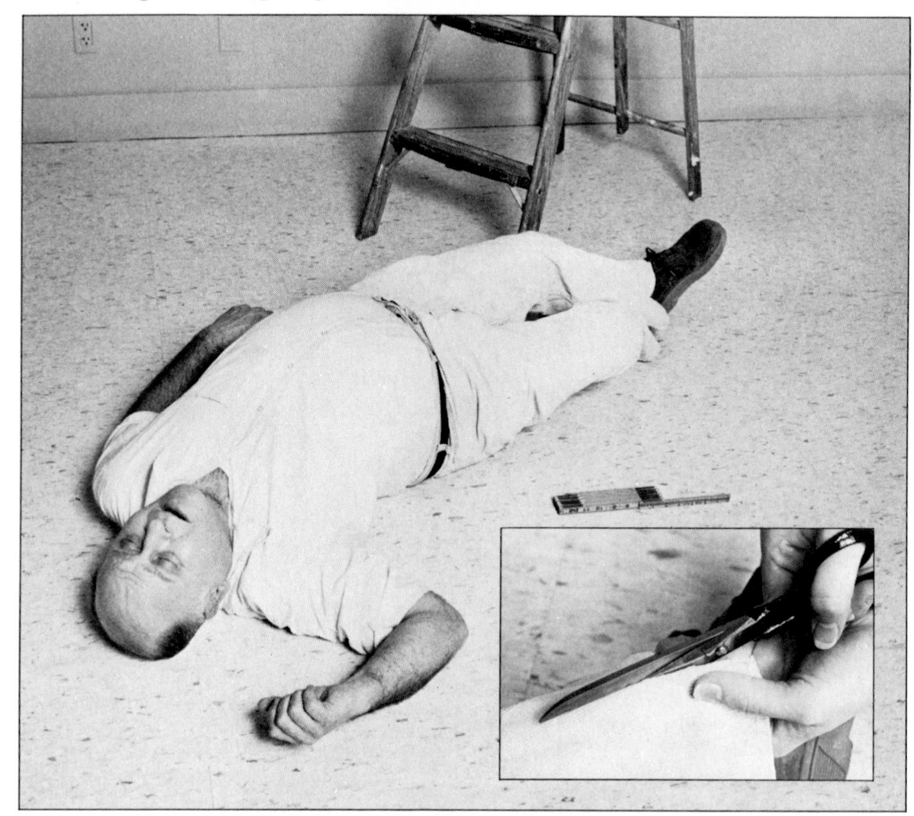

1 *Begin your assessment with a quick visual inspection for life-threatening problems.*

Then, moving your patient's leg as little as possible, cut off any constrictive clothing from it (see inset). Remember, moving the fracture site can cause further damage by increasing bleeding, compressing or tearing nerves, causing muscle spasms, or aggravating swelling.

Note: On an upper extremity fracture, remember to remove rings or bracelets, as well, even if you must cut them off with a ring cutter or metal snips.

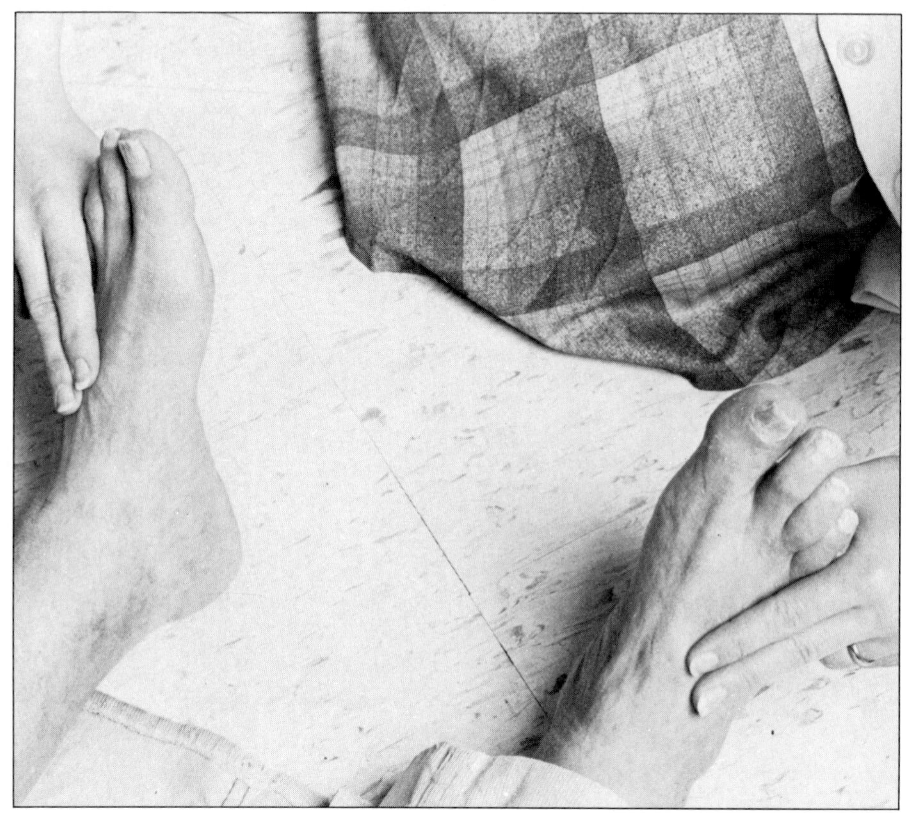

2 Now you're ready to evaluate circulation, sensation, and motion in your patient's injured leg.

Assess circulation by checking bilateral peripheral pulses, as the nurse is doing here.

Nursing tip: Because you'll repeat the assessment after applying the splint, you may mark your patient's pulse with an *X*.

Also check skin temperature and color. Check his nailbeds for capillary refill.

To test motor function, ask your patient to move his toes. Check sensation by gently squeezing the skin on his leg and toes.

3 Now, you're ready to assess Mr. Renner's nerve function in his injured leg. To do so, have him plantarflex (shown here), and dorsiflex his injured leg.

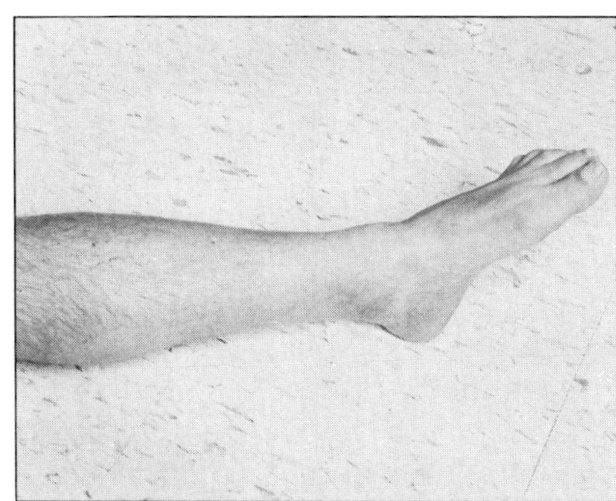

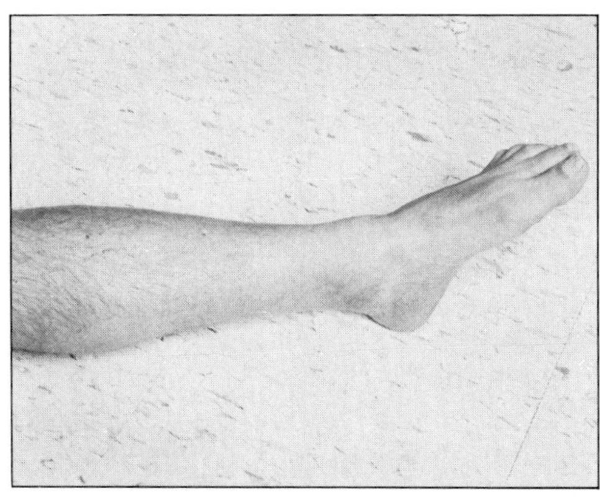

4 Then, inspect and palpate his limb for pain, ecchymosis, deformity, crepitation, or swelling.

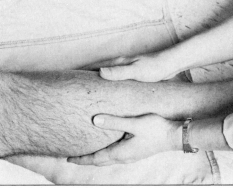

5 Now, check Mr. Renner for additional musculoskeletal injuries. To do so, palpate his body parts quickly. Begin by palpating his seven cervical vertebrae. Make sure they're properly aligned.

Important: Never perform range-of-motion testing on your patient's neck after any traumatic injury, because he may have a spinal fracture or dislocation. Instead, keep his head and neck completely immobilized. Always suspect a spinal injury if your patient's comatose, or if he says he's suffering neck discomfort or arm or leg numbness, tingling, or decreased motor function. In this case, don't even palpate his neck.

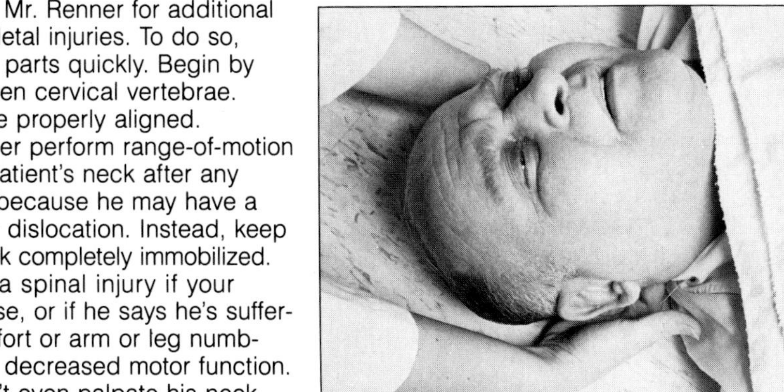

6 Next, palpate the length of his clavicle from his sternum to his scapula.

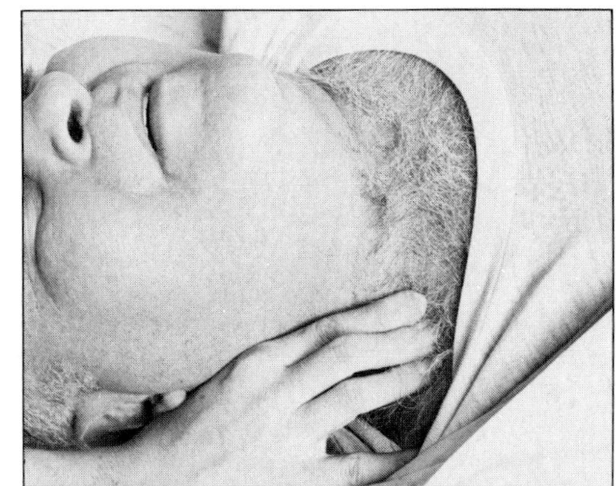

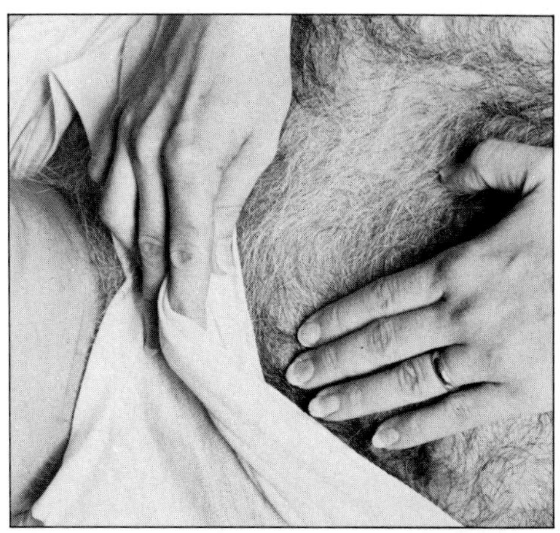

7 Then, palpate his chest and back, working from side to side. *Note:* If he's lying on his back, slip your hands underneath him to palpate it.

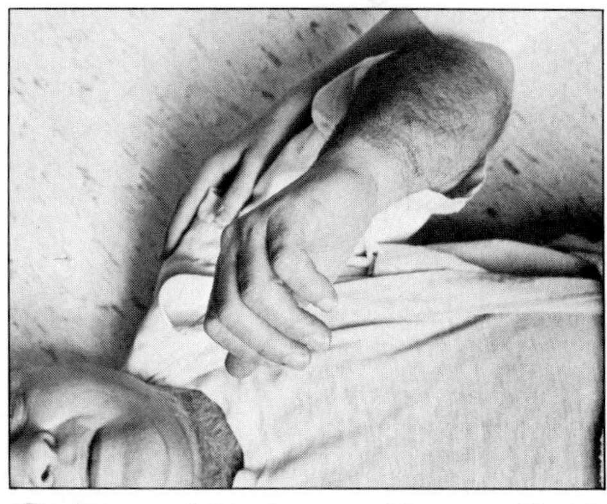

8 Then, ask him to move his arms. Check them for full range of motion. Also, palpate his shoulders and check his shoulder joints for stability.

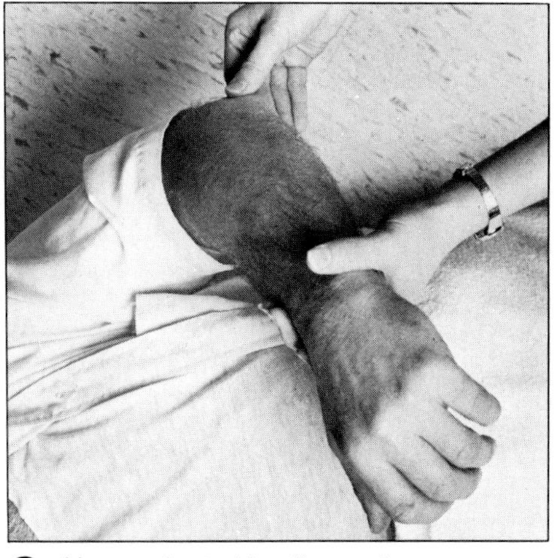

9 Now, palpate his elbows, forearms, hands, and fingers.

Wraps, splints, and slings

10 Palpate his abdomen for tenderness, distention, crepitation, or firmness, as shown here.

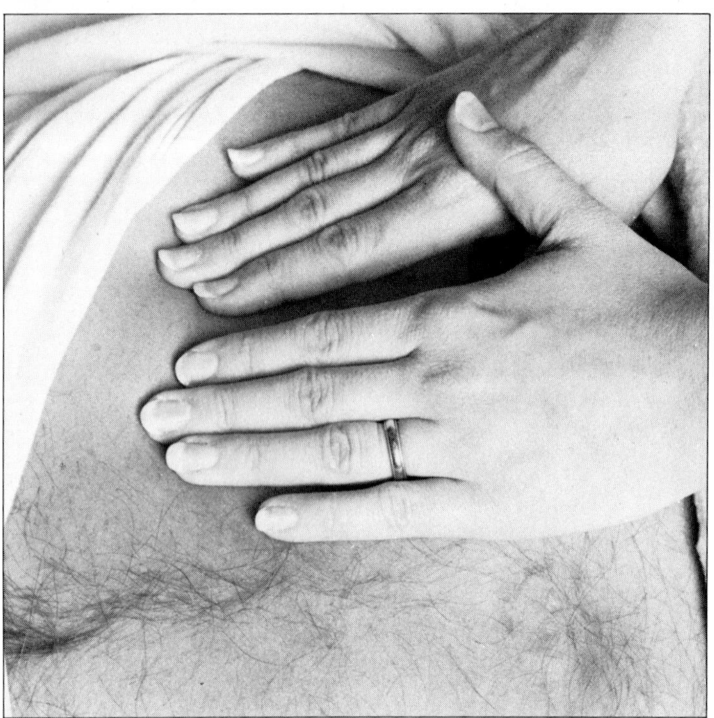

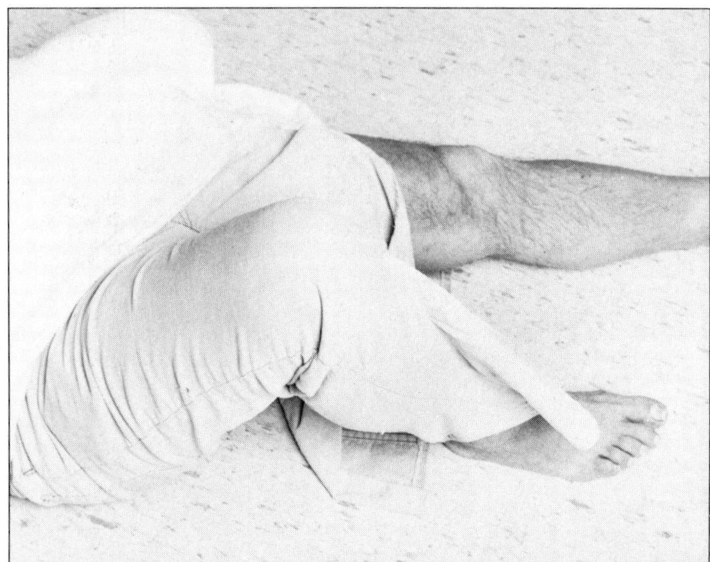

11 Next, palpate his hips. Have the patient rotate his uninjured hip to test for range of motion. *Important:* Tell your patient not to attempt to move his *injured* leg or hip.

Document your findings accurately. Give the information to the ambulance attendants to pass on to the emergency department staff.

To apply the splint, use the appropriate photostory on the following pages, depending on the equipment you have available. Remember, your aim is to immobilize the extremity well above and below the fracture site, without causing neurovascular impairment.

Applying a Jobst-Jet® Air Splint

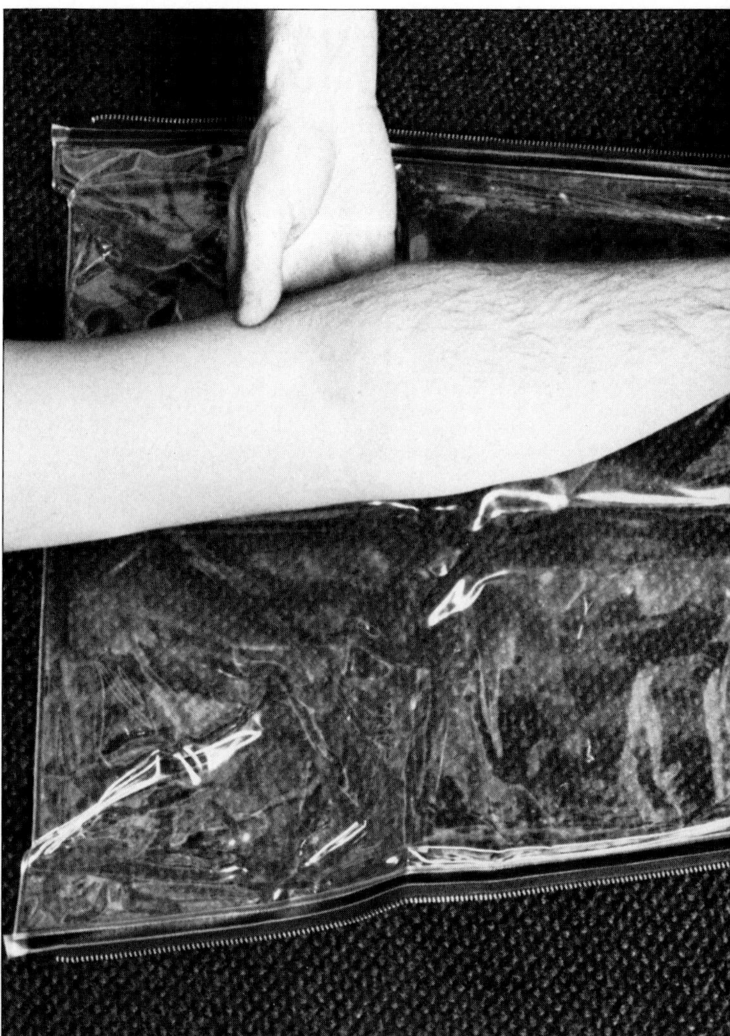

1 *You're an industrial nurse in a large company. An employee, Malcolm Leonard, fractures his arm falling down a staircase. You have a long arm air splint in your first aid box. But, do you know how to apply it?*

First, you should be familiar with some of its features. The air splint is a transparent sheath which inflates to immobilize your patient's injured limb. Use it immediately after an injury occurs, until the patient can be examined by a doctor. Because the splint's transparent, you can monitor skin color, bleeding, and limb position. Also, the splint can remain in place while X-rays are taken. In addition, it acts as a pressure bandage to control superficial venous bleeding.

Here's how to apply the splint:

First, lift your patient's arm slightly, supporting it at his elbow and wrist, as shown here. If possible, have an assistant place the deflated, unzipped, plastic splint under the patient's arm. Arrange the splint so its air nozzle is accessible for inflation. As you place the patient's arm on the splint, extend his fingers, keeping them at least 1 inch inside the distal edge of the splint.

Make sure the splint extends well above and below the actual fracture site.

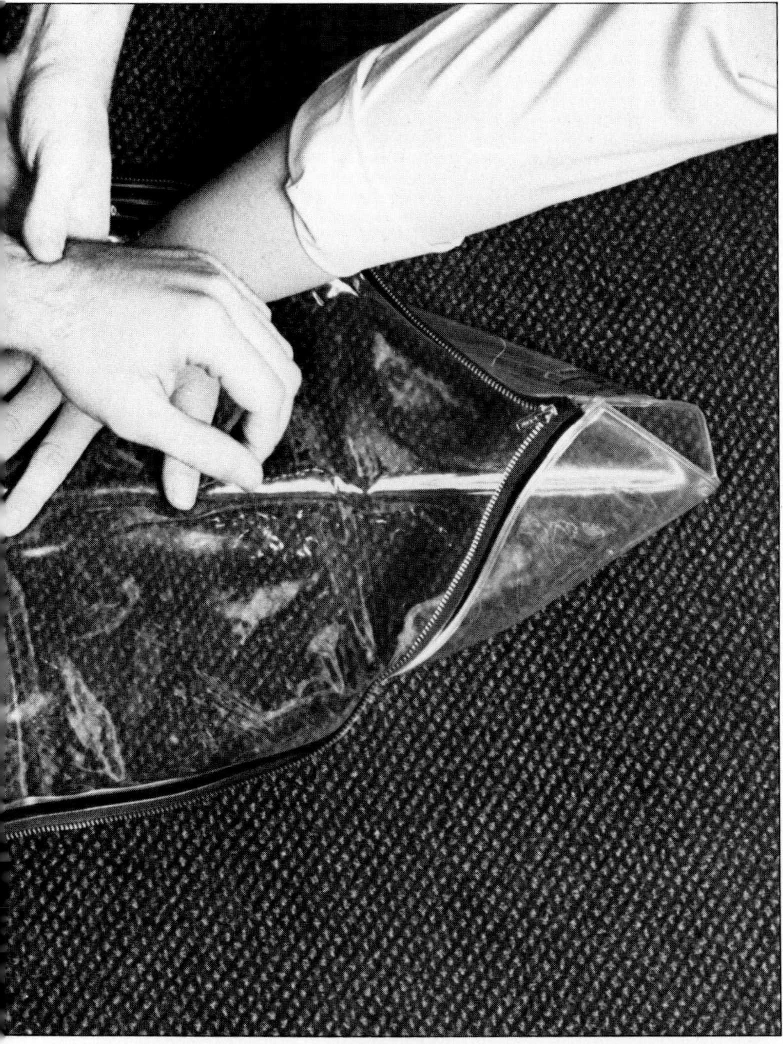

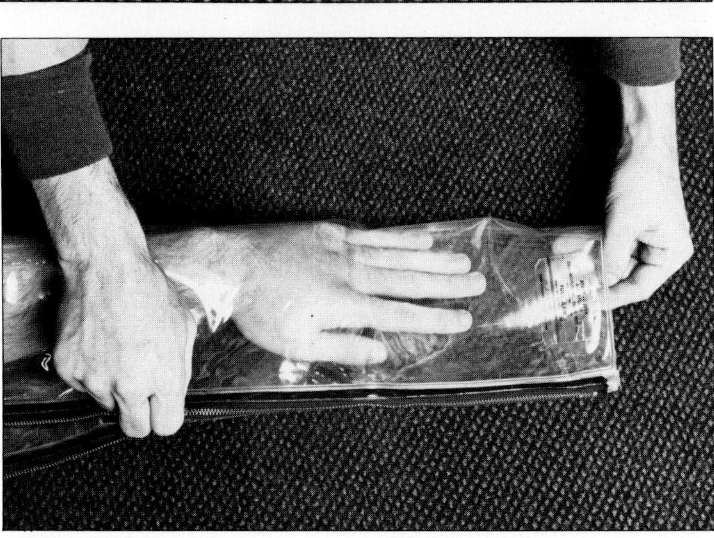

2 When his arm is positioned correctly, zip the air splint completely closed, as the nurse is doing here.

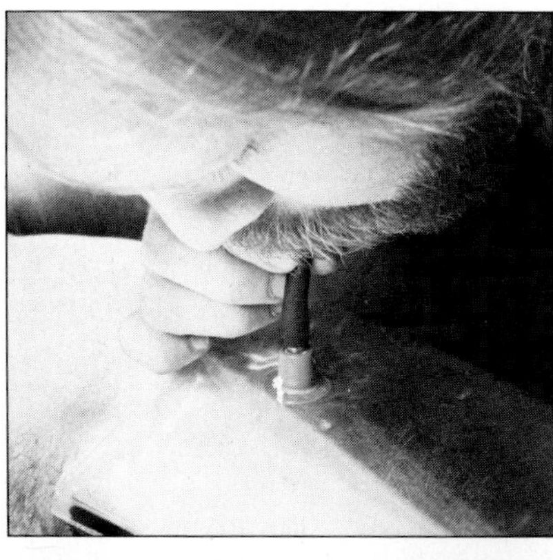

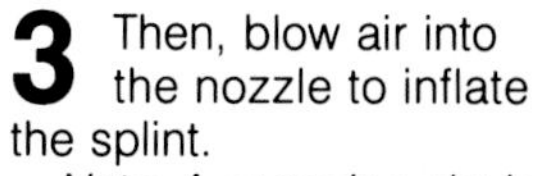

3 Then, blow air into the nozzle to inflate the splint.

Note: A pumping device should only be used by specially trained personnel. If a pumping device is used, the splint should never be inflated more than 40 mmHg.

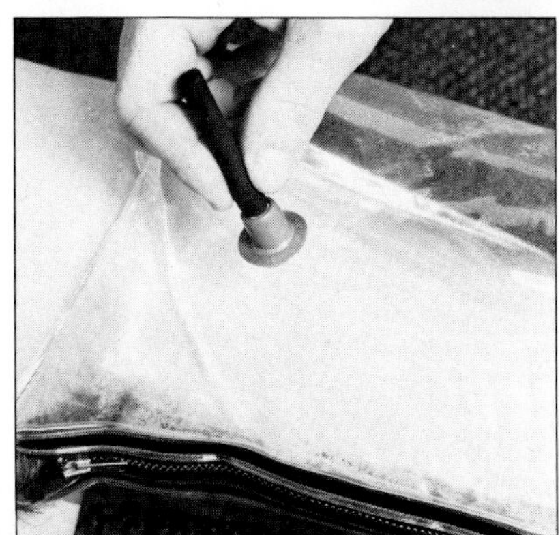

4 Now, screw the air valve closed by turning it clockwise.

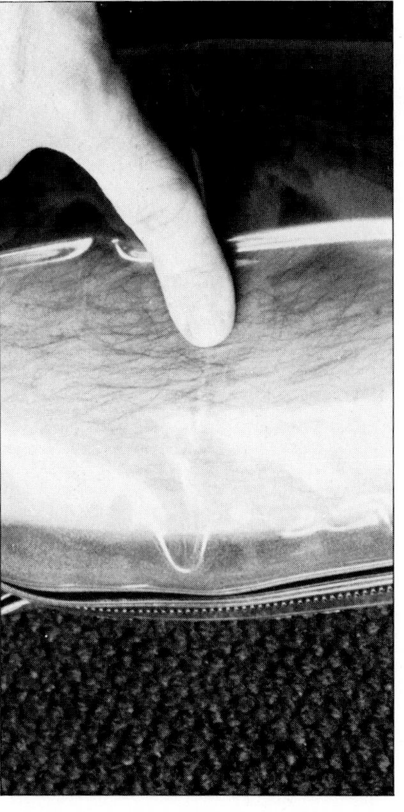

5 Then, check the air pressure in the splint. To do so, depress the inflated splint with your fingertips. If you can indent the plastic approximately ½″ (1.3 cm), the splint is properly inflated. If it's under- or overinflated, open the valve and add or release air. Close the valve and again test for correct inflation.

Document the time you applied the splint, as well as the condition of Mr. Leonard's arm. Call the ambulance and arrange to have Mr. Leonard transported to the hospital for treatment.

To deflate the air splint for removal at the hospital, turn the air nozzle counterclockwise. After some of the air has escaped, open the zipper. Allow the splint to deflate completely.

Wraps, splints, and slings

Applying a Hare traction splint

1 *If your patient in an emergency situation has a hip, femur, tibia, or fibula fracture, you may use a* Hare traction splint *to temporarily immobilize it. Why? Because the legs' strong bones fracture only in response to great force. The effect of this force on the bone causes much associated tissue damage, severe pain, and muscle spasms.*

A traction splint provides countervailing pull against muscle contractions. By immobilizing the broken bone ends, the splint helps reduce pain from bone movement in soft tissue, and helps prevent further injury.

Important: Never use a traction splint for a fracture within 1″ to 2″ (2.5 to 5.1 cm) of the patient's knee or ankle. Doing so could cause further injury.

To apply a Dyna-Med, Inc. Hare traction splint, follow these steps:

First, perform an emergency assessment, as instructed on pages 46 to 48.

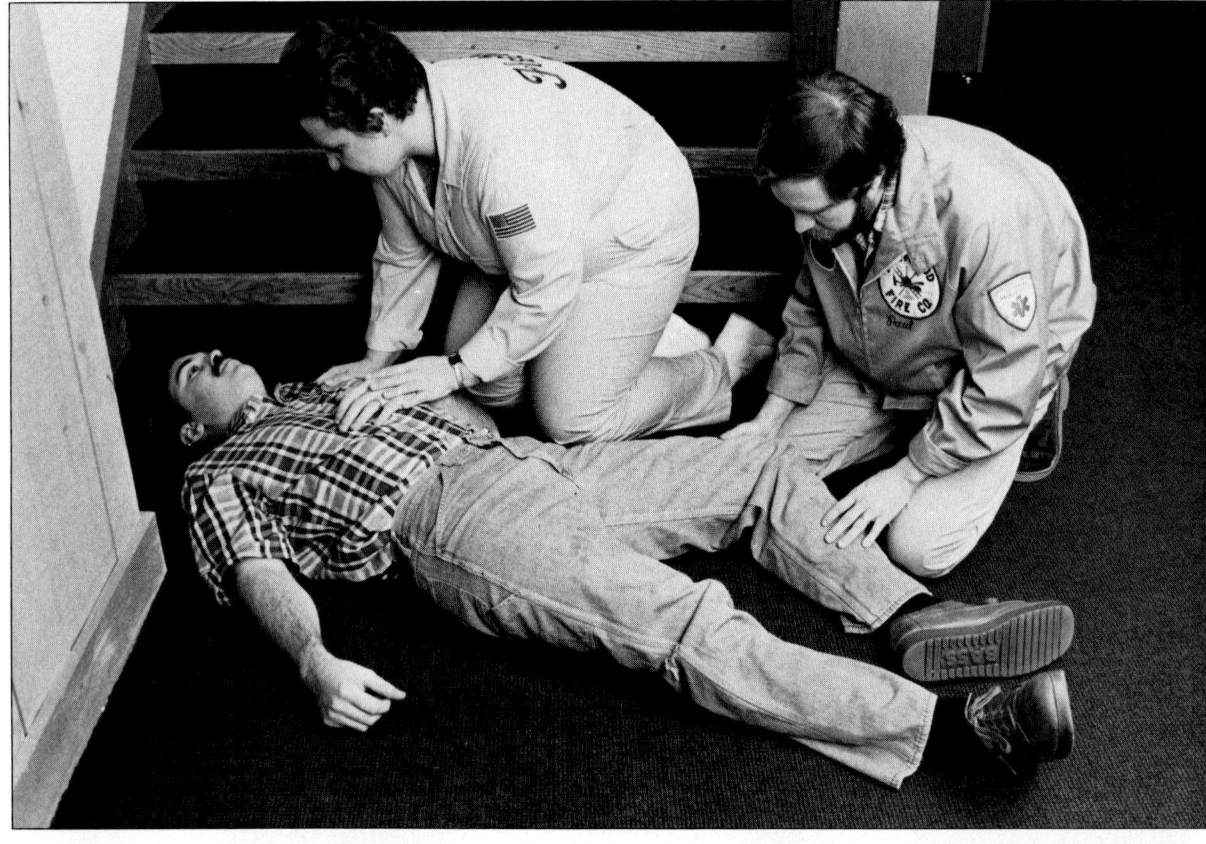

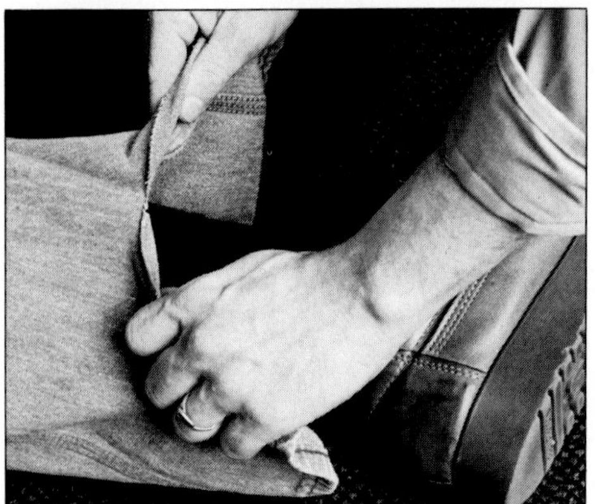

2 Cut away the clothing on his affected leg, as shown, to allow a closer look at his injuries. Also, remove the shoe from his injured leg.

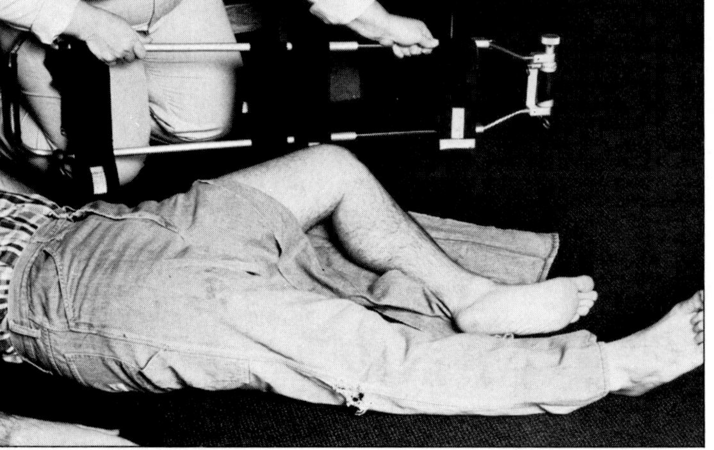

3 Then, place the splint beside the patient's leg and adjust it to the correct length. Open all Velcro support straps.

4 Next, have your assistant arrange the ankle-hitch straps around the patient's foot. To do so, place the side straps around his heel and the center strap under his heel, as shown.

5 Now, lift and support his leg while your assistant crosses the two side straps over your patient's foot. Then, have your assistant pull on the three strap end-rings, to apply traction.

6 While your assistant continues to exert traction on the end-rings, slide the splint under your patient's leg. Position it snugly against his ischium. Set up the three-tailed hitch under his foot.

7 Apply the ischiatic strap around the top of your patient's leg, firmly and securely, but not tightly enough to compromise circulation.

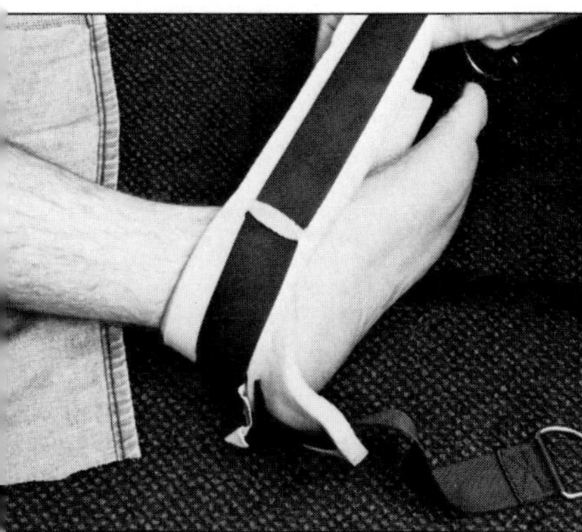

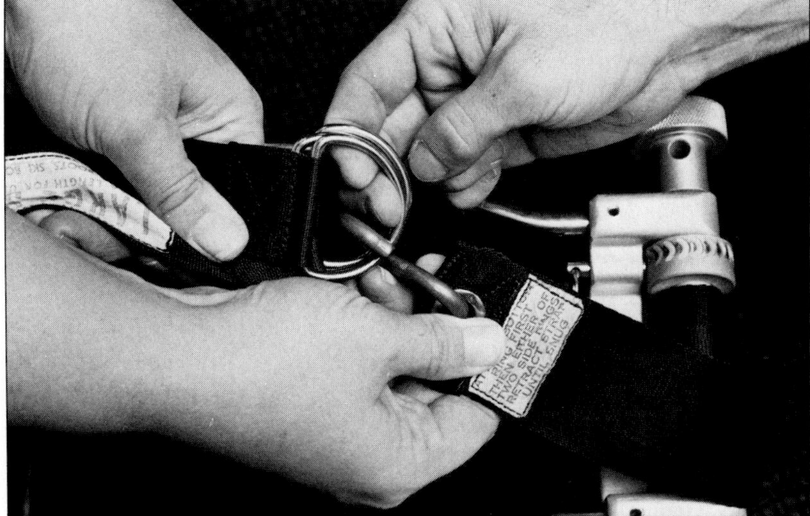

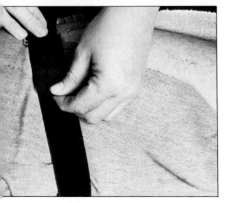

8 While your assistant maintains traction, slip the traction mechanism's webbing-strap hook around the three rings.

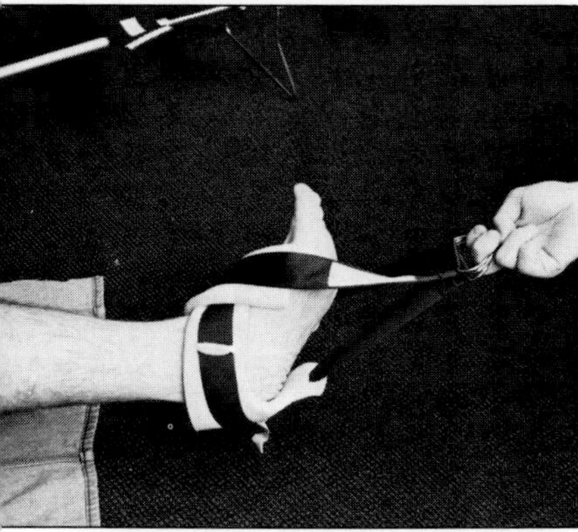

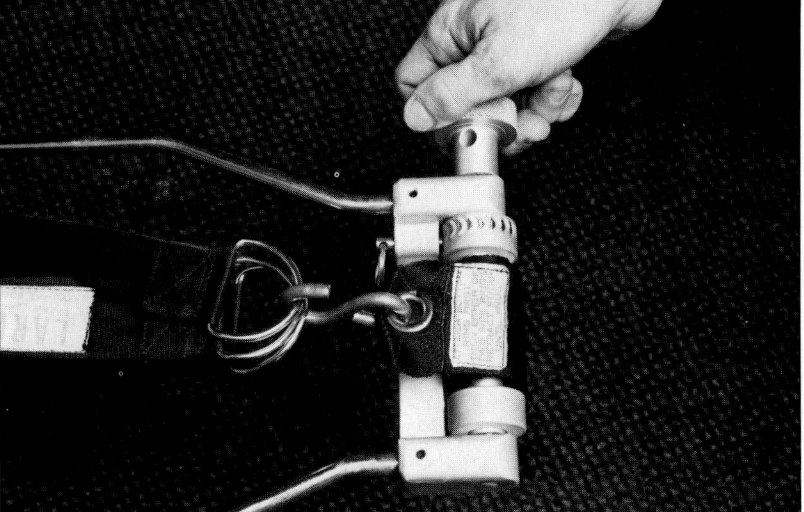

9 Now, have your assistant turn the ratchet wheel with his right hand until it's exerting as much pull as he's been applying manually. As soon as he's done so, release manual traction. Then, have him turn the ratchet wheel to adjust the traction force until your patient indicates that his pain's relieved.

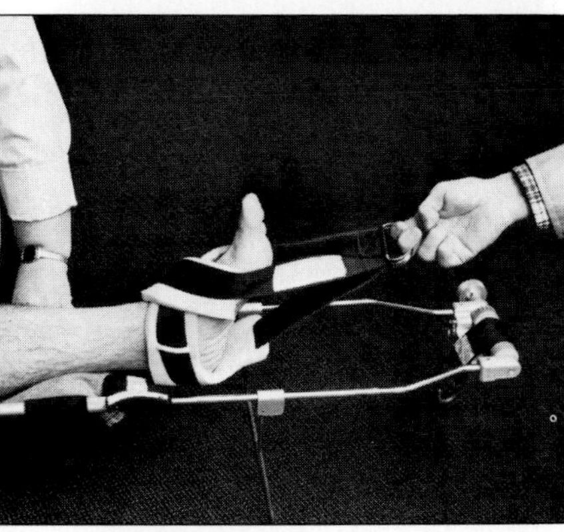

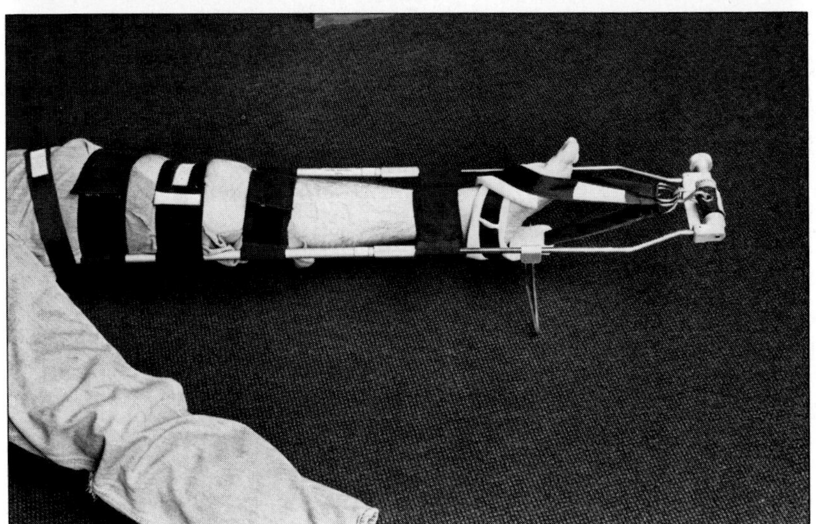

10 After adjusting the traction force, fasten the splint's Velcro straps below his knee. Then, finish fastening the straps above his knee. Check each fastener for proper placement.

Document the procedure. Assist in transporting the patient to the emergency department for further treatment.

Wraps, splints, and slings

Improvising a splint

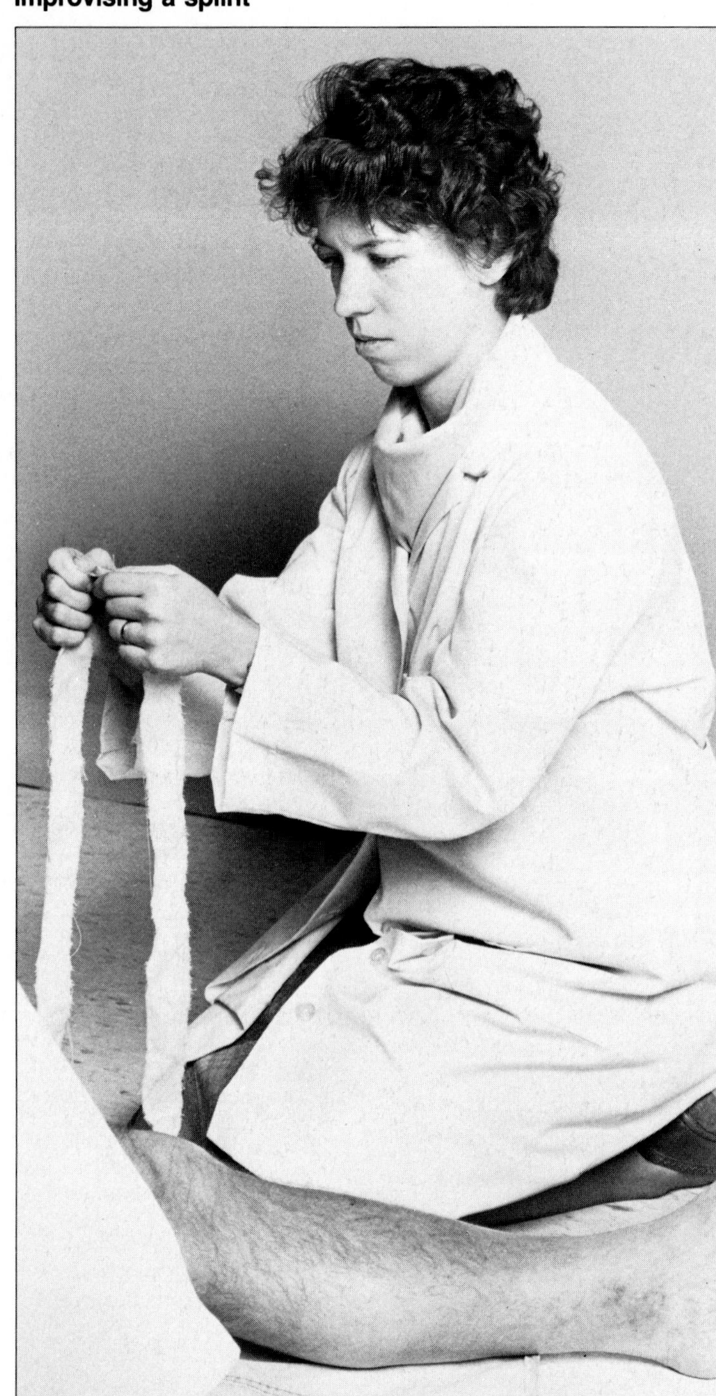

1 *What if your patient needs an arm or leg splinted, but you don't have the proper equipment? Look around you. Do you see magazines, pillows, or some pieces of wood nearby?*

If so, you can use these items to improvise a splint. *Note:* Outdoors, you can use a fallen tree limb, or a cushion from a boat. *Remember:* Your aim is to immobilize the extremity well above and below the fracture site, without compromising circulation or causing further injury. Suppose you're using magazines. First, tear up a sheet for ties.

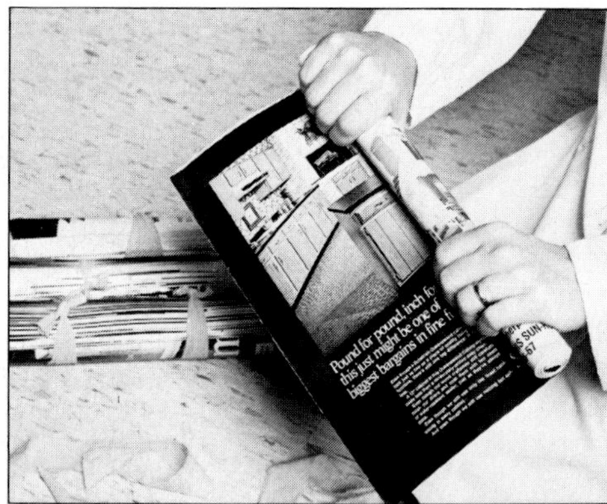

2 Then, roll several magazines up lengthwise into tight, firm rolls, and tie the rolls securely.

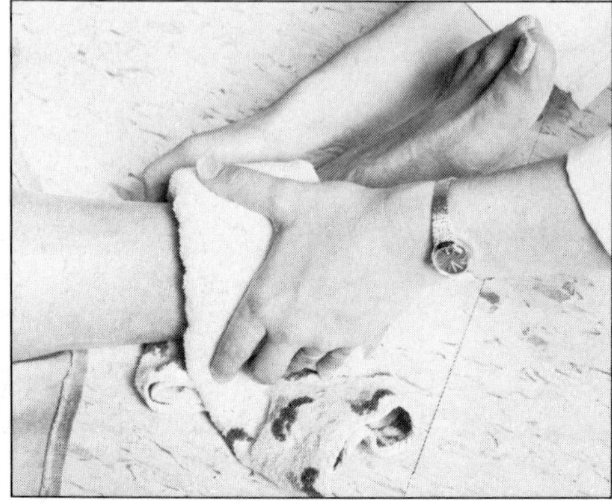

3 Next, pad your patient's affected extremity, (especially over bony prominences), using clothing, towels, or any soft materials. Doing so will help prevent skin breakdown from pressure.

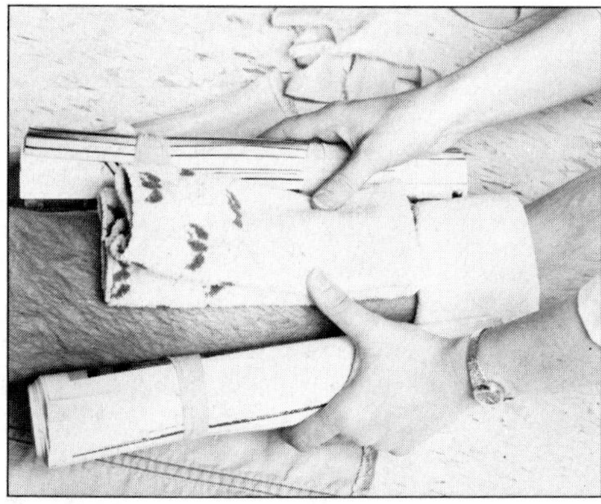

4 Now, place the magazines against the patient's limb, as shown.

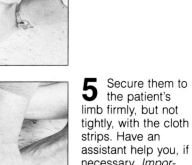

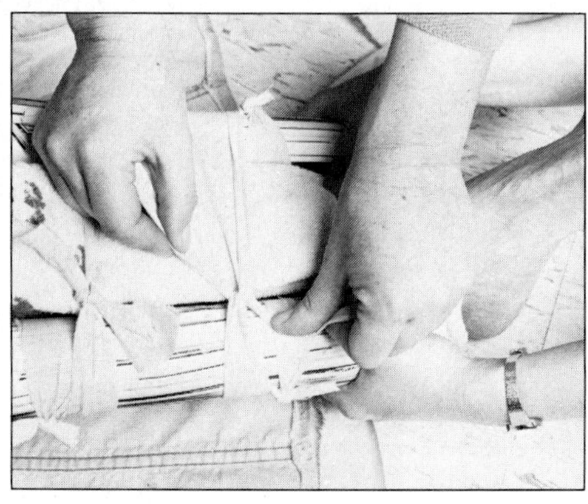

5 Secure them to the patient's limb firmly, but not tightly, with the cloth strips. Have an assistant help you, if necessary. *Important:* Never use rope or twine; these may constrict circulation.

Assist in your patient's transfer to the emergency department.

Nurses' guide to immobilizers

Suppose the doctor orders an immobilizer splint for your patient following surgery. Depending on the affected body part, your patient could be wearing any of the devices shown in the chart at right. Do you know their special features and the specific care they require? Study the chart for this information.

Of course, these are only some examples of immobilizers. They're available in different styles, as well as for other body parts, such as the ankle.

For general care considerations for patients wearing immobilizers, and for detailed information on skin care, see page 55.

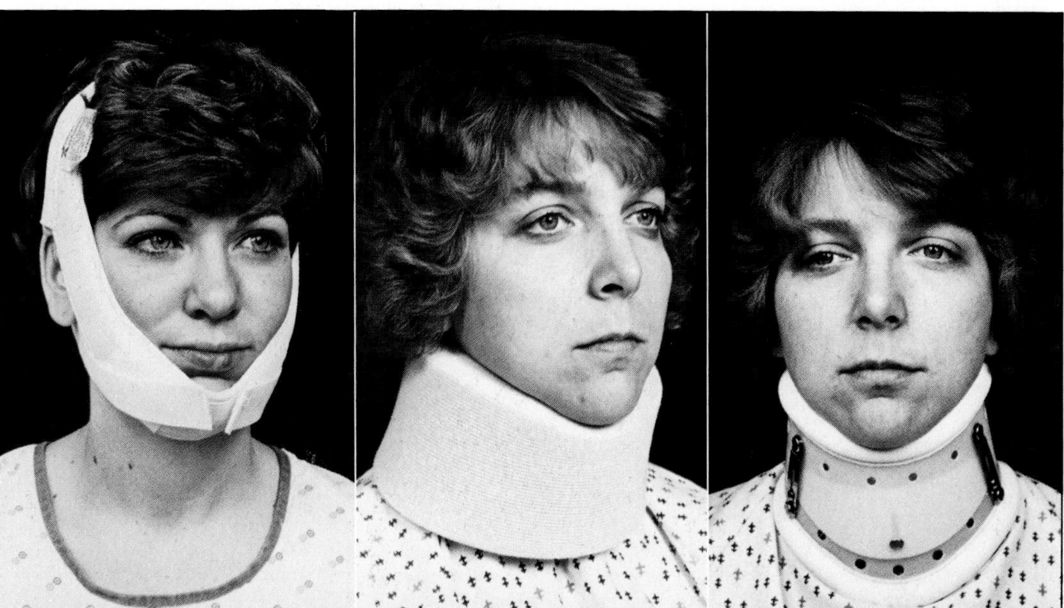

Jaw immobilizer	Soft cervical collar	Hard cervical collar
Jaw immobilizer (All Orthopedic Appliances O'Malley jaw fracture splint) Padded strap fits around chin and over top of head. Velcro straps fasten at top of head and under chin. **Indications** • Fractured jaw • Dislocated jaw **Nursing considerations** • Remove immobilizer for meals and to administer oral medication. • Remove immobilizer at least once every 4 hours. Massage bony prominences vigorously. • To prevent aspiration of vomitus, instruct patient to turn on her side and call you if she feels nauseated. • Check the straps around the patient's ears frequently. If you see any signs of irritation, pad the patient's ears. • Apply immobilizer just tightly enough to prevent jaw movement. Have immobilizer refitted if proper application does not prevent movement.	**Soft cervical collar (Futuro® Patient Aids®)** Felt or foam collar, with optional reinforcing metal stays fastens around patient's neck with a Velcro closure. The collar is usually contoured, being wider at the middle with a depression or cup for the chin, and tapering toward its ends. It provides gentle support and reminds the patient to avoid cervical spine motion. **Indications** • Cervical muscle spasm, ligament separation, tendinitis, or osteoarthritis • Following cervical laminectomy with fusion, although hard cervical collar is used more frequently **Nursing considerations** • Doctor will specify how collar is to be applied. Both patient's neck size and collar design must be considered. • If doctor orders slight degree of flexion, place tapered (closure) end anteriorly. • If doctor orders neutral position, use a collar with gentle contours instead of tapered ends. • To improvise a cervical collar, use a bath towel. Fold it in half lengthwise, and then in half again. To secure the folded towel, pin it behind the patient's neck.	**Hard cervical collar (Richards® Myo)** Rigid molded plastic (or metal-and-leather) collar fastens around patient's neck. Most types conform to contours of chin as well as neck. **Indications** • Cervical muscle spasms, ligament separation, tendinitis, or osteoarthritis • Following cervical laminectomy with fusion **Nursing considerations** • Collar must be fitted specifically for the patient by an orthopedic supply company. • Hard cervical collar provides more stability and immobilization than soft collars.

Wraps, splints, and slings

Nurses' guide to immobilizers continued

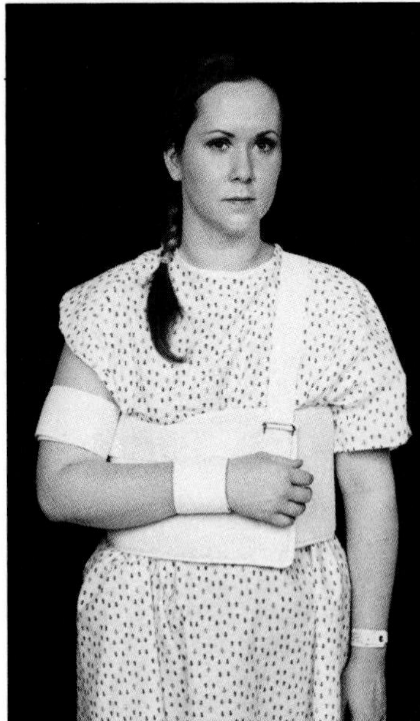

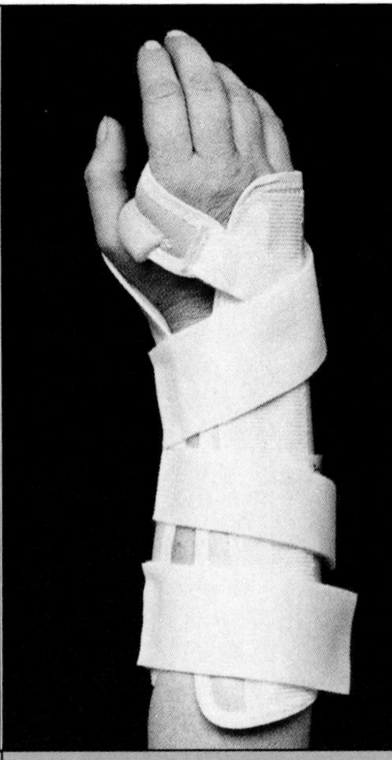

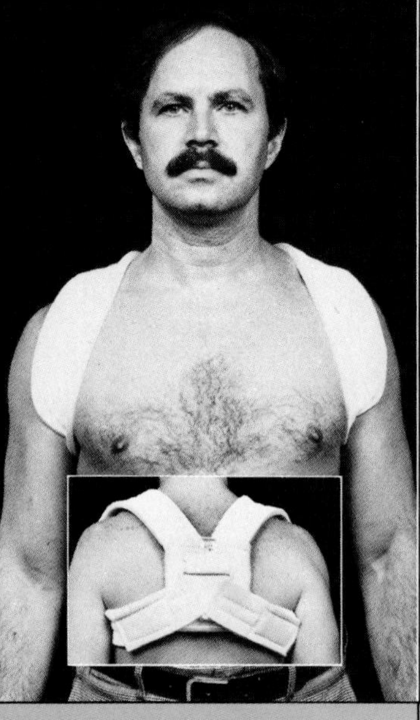

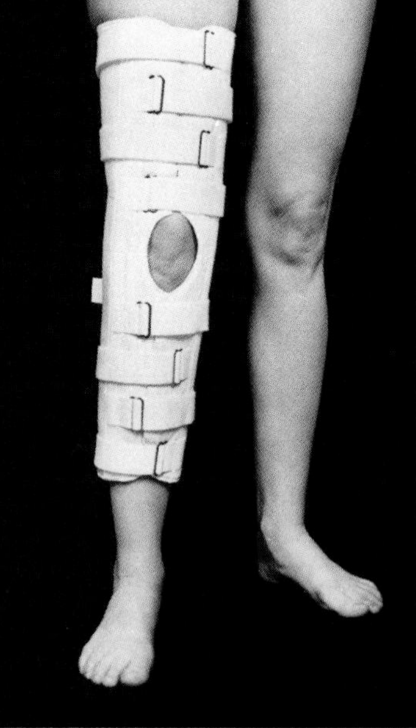

Belt-type shoulder immobilizer (Richards Universal)
Wide, foam-padded belt, like a rib belt, fits snugly around patient's chest. The belt fastens with a Velcro closure. Two attached cuffs encircle the patient's arm, one just above her elbow, and the other around her wrist. The cuff above her elbow keeps her upper arm abducted. The cuff around her wrist supports her lower arm across her chest.

Indications
- Shoulder dislocation
- Clavicle fracture

Nursing considerations
- Wrist cuff may be released to allow modified lower arm range-of-motion exercises, while upper arm remains abducted.
- Placement of arm in horizontal position may be therapeutic or primarily for comfort and support.
- Assess your patient's respiratory status frequently to make sure ventilation is not being impaired by strap tightness.

Wrist immobilizer (Richards vinyl wrist-forearm splint)
Padded vinyl covering with metal stays and Velcro straps extends from midpalm halfway up forearm. A strip of foam padding lines thumb opening.

Indications
- Following wrist surgery
- Severe wrist sprains

Nursing considerations
- Splint maintains wrist in dorsiflexion, to relieve tension on wrist nerves and arteries.

Padded clavicle strap (Comfort Care Pontotoc®)
Forms a figure eight around your patient's shoulder, and is fastened in the middle of his upper back with a Velcro closure. Strap is padded to provide firm compression in the clavicle area.

Indications
- Clavicle fracture

Nursing considerations
- Check to make sure the strap does not apply too much pressure under the patient's arms, which may cause nerve damage.
- Encourage good posture.

Knee immobilizer (Dillon Mfg. Co.'s bunny line®)
Padded canvas wrap fits around entire leg in knee area; contains steel stays that are either straight or contoured, depending on degree of knee flexion desired; provides a foam insert behind the knee for support; features a circular cutout centered over the patella.

Indications
- Following knee surgery, such as meniscectomy, arthroscopy, or total knee replacement
- Sprains or strains

Nursing considerations
- Cutout over patella allows snug fit without excessive pressure on the patella. Also provides a landmark for fitting immobilizer properly.
- Patient usually returns from surgery with immobilizer in place. If she doesn't, you must obtain and apply the immobilizer. The doctor's order will indicate immobilizer length and whether it should be straight or contoured. Measure patient's thigh and calf circumference. Then, consult the manufacturer's chart to obtain the correct size immobilizer.
- Patient may require crutches or a walker for ambulation.

Caring for a patient wearing an immobilizer

If your patient is wearing an immobilizer, follow these guidelines in caring for him:

- Check the immobilizer frequently for correct fit.
- Assess his neurovascular status at least once every 4 hours, using the guidelines on page 24.
- If the immobilizer covers a wound dressing, check the dressing every 4 hours to make sure it's dry and intact. If drainage is present, mark the dressing, and reinforce or change it as ordered. Document your assessment.
- Check all adjustable straps and other parts of the immobilizer frequently to make sure they're not too constrictive or too loose. If you applied the immobilizer while the patient was supine, remember to adjust it as his position changes; for example, when he sits or walks.
- If your patient is confused or combative, suggest a cast or other more permanent immobilizing device to the doctor.
- At least once every 8 hours, remove the immobilizer. Note any reddened areas or soft spots that might indicate formation of a decubitus ulcer. Then, provide the skin care described below.
- If available, attach the manufacturer's information to the patient's care plan to ensure proper use of the immobilizer.
- If your patient's going home with an immobilizer, give the patient or a family member instructions for skin care, for care and cleaning of the device, and for removal (if permitted) and reapplication. Also, teach him and a family member to perform a neurovascular assessment. If the manufacturer supplies instructions for the patient, be sure to give them to him.

Document all patient teaching in your nurses' notes.

Performing skin care

Suppose your patient's wearing a roller bandage, an immobilizer, or any other orthopedic equipment that covers her skin. If so, she'll require meticulous skin care to prevent skin irritation or decubitus ulcers. *Remember:* Decubitus ulcers don't inevitably result when a body part is immobilized or covered. They develop if the patient's skin is poorly cared for, she's positioned improperly or turned infrequently, her nutrition is inadequate, or she has poor circulation. Provide good skin care at least once every 8 hours, but preferably once every 4 hours. To do so, use the following guidelines:

- First, remove the immobilization device, unless contraindicated.

Note: Only specially trained staff members should remove a cervical collar.

- Now, closely inspect your patient's skin for signs of pressure, such as soft areas, or areas of skin-color change.
- Next, wash her skin with mild soap and water. Then, rinse her skin thoroughly and pat it dry.
- Now, you may apply lotion to your patient's skin to help conserve skin moisture. If you do, apply it sparingly, and be sure it's completely absorbed before reapplying the roller bandage or other skin covering to your patient.

Note: Avoid using powder on your patient's skin. However, if her skin is very irritated, you may use a light dusting of cornstarch. Or, use cornstarch in the bathwater.

- Next, massage all bony prominences on the affected body part. Then, *gently* massage fleshy areas. *Caution:* Never massage a patient's calves. You could dislodge any blood clots present and inadvertently cause pulmonary embolism.
- For a patient whose skin comes into contact with rigid material, such as the hard cervical collar shown in the photos, toughen her skin at bony prominences to develop a protective callus. To do so, rub her skin briskly with a terry cloth towel each time you perform skin care. Or, you may apply either alcohol or tincture of benzoin and allow it to dry thoroughly.

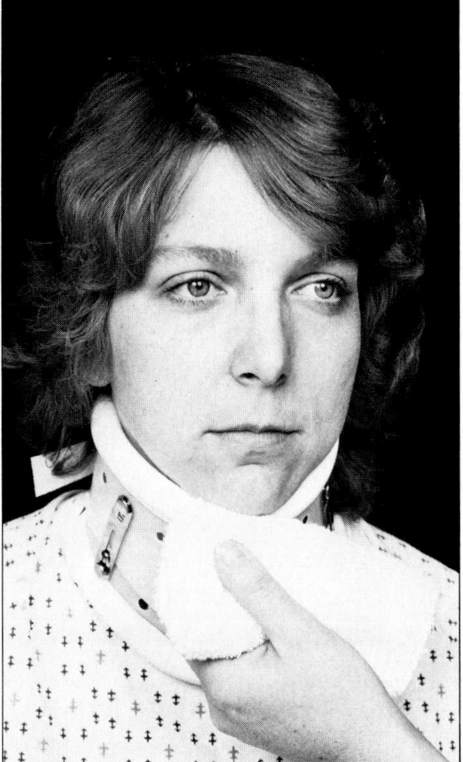

Note: Avoid using preparations with adhesive qualities (such as tincture of benzoin) on a patient with friable, easily damaged skin; for example, an elderly patient or patient on long-term steroid drug therapy.

- If any adjustment of a custom-fitted immobilizer is necessary, call the orthopedic supply company that fitted it. Until the company's representative can make the adjustment, you may temporarily pad the immobilizer. However, be sure to pad the area of incorrect fit, rather than the chafed or irritated area.
- After performing skin care, turn your patient to relieve pressure areas. Be sure to turn her at least every 4 hours. If she's wearing a limb immobilizer, reposition the limb every 2 hours.
- Document in your nurses' notes the skin care you've provided and any position changes. Record any changes in the condition of your patient's skin.

Wraps, splints, and slings

How to apply a sling

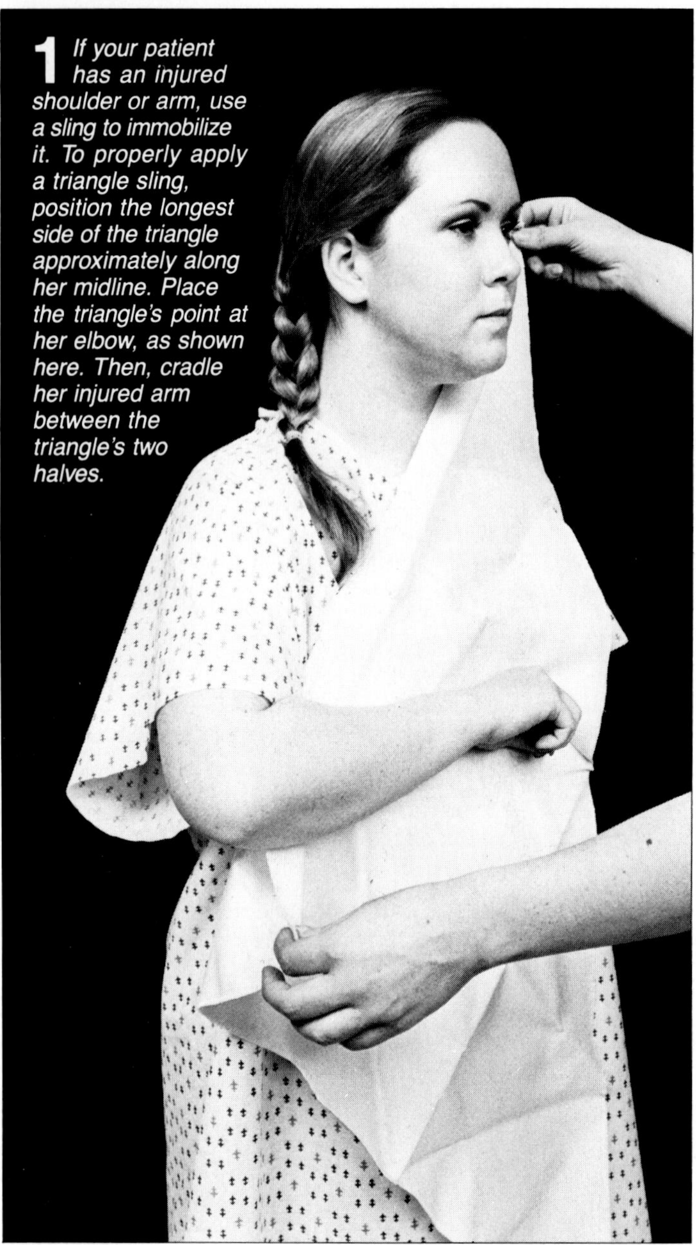

1 *If your patient has an injured shoulder or arm, use a sling to immobilize it. To properly apply a triangle sling, position the longest side of the triangle approximately along her midline. Place the triangle's point at her elbow, as shown here. Then, cradle her injured arm between the triangle's two halves.*

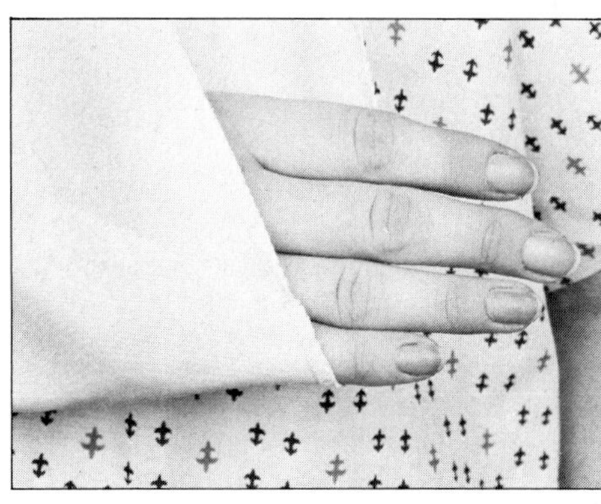

2 To prevent nerve damage leading to wrist drop, make sure the sling's midline edge extends to her finger's first interphalangeal joints.

Also, to help reduce swelling, arrange the sling so that her hand is elevated slightly above her elbow.

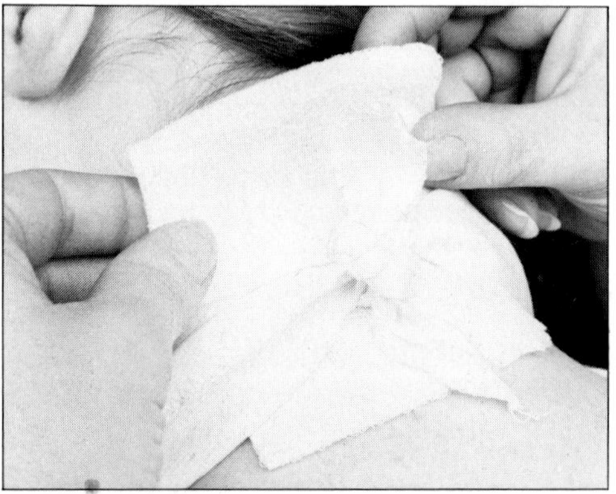

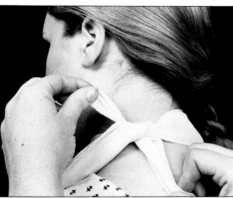

3 Now, knot the two ends of the sling loosely, but securely, around your patient's neck.

Important: Never position the knot over the cervical vertebrae, or you may cause nerve damage.

4 To keep the knot securely positioned, as well as to protect the patient's skin, pad her skin under the knot with a 4″x4″ gauze pad.

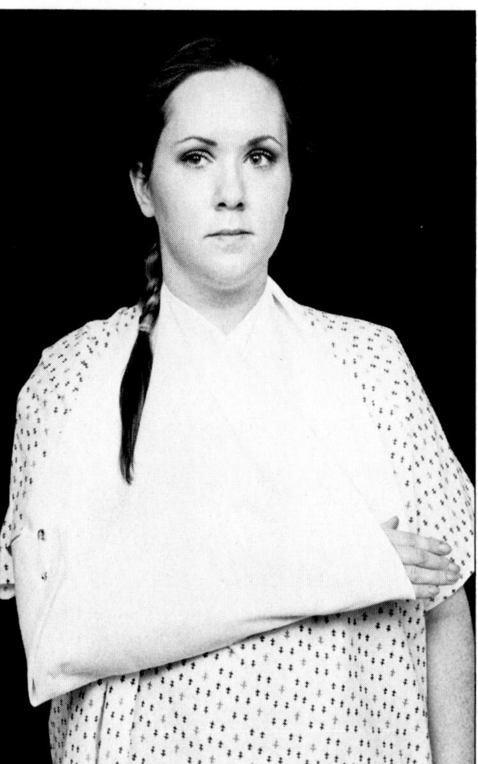

5 Use a safety pin to fasten the sling at her elbow.

When the sling's applied properly, the patient's injured arm should be immobilized so that the elbow is at a 90° angle, as shown here.

Encourage your patient to maintain muscle tone in her injured arm by flexing her hand or squeezing a tennis ball.

Document the procedure.

How to apply a swathe and sling

1 *To immobilize your patient's dislocated shoulder in an abducted position, apply a swathe and a sling to his upper body.*

To do so, position the patient's injured arm or shoulder as close as possible to his body.

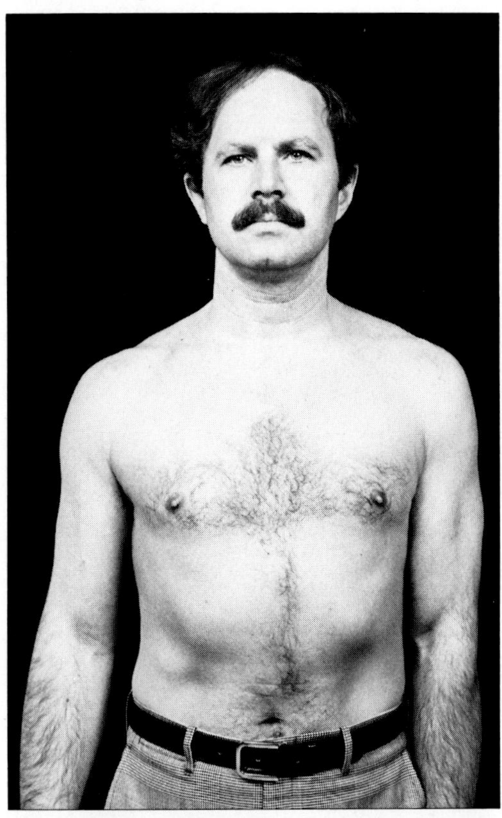

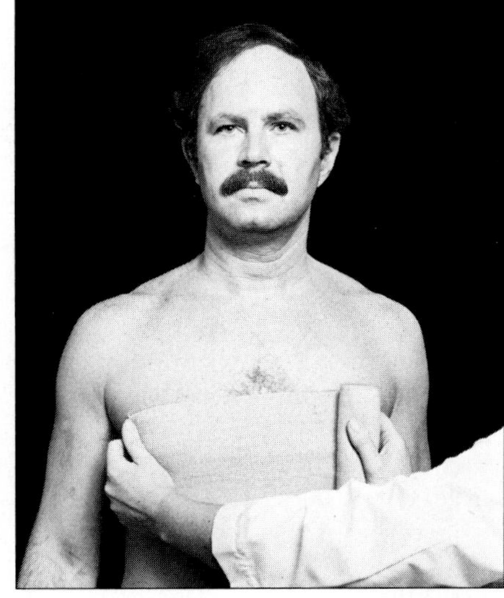

3 Now, wrap two 6″ (15.2 cm) elastic roller bandages several times around his upper arm and torso. Start from his chest, just below shoulder level, on his uninjured side.

Important: Take care to leave his uninjured arm free. Also, never cover his hand or wrist, or you might impair circulation.

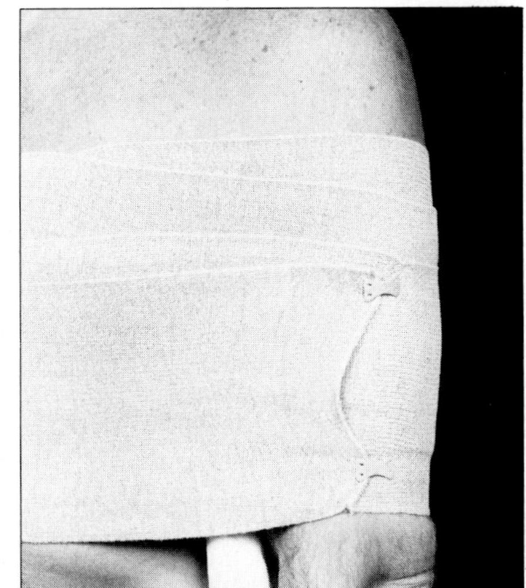

4 Anchor the wrap over the soft tissue on the front surface of his arm, using two clips.

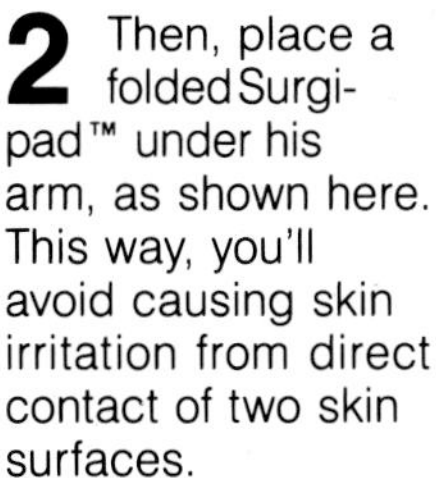

2 Then, place a folded Surgi-pad™ under his arm, as shown here. This way, you'll avoid causing skin irritation from direct contact of two skin surfaces.

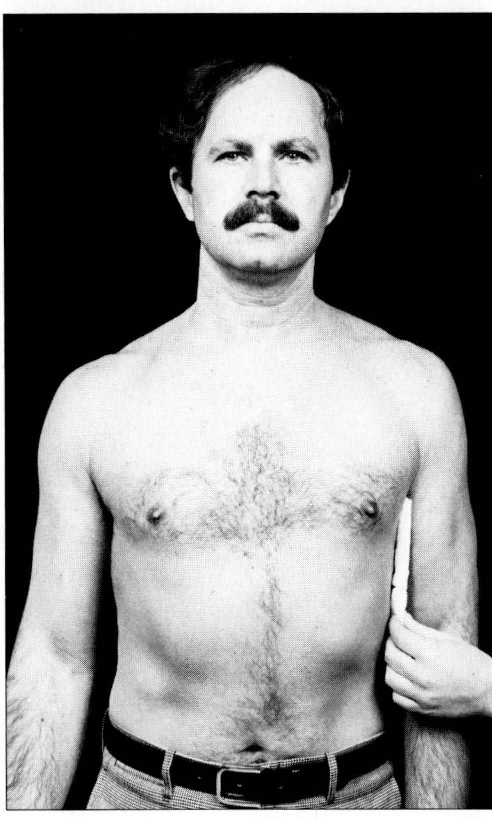

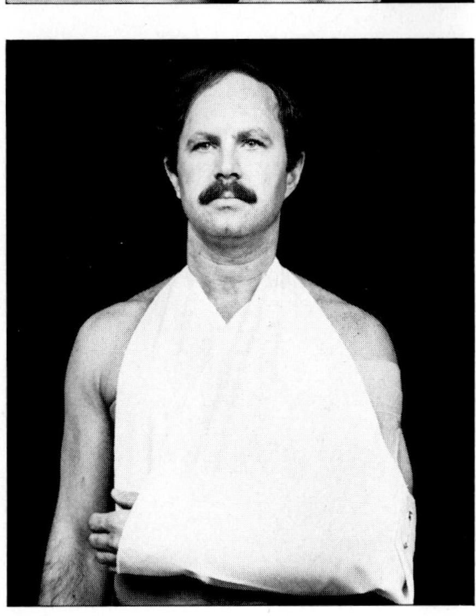

5 Finally, support his lower forearm in a sling, as described on the preceding page.

Remember to document the procedure.

Wraps, splints, and slings

Putting a patient in a double sling

1 *If your patient has a long leg or arm cast, the doctor may order that you keep it suspended in a sling. Elevating the limb will help reduce swelling, which could lead to compartment syndrome. Sling suspension elevates a heavy cast more effectively than propping it on pillows.*

If your patient has a long leg cast, you'll use two slings, one under his thigh and one under his calf. You'll attach the slings to ropes, which run through pulleys suspended from an overhead traction frame. (For detailed information about traction equipment, including knot-tying instructions, see pages 69 to 72.)

Before applying the sling, check the cast to make sure it's fully dry. You may have an assistant help you apply the double sling, or you may apply it by yourself. If the patient's able, have him help you by lifting his casted leg with his hands. Perform the following steps.

First, explain the procedure to your patient.

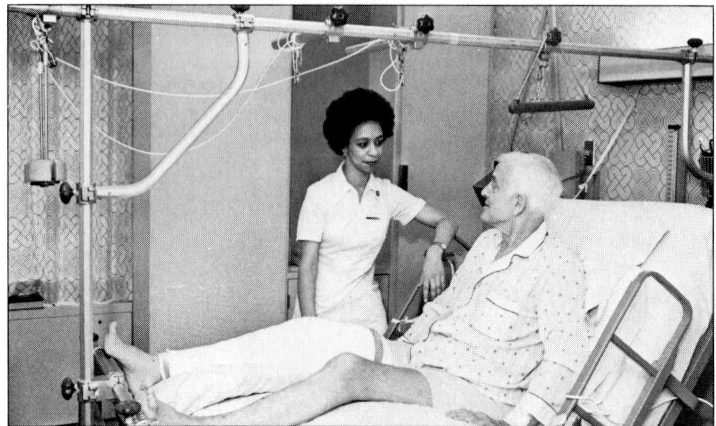

2 Then, attach two equal weights to the ropes from which you'll suspend the slings, and hang the weights temporarily on the bed frame. *Note:* The doctor will probably prescribe 3 to 7 pound (1.4 to 3.2 kg) weights, depending on the size of your patient.

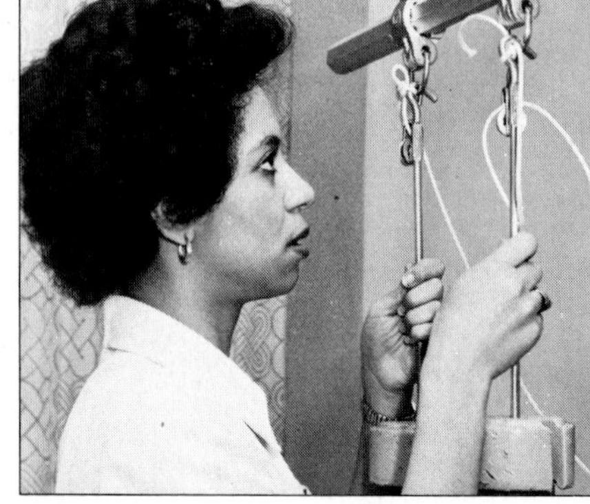

3 Next, place one sling under his thigh and a second under his calf. Arrange the top sling so that both its edges are under the patient's thigh. They should not constrict his groin area or his popliteal space.

Arrange the second sling so its edges don't constrict his popliteal space or his heel.

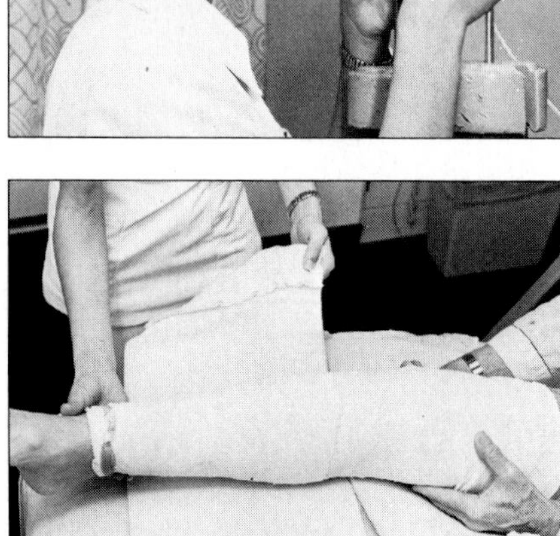

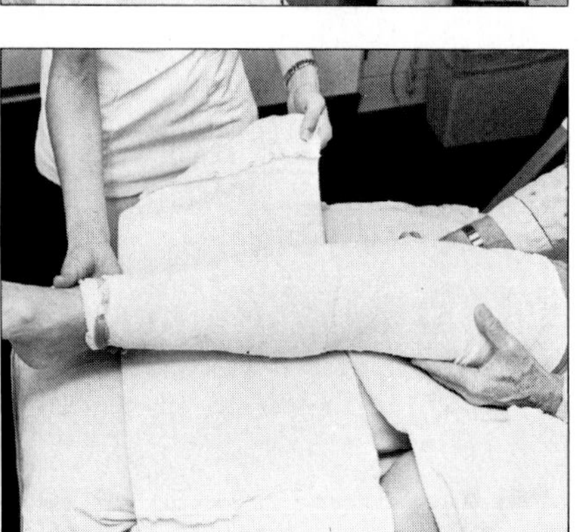

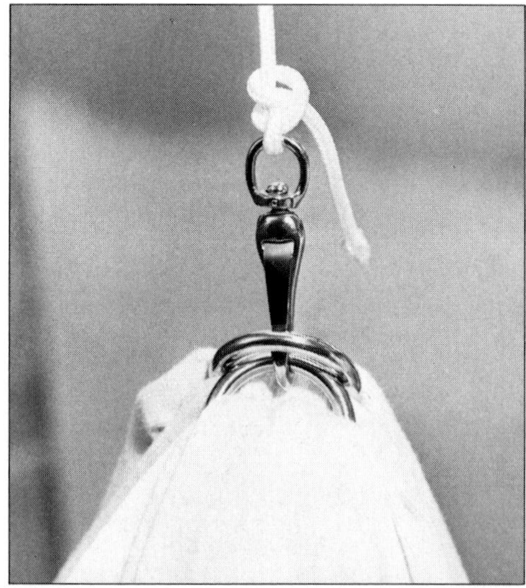

4 Now, you're ready to attach the thigh sling to the weight rope. To do so, hold both ends of the sling together.

Then, insert the rope clip through one sling ring and clip it to the second sling ring. Attaching the sling this way (instead of inserting the clip through both rings and clipping the rope) helps prevent slippage. Now, attach the second sling.

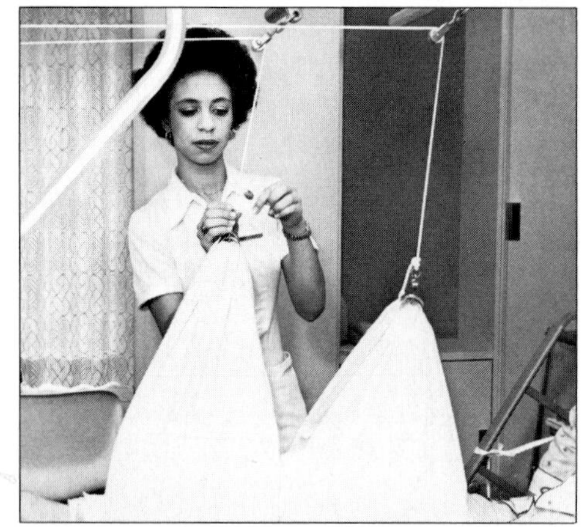

5 Next, check to see that the weight knots are secure. Then, to prevent slippage, tape the knot ends (not the knots themselves) with adhesive tape, as the nurse is doing here.

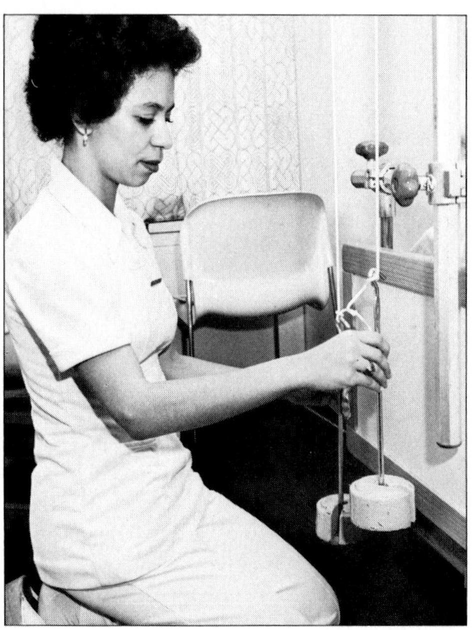

6 Now, release the weights, and lower both gently at the same time. Be sure the weight ropes hang free of the bed frame and that the weight doesn't pull your patient's hips off the bed.

Document the procedure on the appropriate forms.

To remove the double sling, carefully remove both weights at the same time, as your patient supports his cast. Then, reverse the procedure you just performed.

Casts

Let's suppose you're caring for a patient with a newly applied cast. Do you know how to position the cast as it dries? Do you know how to finish rough cast edges? Or how to teach your patient to clean the skin areas above and below his cast?

Do you really know all you should about casts, including how to help prepare your patient for cast removal? What to suspect if your patient complains of a burning sensation under his cast? Or how to instruct your patient in home cast care?

For the answers to these questions, read this section. In addition to helpful charts to familiarize you with cast types and materials, and photostories on various aspects of cast care, we've included a home care aid for you to photocopy and give to your patient.

Casting materials: How they differ

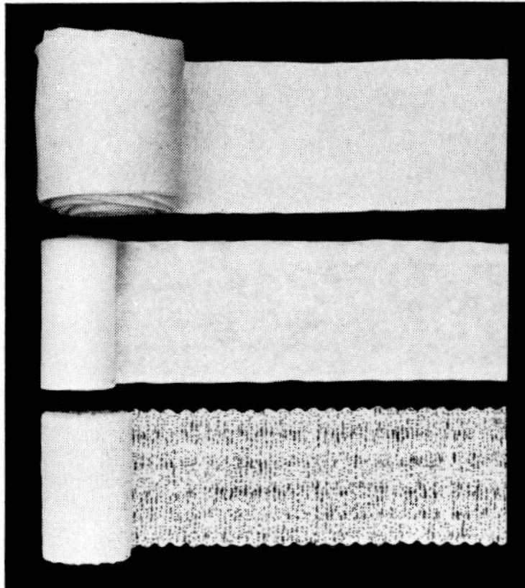

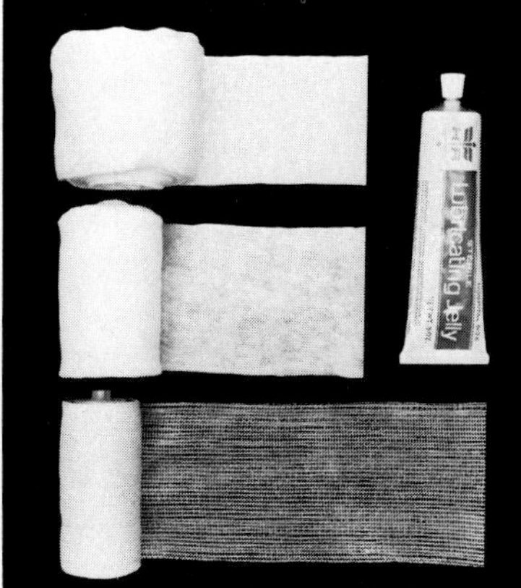

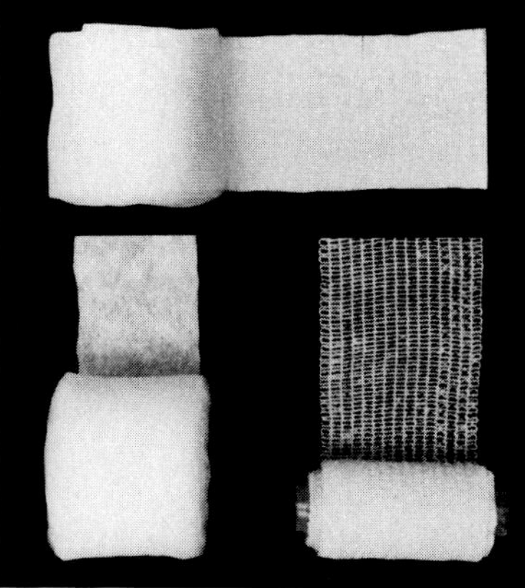

You've been instructed to prepare your patient for a cast application, so you'll need to know which casting materials the doctor may use. Are you familiar with the various casting materials? If not, review the following information.

Plaster (Specialist™ plaster bandage)

Open weave cotton rolls or strips saturated with anhydrous calcium sulfate (chalky white powder made from gypsum crystals)

Advantages
- Maintains rigid immobility
- Can be used for severely displaced fractures
- Easily molded to fit limb's contours
- Radiolucent
- Inexpensive; an advantage when limb position change or change in degree of edema necessitates recasting

Disadvantages
- Messy to apply
- Dries slowly
- Heavy, bulky, cumbersome
- Easily weakened by moisture

Nursing considerations
- Immerse rolls in water before use.
- Wear protective gloves when handling plaster tape.
- Protect floor during application.
- Protect pillows with bed-saver pads or rubber sheeting during drying.

Fiberglass (Scotchcast™ casting tape)

Open weave fiberglass tape saturated with polyurethane resin

Advantages
- After initial application, tape dries quickly, within 10 to 15 minutes; can bear body weight within ½ hour after application
- Maintains rigid immobility
- Lightweight and porous, but durable
- Maintains integrity when immersed in water
- Radiolucent

Disadvantages
- Can't be used for severely displaced fractures or where unusual edema is present
- Increased chance of skin maceration from wet cast when cast isn't dried properly
- Expensive

Nursing considerations
- Use only rayon stockinette and padding, and lubricant provided by the manufacturer, or K-Y Jelly.
- Open each roll immediately before using it.
- Wear protective gloves while handling tape.
- Remove resin from metal instruments with nail polish remover, immediately after use.
- Don't encourage patient to wet cast, because of difficulty in thoroughly drying cast padding. If doctor permits swimming or bathing with cast, teach patient proper drying procedures, according to manufacturer's instructions. However, patient should avoid beach swimming because sand may be trapped under cast, creating irritation that can lead to skin breakdown.

Synthetic (delta-lite™ casting tape)

Polyester and cotton open-weave fabric impregnated with water-activated polyurethane

Advantages
- After initial application, tape dries in 7 minutes; can bear body weight in 20 minutes
- Less sticky than fiberglass to apply
- Maintains rigid immobility
- Lightweight and porous, but durable
- Moisture resistant
- Radiolucent
- Can be removed with cast scissors
- Bonds to plaster for easy repair of plaster casts

Disadvantages
- Requires immersion in 70° to 80° F. (21.1 to 26.6° C.) water just before application
- Increased chance of skin maceration when wet cast isn't dried properly
- Expensive

Nursing considerations
- Open each roll immediately before using it.
- Wear protective gloves when handling tape.
- Be sure immersion water doesn't exceed 80° F. (26.6° C.) or excess heat production will result, causing patient discomfort.
- Don't squeeze water from roll before application or water's cooling effect will be lost.
- Use only cotton stockinette and padding before applying tape.
- To remove resin from skin, swab skin lightly with alcohol or acetone.
- Cast may be reinforced or patched by adding more tape.
- Don't encourage immersion of cast in water. If doctor permits cast immersion, teach patient proper drying procedures, according to manufacturer's instructions.

Casts

Assisting with fiberglass cast application

Forty-eight-year-old Diane LaCava has left elbow tendinitis aggravated by spasticity. To help relieve her condition, the doctor has decided to immobilize her elbow with a long arm fiberglass cast. He asks you to assist with cast application.

- Begin by explaining the casting procedure to Ms. LaCava. Encourage her to relax. To provide privacy and protect her clothing, drape her with bed-saver pads. Or, help her put on a disposable gown. Then, as the doctor assesses Ms. LaCava's arm, gather the equipment he'll need: two pieces of rayon stockinette, rayon padding, two 2″ (5.1 cm) rolls of Scotchcast™ casting tape, two pairs of unsterile gloves, a bucket filled with water at room temperature, and water-soluble lubricant, such as K-Y Jelly.
- To provide neater cast edges, the doctor will place one of the stockinette pieces around Ms. LaCava's hand, and the other around her upper arm (see photo below). Later, after two layers of fiberglass tape are applied, the doctor will turn down the stockinette edge and anchor it with more fiberglass tape.
- After applying the stockinette, he'll wrap the length of her arm with the rayon padding (as shown in the top right photo). Be sure to support her arm, as the nurse is doing here. To prevent complications, he'll take care not to fold or wrinkle the padding.
- Now, slip on a pair of gloves. As you know, the casting tape becomes sticky when moistened.

As the doctor puts on his gloves, you'll open

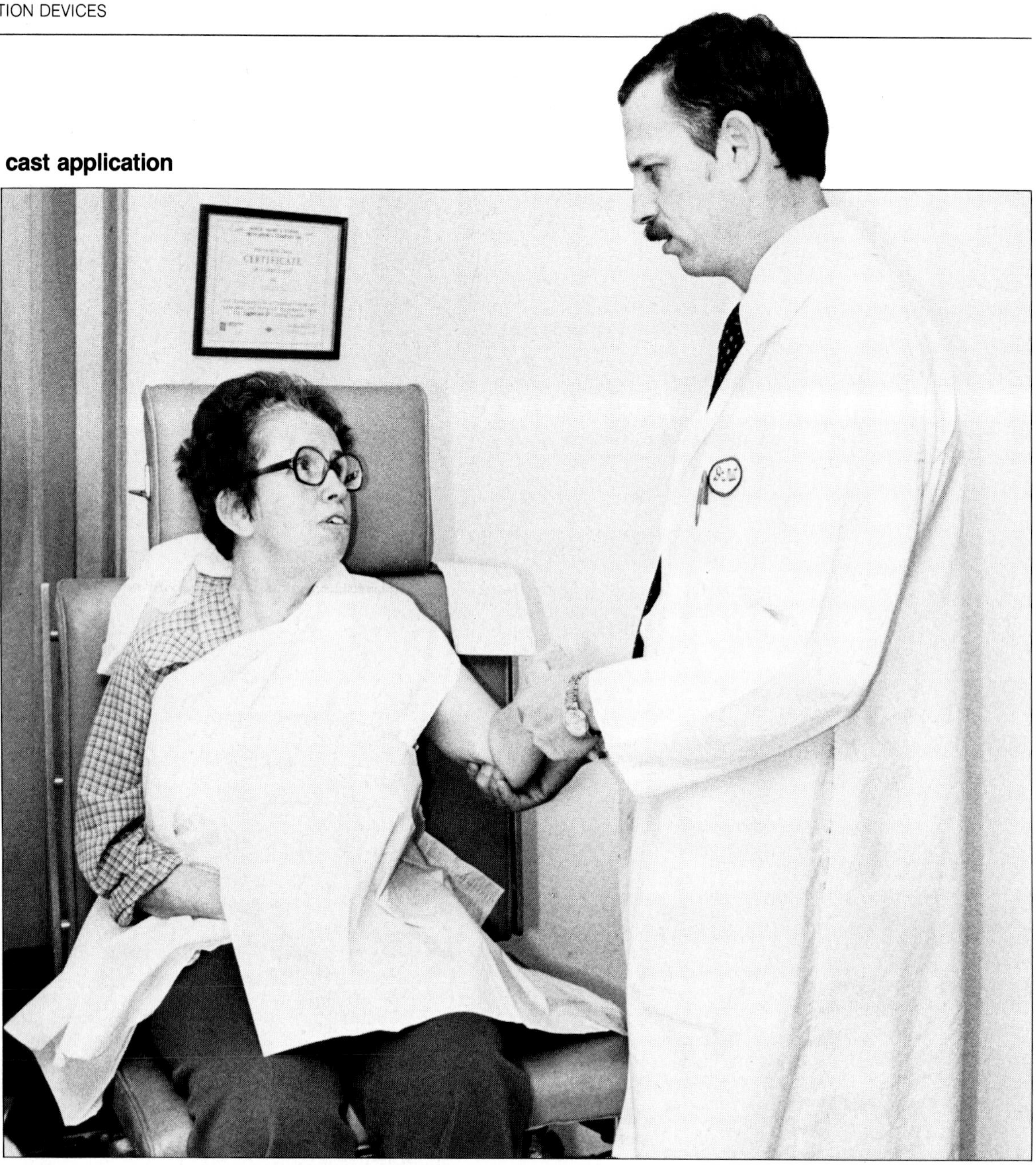

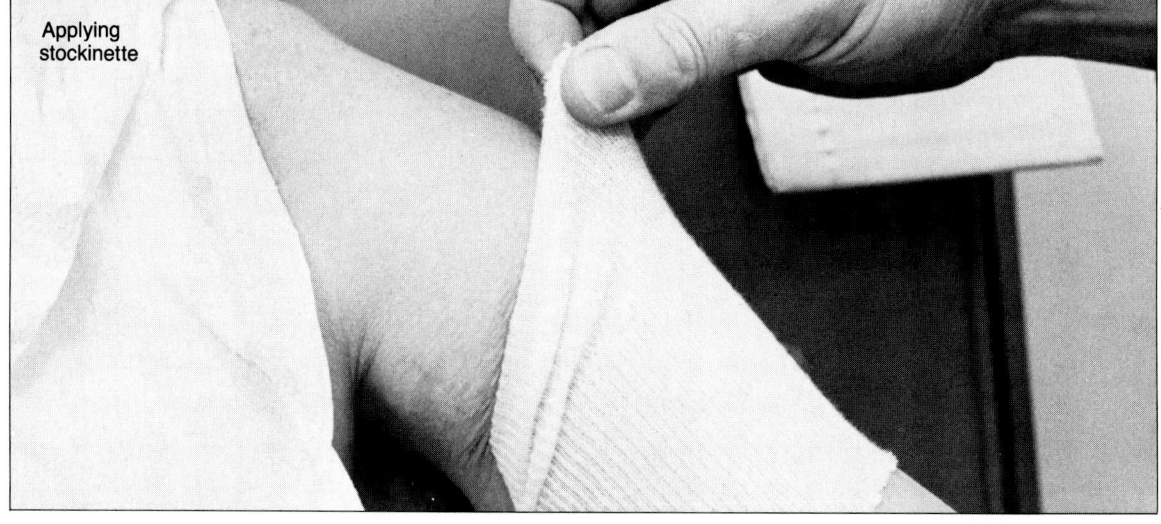

Applying stockinette

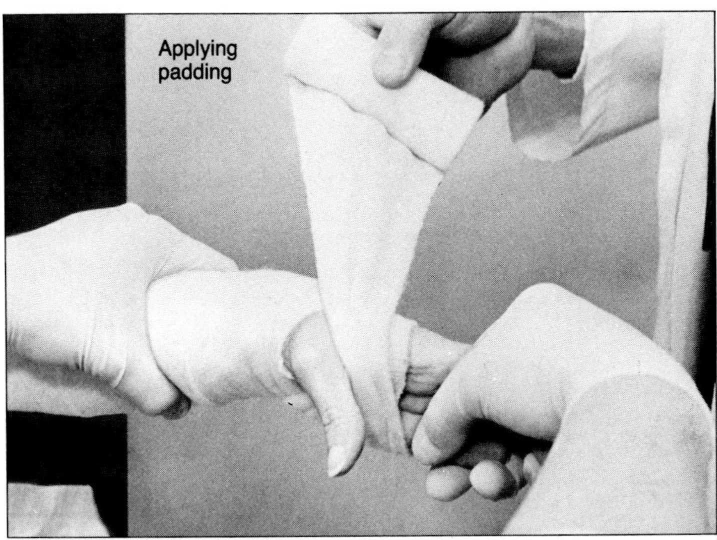
Applying padding

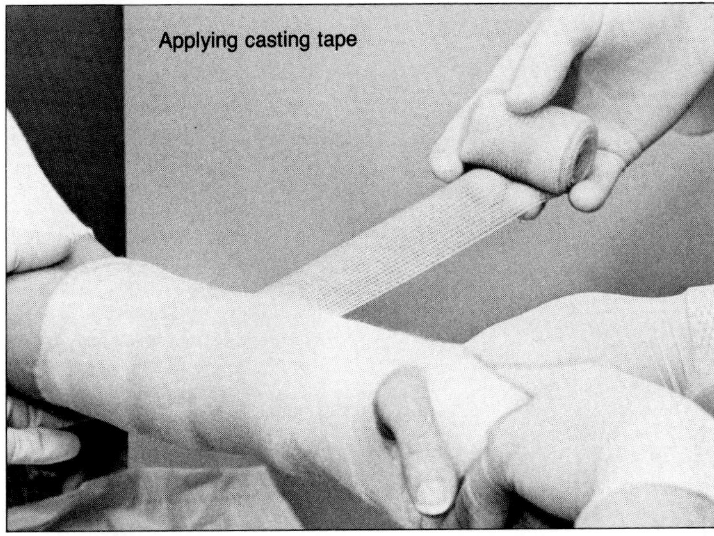
Applying casting tape

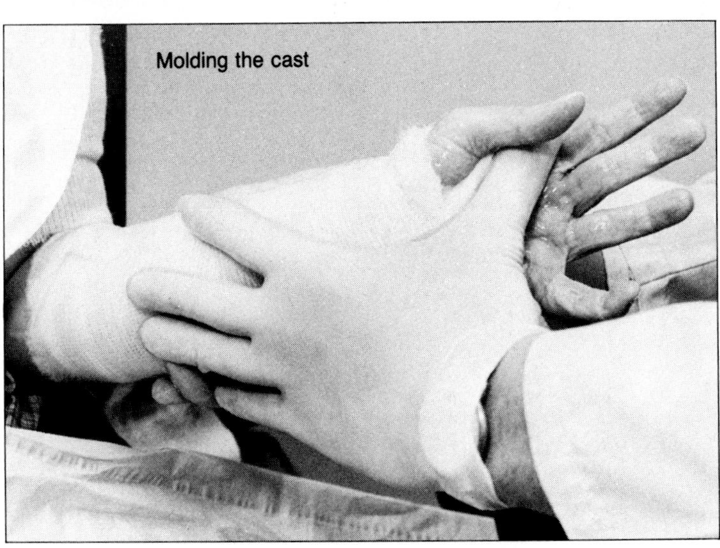
Molding the cast

one roll of casting tape. *Remember:* To keep the tape from hardening, open one roll at a time.

Immerse the tape in lukewarm water for 10 to 15 seconds. Shake out any excess water.

- The doctor will apply the long arm cast in two parts because of Ms. LaCava's spasticity. He'll begin wrapping her lower arm with casting tape, using a spiral motion. Support her arm at her elbow and fingers (see middle photo).
- When the doctor's applied three to four layers of casting tape, he'll smooth the cast to ensure proper contact between tape layers. Assist him by squeezing a small amount of water-soluble lubricating jelly onto his glove.
- After smoothing the lower cast with the lubricating jelly, he'll mold the cast (see bottom photo). *Remember:* About 6 minutes after immersion in water, Scotchcast hardens in the molded position.
- Now he'll apply the cast's upper portion.
- When 15 minutes has elapsed, the cast will be completely hardened. To check cast fit, slip two fingers inside the cast edge. If you can fit more than two fingers, the cast may be too loose. Consider the cast too tight if you're unable to get your fingers into the cast.
- Now, check the circulation in your patient's casted arm. To do this, check her thumb and fingernails for capillary refill. If you note a sluggish color return, notify the doctor. The cast may be too tight.

Finally, document the procedure, and your patient's reaction to it, on the appropriate forms.

Cast drying: Caring for the patient

Your patient just had a short leg cast applied. You'll need to care for him as the cast dries. Do you know how? Follow these steps:

- First, explain the drying procedure to your patient. Tell him or a family member he can speed the drying process by keeping his cast exposed to the air and repositioning it frequently.
- Then, place two regular-size firm pillows (or a Span+Aids® cast elevator) next to his cast. If you're using pillows, check to be sure they have rubber or plastic covers under the linen case. Place bed-saver pads between the cast and the pillows to absorb moisture.

Important: To ensure proper drying, never place a wet cast directly onto plastic.

- Have the patient lift his casted limb up on the pillows, if possible. Stress the importance of using his palms–not his fingers—to lift the cast. Remember, fingertip pressure on the cast may cause indentations in the plaster, resulting in potential pressure areas.

As the cast is lifted, check its underside. If you see any dents or flat spots, notify the doctor.

- Position the cast on the pillows. Check to be sure the cast is elevated above heart level and that the pillows extend above and below the cast.
- After 2 hours, reposition your patient's cast on the pillows, alternating between the supine, side-lying, and prone positions. Doing so allows the cast to dry evenly. When you reposition your patient, make sure his popliteal areas, heels, toes, ankles, wrists, and elbows are pressure-free. Also, take this opportunity to perform the neurovascular check described on page 24, and the nerve-function check on page 25.
- Continue to assess and reposition your patient's cast every 2 hours, or as ordered.

Important: A plaster cast should dry from the inside out in approximately 72 hours. Don't use lamps, hair dryers, or fans to hasten the procedure because they won't penetrate to the cast's interior.

- Document the procedure, including your assessment, on the appropriate forms.

Casts

How to trim a cast

1 *Now, Diane LaCava's cast is completely dry. You'll want to check for—and finish—rough cast edges. Finishing a cast creates a smooth surface next to the skin, helping prevent skin irritation and breakdown. Also, a finished edge will hold the cotton cast padding or stockinette better.*

Suppose one edge of your patient's cast is extremely rough. Carefully smooth or trim the edge with a cast knife or scissors. Or, pull rough edges away from the skin using duck bill forceps, as shown here.

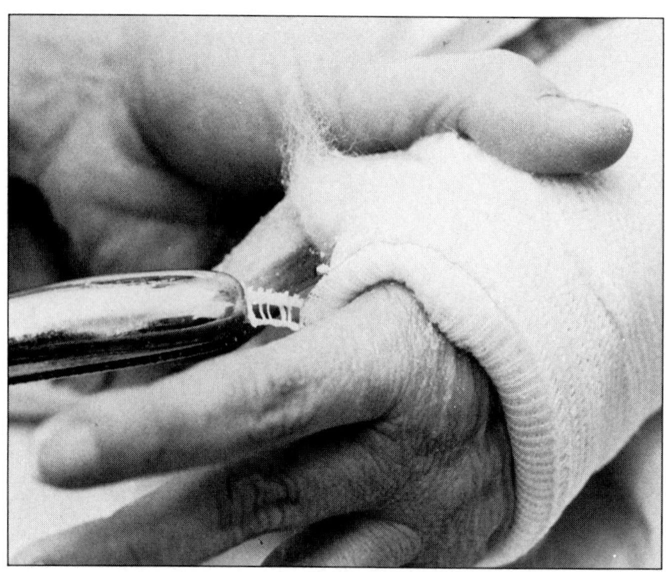

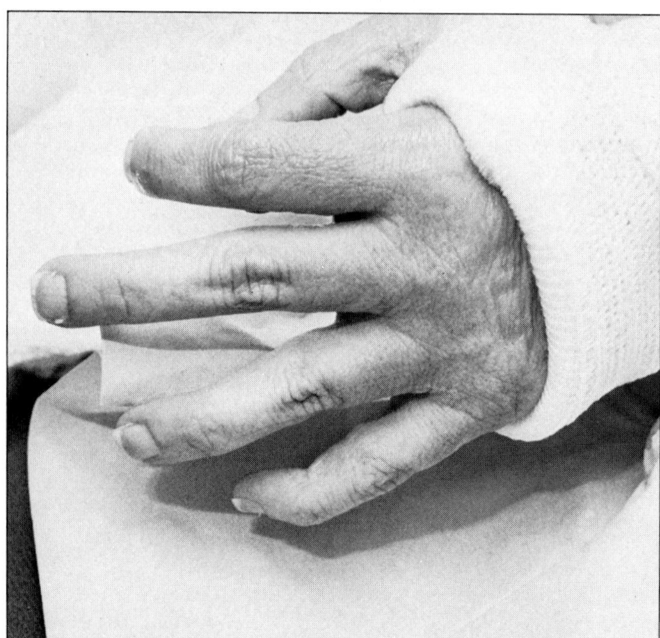

2 When you're finished, pull the padding over the cast edge. Then, petal the edge as instructed at right.

Finally, teach your patient how to assess her cast. Emphasize the importance of routinely checking her cast for rough edges, and petaling any she may find. (For more cast care information, see the opposite page.)

How to petal a cast

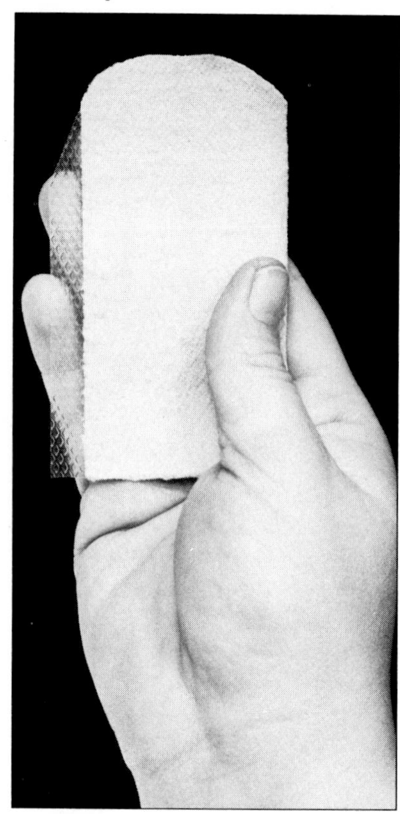

1 *To cover an edge you've trimmed (or a rough edge that doesn't need trimming), petal it with adhesive tape or moleskin. To do this, first cut several 4"x2" (10.2x5.1 cm) strips. To keep the strip corners on the outside of the cast from rolling, round them, as shown here.*

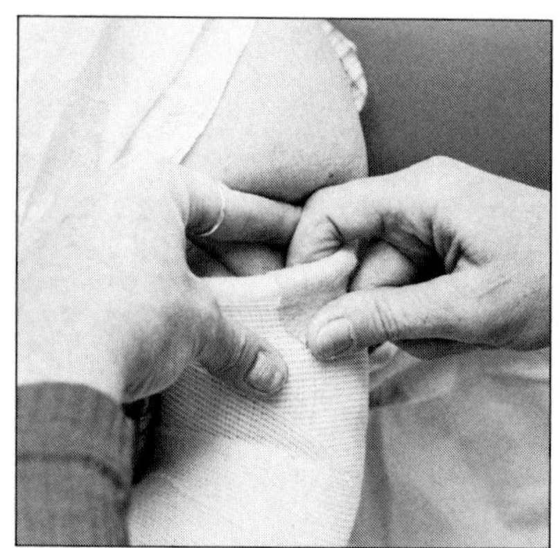

2 Now, you're ready to teach your patient or a family member how to apply the moleskin strips to her cast. Making sure that the rounded end of the strip is on the outside of the cast, tuck the straight end just inside the cast edge. Smooth the moleskin with your finger until you're sure it's firmly secured. To avoid skin irritation and breakdown, always take care not to crease the moleskin.

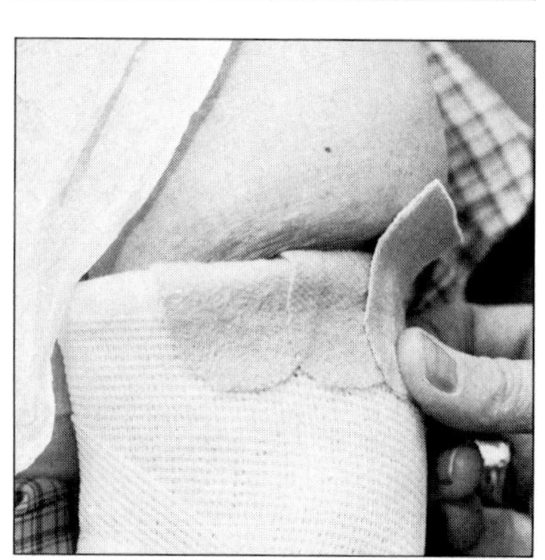

3 After you've applied two strips to the cast, repeat the procedure, applying overlapping pieces over the cast edge until all roughened edges are completely covered. Or, your patient may complete the petaling.

Document the procedure on the appropriate forms.

Caring for a patient with a cast

If you've ever cared for a patient with a cast, you know that you'll have to position him properly and assess his condition frequently. Always keep your patient's extremity elevated above heart level. For specific positioning guidelines, see page 64. Also, here are some assessment considerations to keep in mind:

- Perform the neurovascular check described on page 24. When you perform the check, be sure to observe and palpate the areas around the cast for swelling, redness, cyanosis, blister formation, and broken skin. Also, note skin temperature. As you know, swelling, loss of color, and cool skin in these areas may indicate neurovascular impairment.

Note: Because of cast location, comparing bilateral pulses may be impossible to perform properly. If so, be sure to perform bilateral skin color and capillary refill checks carefully.

- Instruct your patient in an arm or leg cast to touch, flex, and extend his fingers or toes at least four times a day. Have him perform the simple nerve damage tests indicated on page 25.
- Observe the cast for drainage as explained at right.
- If your patient's on bed rest, inspect all skin areas (especially bony prominences such as back, iliac crests, elbows, heels, and Achilles tendons) twice daily, when you turn your patient. Look for signs and symptoms of pressure sores; for example, redness and swelling, as well as pain and restlessness. Perform the skin care indicated on page 55.
- Smell the cast edges every 8 hours. Foul odors (besides perspiration and elimination soilage odors) may indicate complications, such as wound infection or pressure necrosis.

In addition to assessing your patient, follow these general care guidelines:

- Finish any rough cast edges, following the steps on the previous page.
- Protect the cast from getting wet and stained.
- If your patient has a hip spica or body cast, place waterproof material, such as plastic wrap, around the cast's perineal edge to prevent elimination soilage. After elimination, clean the plastic by wiping it with a washcloth. Replace the plastic wrap as necessary.
- Encourage your patient to participate as much as possible in his daily care. Praise him for his efforts. Involve the physical or occupational therapist in teaching your patient daily living activities while he's in a cast.
- Provide good skin care. For example, have the patient bathe daily, assisting as necessary, and be sure to dry his skin thoroughly. Give frequent alcohol or lotion rubs, and check that his bed linen is free of wrinkles, food crumbs, and plaster particles. Encourage the patient to turn and change position every 2 hours.
- Make sure the patient performs range-of-motion exercises of all uncasted joints at least three times a day.

Assessing cast drainage

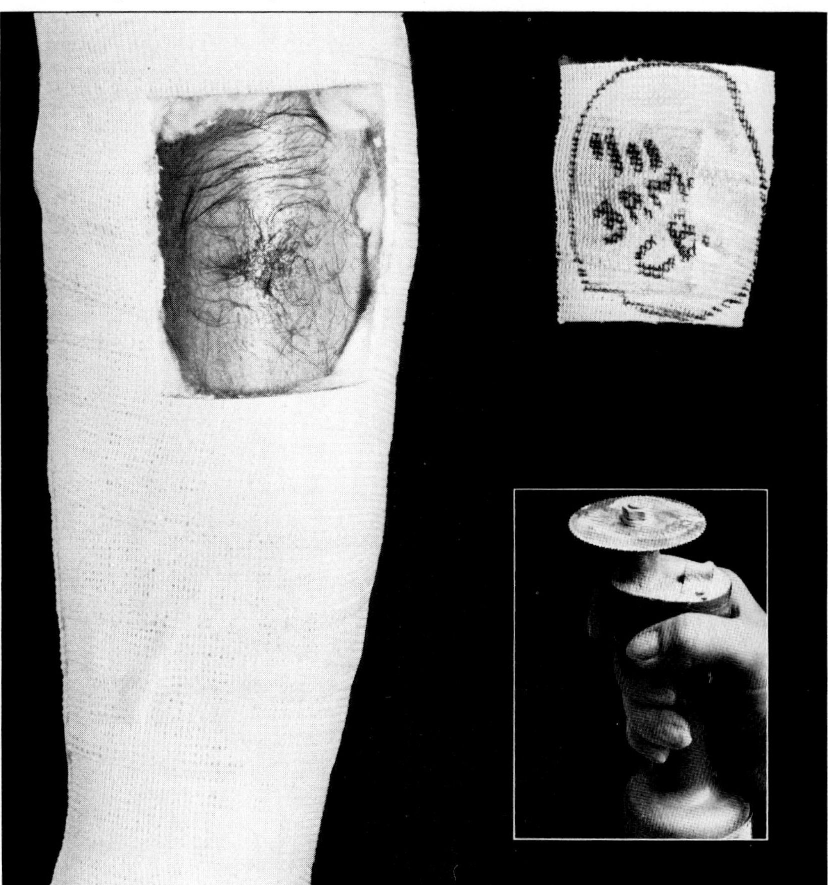

Anytime a patient has drainage that visibly stains his cast, you must try to determine the source. First, check your patient's records. Does his cast cover an open wound? If the drainage occurs within 48 hours after casting, it may be normal. But, if your patient's had the cast for more than 48 hours, suspect complications such as a reopened wound. Or if his cast doesn't cover a wound, suspect skin breakdown from pressure or a blister.

Notify the doctor immediately if any of the following occur:

- Drainage from a wound increases significantly during the first 48 hours after the cast is applied.
- Drainage stains the cast bright red.
- Drainage occurs even though no wound was present when the doctor first applied the cast.
- Drainage odor has changed. (This may indicate infection.)

If drainage does occur, assess its amount, color, and odor at least once every 2 hours. Using a felt-tipped pen, outline the drainage on the cast, as shown in the photo. Record the date, time, and your initials within the outline. Document your findings.

Note: Drainage won't necessarily stain the patient's cast. Be sure to check your patient's bed linens (especially under the cast) for drainage leaking from the cast ends.

If drainage is heavy, the doctor may order a window cut in the cast (see photo) so he can observe and treat the open area. *Important:* Save the window piece. He may replace it later, after the open area's healed.

Trim and petal the window edges on the cast. Protect the cast edges by covering them with plastic wrap. Secure the plastic with adhesive tape.

Remember: The window will be a weak point on the cast. Always handle this portion of the cast carefully, to prevent the cast from cracking.

Casts

Dealing with special positioning problems

Keeping your patient's cast positioned properly is part of your nursing responsibility. In most cases, you'll elevate the casted arm or leg above heart level. However, the way you position and support your patient and his cast will depend on his condition, and the equipment available. Here's how to deal with a variety of different casts:

Patient with an arm cast

• Use two or three firm pillows or a Span + Aids® cast elevator to elevate the cast.

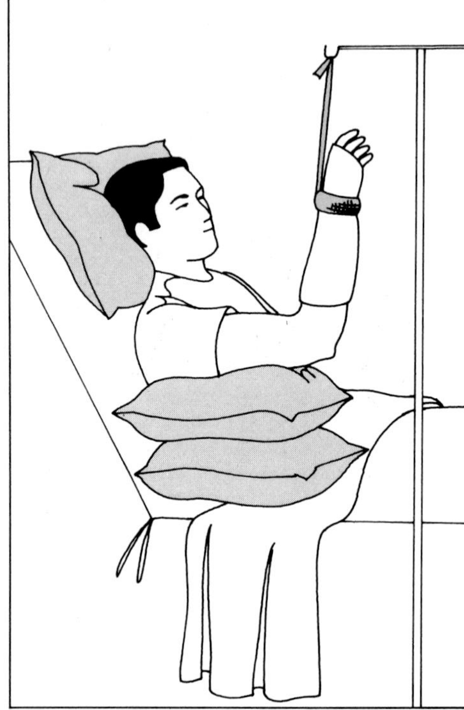

• If ordered or indicated, attach the cast to an I.V. pole, using stockinette or gauze. Support the cast by placing pillows underneath it. *Important:* Be sure the elbow portion of the cast hangs clear of the bed and isn't supported by a pillow.

Nursing tip: If your patient experiences numbness or tingling in his elbow, check to make sure the elbow isn't pressing against the pillow.

• If your patient's restless or on seizure precautions, tie a pillow around the cast to reduce possible cast damage from banging or bumping.

• If your patient's comatose, position a pillow against his arm laterally to prevent arm rotation.

• When your patient can move around, apply a sling to keep the cast in the proper position (see page 56).

• If your patient has a *hanging cast,* which is used to maintain traction on a fractured humerus or ulna, have him rest and sleep in a high Fowler's position. Do not support a *hanging cast* on a pillow or I.V. pole.

Patient with a leg cast

• Use two to three firm pillows or a Span + Aids cast elevator to elevate cast. Reposition pillows, as necessary. Be sure to keep patient's heel and toes (if he's in a prone position) off pillows and mattress.

• Place pillows on both sides of your patient's thigh to prevent hip rotation.

• If your patient's in a wheelchair, pad the legrest with a pillow. Then, elevate the cast on the legrest. Secure the cast to the legrest with a belt.

• Does your patient need a bedpan? Keeping his casted leg elevated on pillows, place a fracture bedpan under his buttocks, from the side of his body opposite the cast. If your patient's able to assist, have him use the trapeze to lift his buttocks off the mattress while you slide the bedpan under them.

• Elevate a long leg cast with a double sling, as ordered (see page 58).

Patient with a hip spica cast

• To support a unilateral cast, place the pillows crosswise, at your patient's lumbar region, and lengthwise along the outside of casted leg.

• Never use the bar on a spica cast for lifting or turning.

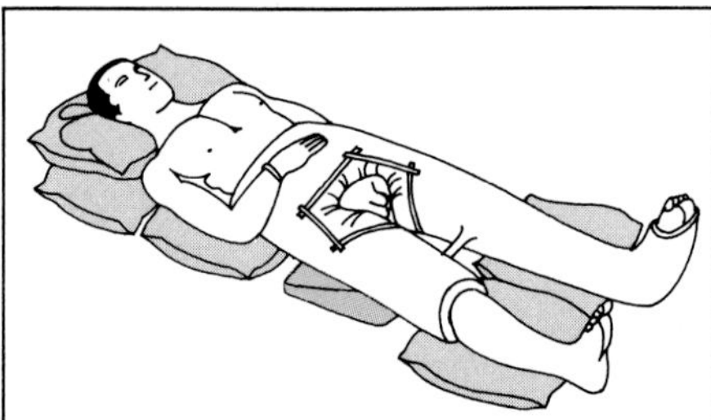

• For elimination, position fracture bedpan so the posterior lip is under patient's buttocks. If the spica cast's unilateral, slide the bedpan under the patient's buttocks from his uncasted side.

Patient with a body cast

• Place a small pillow crosswise under patient's lumbar region.

• Provide a pillow for patient's head and shoulders, unless contraindicated.

• Check to be sure patient's heels and toes are pressure-free.

PATIENT TEACHING

Sending your patient home with a cast

The home care aid that follows will help you teach your patient (or a family member) how to care for his cast at home. Keep in mind that a cast—regardless of type or size—will cause a disruption in your patient's day-to-day activities. Reassure him and offer encouragement. Explain as much as possible about his cast and its care.

Instruct your patient to keep the cast elevated on two pillows and uncovered for at least 48 hours (or as ordered), as the cast dries. In addition, tell him to use his palms—not his fingertips—to frequently change the cast's position on the pillows. Remind him that all these measures promote even cast drying and help reduce swelling. Warn your patient that the wet cast will feel heavy. But, reassure him that as the cast dries, it will get lighter. Also, tell him not to poke at the wet cast with his fingers.

Discuss with your patient the observations necessary to ensure comfort and prevent complications. For example, show him how to move his fingers and toes to assess motion.

Because your patient will have the cast on for some time, explain the importance of exercise in preventing complications. (See the last section for more information on preventing complications.) Also, show him how to perform any special exercises ordered by the doctor.

Emphasize to your patient that cast care, as described on the next two pages, must continue as long as he's wearing the cast.

Finally, give your patient a copy of the home care aid and review the instructions with him and his family. Be sure to indicate on the home care aid the type of cast your patient's wearing (mark step 4 or 5).

Home care

Caring for your cast at home

1

Dear Patient:
As you know, the doctor has immobilized your injury site with a cast. Of course, proper healing depends on your cooperation.

Contact your doctor immediately or return to the emergency department at once if you note any of the following in your casted arm or leg:

- increasing pain
- pain unrelieved by prescribed medication
- swelling unrelieved by elevating cast above heart level for 1 hour
- a change in sensation
- numbness, tingling, or burning
- decreased movement or loss of movement in your fingers or toes
- a change in skin color above or below the cast
- a bad smell coming from inside the cast
- a warm area or fresh stain on the cast
- an object dropped into or stuck in the cast
- a weakened, cracked, loose, or tight cast.

To care for your casted arm or leg, follow these guidelines:

To prevent excess swelling, keep your casted arm or leg elevated on pillows, above chest level, as much as possible (see the illustration). Check for swelling above and below the cast several times a day. To do this, compare your casted arm or leg with your other arm or leg. Consider a little swelling normal. Apply ice to swollen areas.

2 Now check for numbness, tingling, or pain by touching the area above and below your cast. Repeat this check several times a day. *Note:* You may feel pain even without touching your limb.

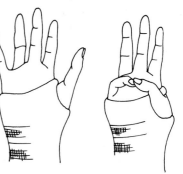

Perform the movements shown in the illustration (depending on the location of your cast). These exercises test nerve function. If you can't move your fingers or toes, or if you have more pain when you move them, notify the doctor.

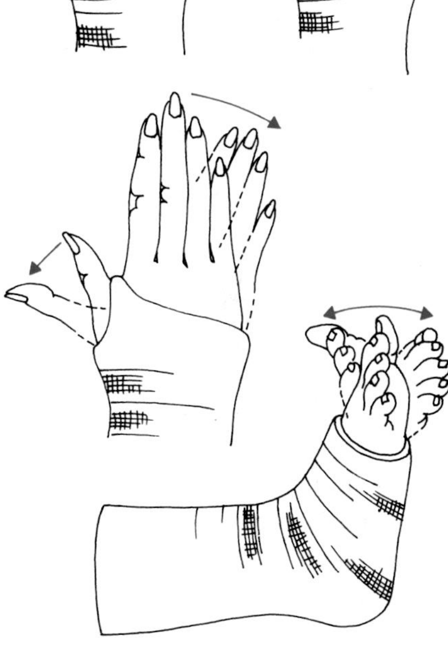

3

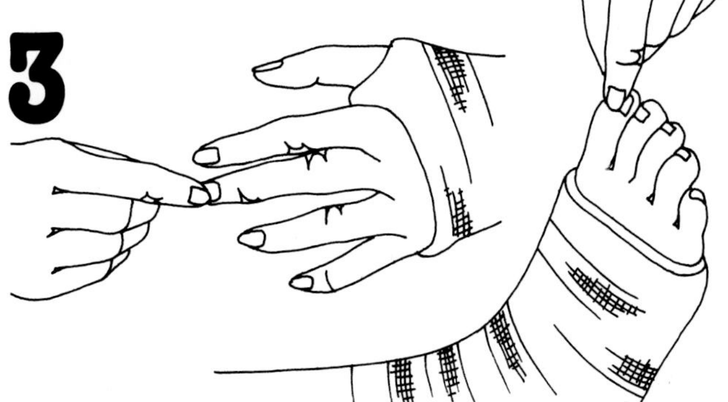

To check your circulation, press briefly on your middle fingernail (on a casted arm) or large toenail (on a casted leg) until it turns white. Then, let go. If normal pink color doesn't return quickly, notify your doctor at once. Repeat this check at least three times a day.

If your fingers or toes are cold, cover them. If that doesn't warm them, notify the doctor.

Casts

Home care

Caring for your cast at home continued

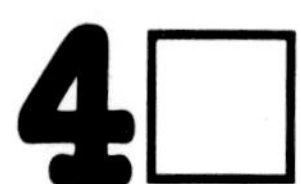

If the nurse has checked this box, you're wearing a plaster cast. That means that if you're planning to bathe or go out in wet weather, you'll need to encase your cast in a plastic bag; for example, a garbage bag. Tie the bag securely above the cast. Do not use rubber bands.

Important: Don't let a plaster cast get wet. Moisture will weaken or destroy it. If the cast does become wet, allow it to dry naturally; for example, you may sit in the sun. Do not cover the cast until it's thoroughly dry.

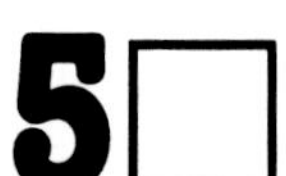

If the nurse has checked this box, your cast is made of one of the new casting materials. Check with your doctor to find out if you may shower or swim with your cast. He'll also give specific instructions about drying it.

He'll probably want you to let your wet cast dry naturally in the air. Because your cast dries from the inside out, a hair dryer or fan will not hasten the drying.

6 When your cast becomes soiled, clean it with a damp cloth and dry cleanser, such as Comet®. Be sure to wipe off any excess moisture. Or, follow these special instructions: ______

______

______

______

______

______

7

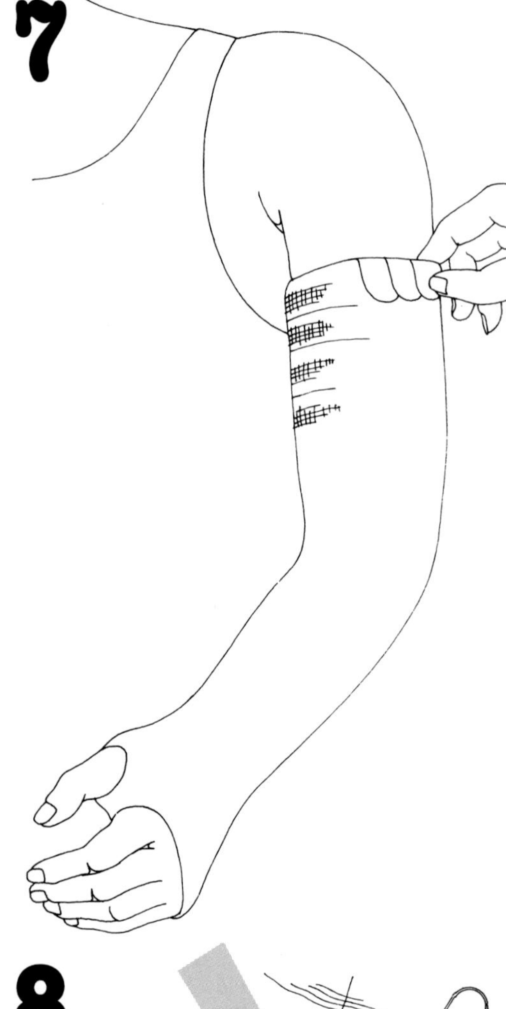

Wash the skin along the edges of your cast with mild soap and water every day. First, protect the cast edge with plastic wrap. Then, use a damp cloth to clean the skin you can reach inside the cast. Take care not to get the cast wet when you wash. Dry your skin thoroughly with a towel. Then, massage the skin at the cast edges and under the cast with a towel or a pad saturated with rubbing alcohol. This helps toughen the skin. To avoid skin irritation, remove loose plaster particles daily by reaching an inch or two inside the cast.

Also, feel the cast for rough edges each day, and cover them with moleskin. To do this, cut several 4″ long, 2″ wide (10x5 cm) strips of moleskin and round their edges. Attach these strips around the cast edges, as shown in the illustration.

8

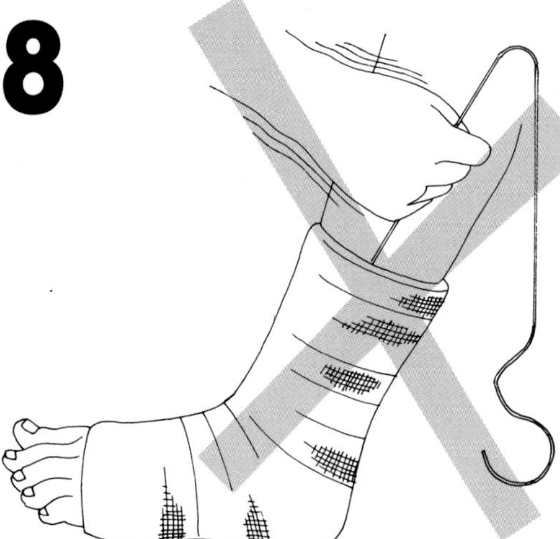

Occasionally, the skin under your cast will feel itchy. *But, don't insert any object into the cast to try to relieve the itching (or for any other reason).* Doing so could damage your skin and lead to infection.

Finally, return to your doctor on the following date to have your cast removed:

______

Don't ever try to trim or remove the cast yourself.

Removing a cast

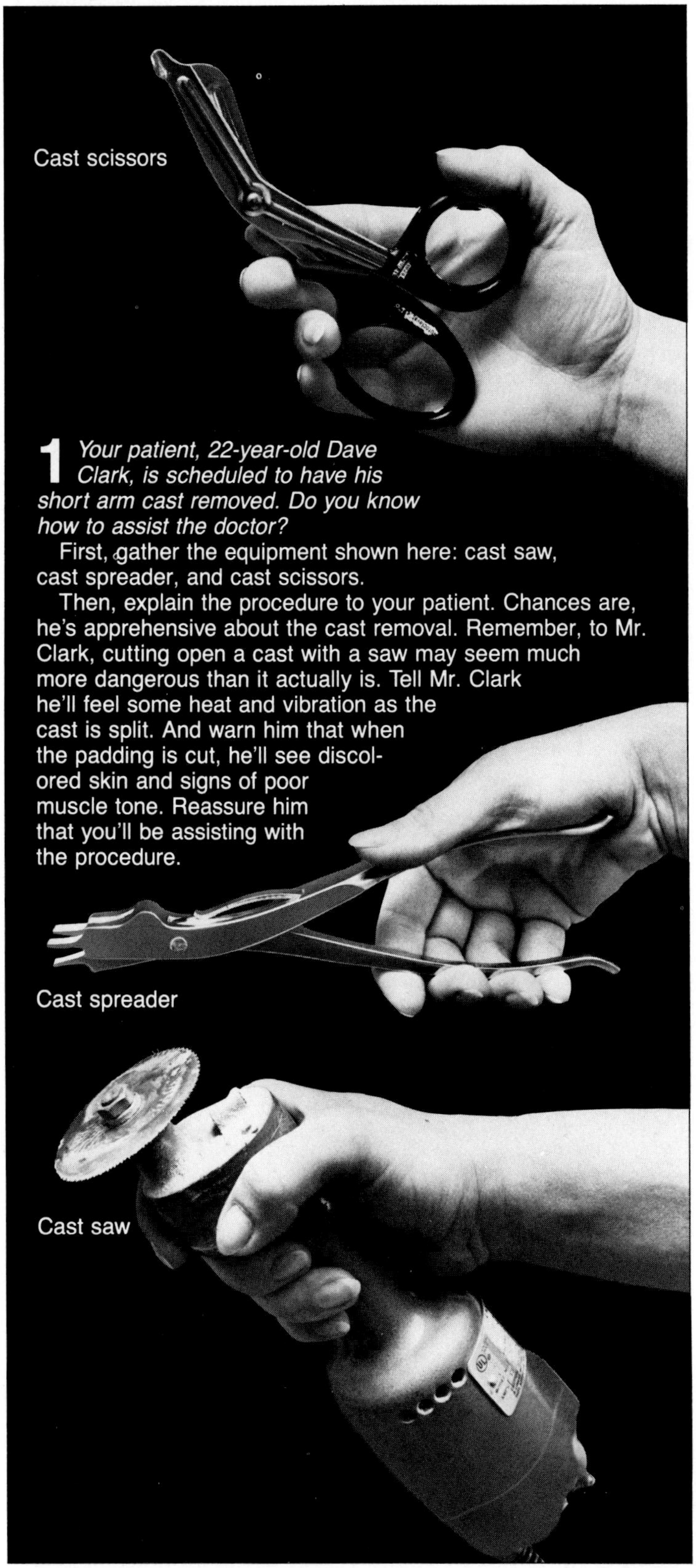

Cast scissors

1 *Your patient, 22-year-old Dave Clark, is scheduled to have his short arm cast removed. Do you know how to assist the doctor?*

First, gather the equipment shown here: cast saw, cast spreader, and cast scissors.

Then, explain the procedure to your patient. Chances are, he's apprehensive about the cast removal. Remember, to Mr. Clark, cutting open a cast with a saw may seem much more dangerous than it actually is. Tell Mr. Clark he'll feel some heat and vibration as the cast is split. And warn him that when the padding is cut, he'll see discolored skin and signs of poor muscle tone. Reassure him that you'll be assisting with the procedure.

Cast spreader

Cast saw

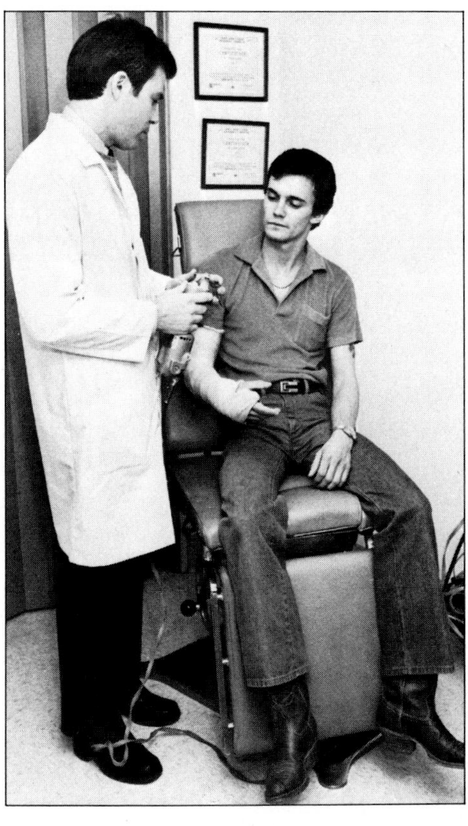

2 Now, begin the procedure following these guidelines:

First, position Mr. Clark on a reclining chair.

Then, the doctor will explain exactly what he'll do. He'll show Mr. Clark what the cast saw looks and sounds like. He'll also demonstrate how it works. At this point, be sure to emphasize to your patient that the saw will not cut into his skin.

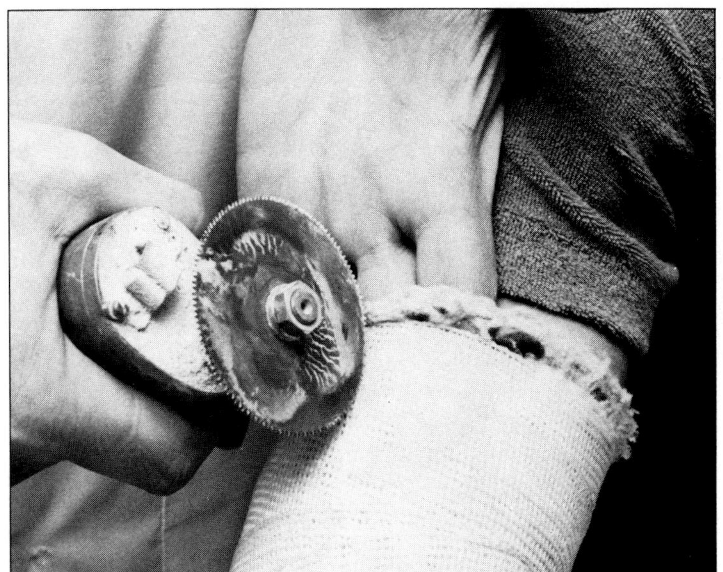

3 Now, the doctor's ready to remove the cast. Cover the patient's lap with a protective pad.

The doctor will position the saw at the cast edge, avoiding wounds or bony prominences, and apply gentle downward pressure. He'll place one hand under the cast edge, as shown here, to help reassure the patient. When he feels the saw penetrate the cast, he'll lift the saw and place it over the next surface to be cut. Repeating this procedure, he'll completely cut one side of the cast.

Casts

Removing a cast continued

4 After he finishes cutting one side, he'll cut the cast's opposite side. As the doctor continues cutting into the cast, closely monitor Mr. Clark's condition. Check his pulse periodically and instruct him to breathe slowly and deeply. If he begins to feel faint, have the doctor stop the procedure. Then, quickly raise Mr. Clark's feet and lower his head. Encourage him to breathe slowly and deeply. Administer aromatic ammonia, as needed.

When your patient feels better, and his vital signs have returned to normal, the doctor will resume cutting the cast. But remember, *keep your patient flat* for the rest of the procedure.

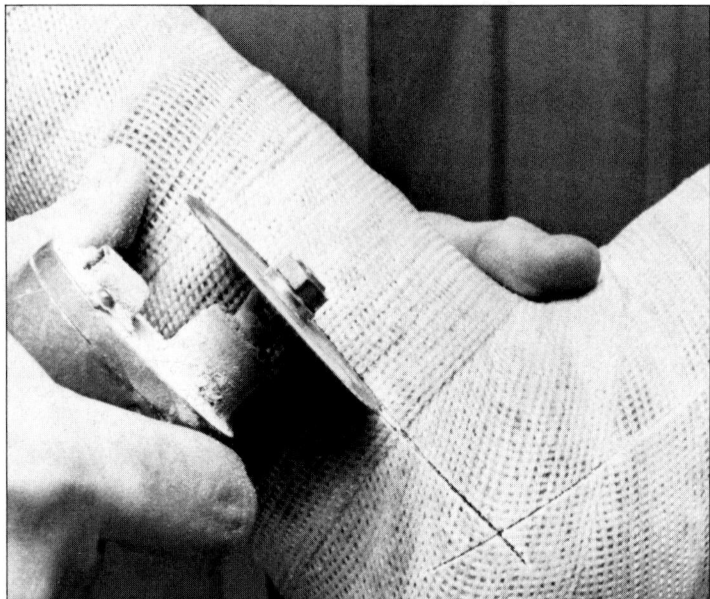

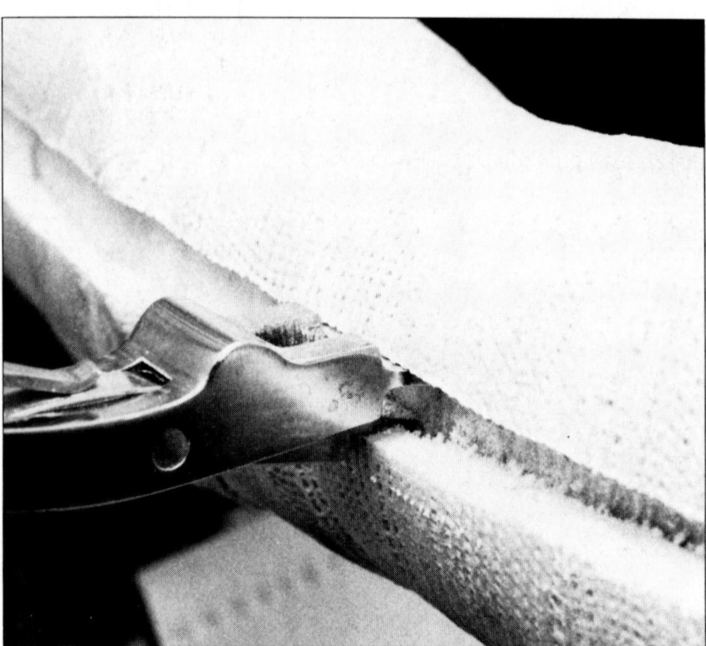

5 When the doctor's finished cutting both sides of the cast, he'll use a spreader to open the cast pieces, as shown in this photo.

6 Using cast scissors, the doctor will cut through the cast padding. As he does so, remind your patient of what he'll see.

Explain that the yellow or gray scaly covering over his skin is caused by an accumulation of dead skin and oil from the glands near the skin surface. Remind Mr. Clark that the previously casted arm will probably appear thinner and flabbier than the uncasted one. Tell him his arm may also ache and feel weak. Reassure him that with exercise and good skin care, his arm will return to normal.

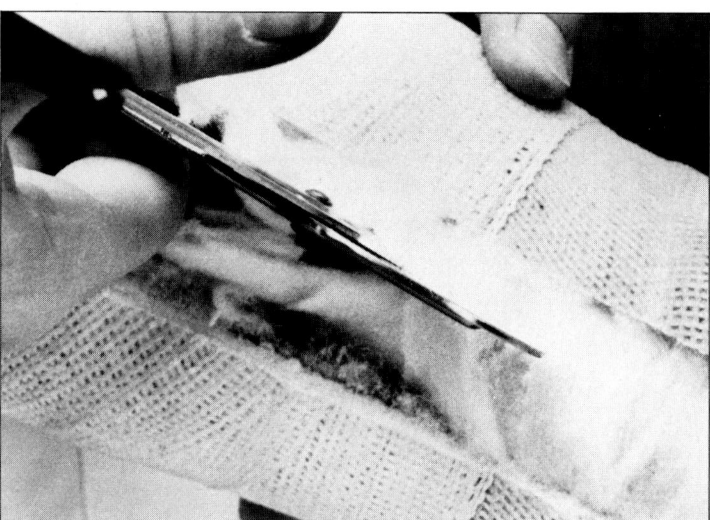

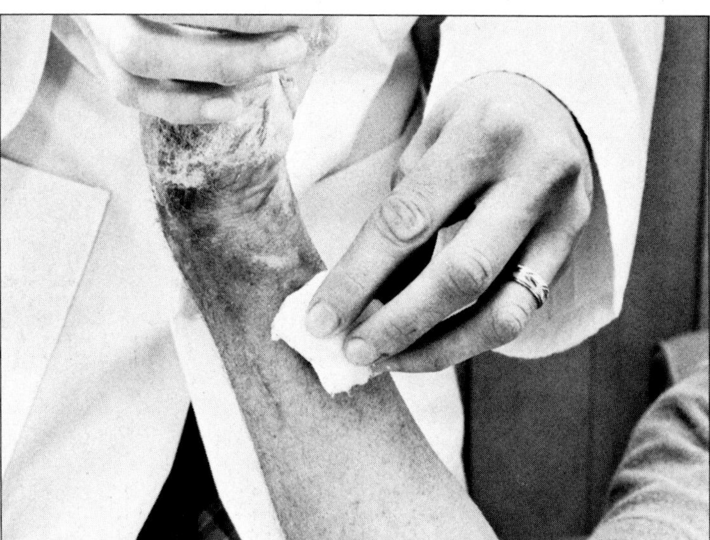

7 Now, using an alcohol-saturated pad, wipe his arm, as the nurse is doing here. This helps loosen accumulated dead skin.

Also, take this opportunity to teach him how to care for his arm at home. Tell him to gently wash it with mild soap and water, dry it thoroughly, and wipe it with an alcohol-saturated pad daily. Emphasize that proper skin care will gradually loosen all the accumulated skin and help his arm return to its normal appearance.

To confirm proper bone alignment and healing, the doctor will order an X-ray of Mr. Clark's arm.

Finally, document the procedure, your patient's reaction to it, and any patient teaching, on the appropriate forms.

Traction

If you're like most nurses, you probably dread caring for a patient who's in traction. The bulky equipment and complex setup can be frightening.

However, they don't have to be. We'll simplify what you need to know in the following pages. For example, we'll show you:

- traction components and their function in a traction setup.
- how to apply traction with a Buck's extension device, pelvic belt, and cervical halter.
- how to care for a patient in cervical spine or halo traction.

For a thorough introduction to traction therapy, study the following illustrations, photos, and text.

Understanding traction

Traction is an important form of orthopedic immobilization. It's applied as an alternative to surgery, and is also used to ensure proper positioning of the affected limb, alignment of a fracture, and correction of deformities, pre- and postoperatively.

Traction therapy restricts movement of a patient's affected limb or body part, and may confine the patient to bed rest over an extended period of time. The limb's immobilized by applying opposing pull at both ends of the injured area: an equal mix of traction and countertraction. Weights provide the traction pull. Countertraction may be produced by other weights, or by positioning the patient's body weight against the traction pull.

Although traction often requires confinement to a hospital bed, it does allow the patient limited motion of his affected extremity, and permits exercise of his unaffected body parts.

A doctor may order traction for any of the following reasons:

- to reduce a fracture and realign bone fragments, by pulling the broken bone ends into the anatomically correct position
- to immobilize a fracture and maintain fracture alignment until callus begins mending the broken bone ends together
- to reduce, relieve, and prevent skeletal muscle spasms caused by orthopedic injuries. As you know, muscles may spasm in an attempt to splint an area of bone displacement and angulation.
- to overcome joint deformities and contractures by stretching muscles, either to avoid or precede surgery
- to rest a diseased joint, as in arthritis.

The three basic types of traction are shown at right:

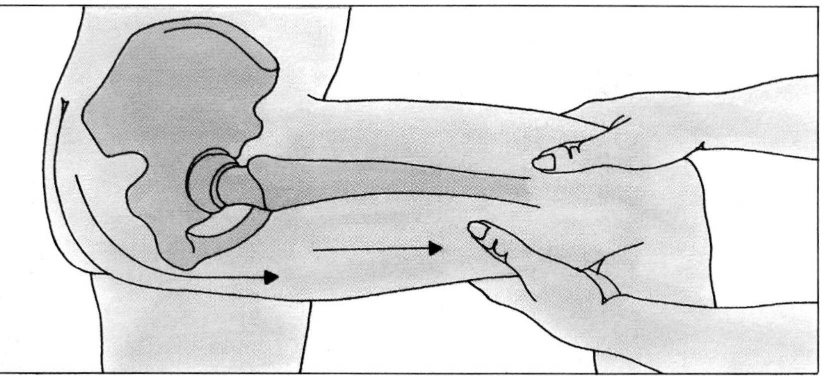

- *Manual traction* temporarily immobilizes an injured area, through hands pulling on the injured body part. Manual traction can be used before more permanent traction, and while applying a cast.

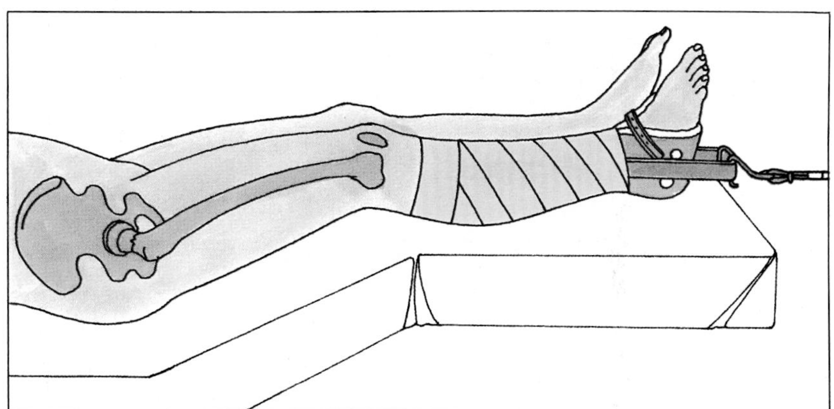

- *Skin traction* immobilizes a body part intermittently over an extended period, through direct application of a pulling force on the patient's skin. The force may be applied using adhesive or nonadhesive traction tape or other skin traction devices such as a boot, belt, or halter. Adhesive attachment allows more continuous traction, while nonadhesive attachment allows easier removal for daily care.

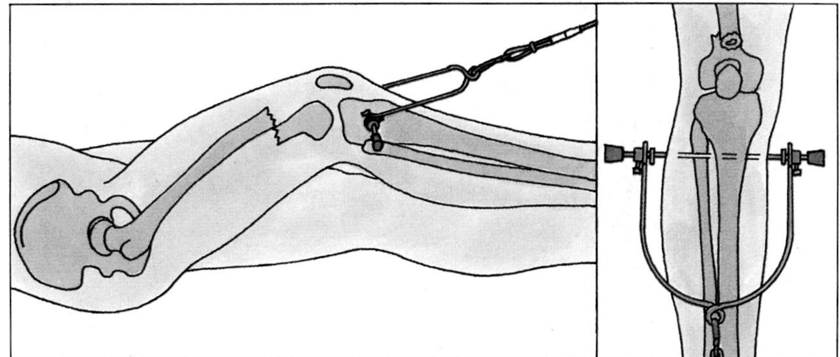

- *Skeletal traction* immobilizes a body part for prolonged periods by attaching weighted equipment directly to the patient's bones. This may be accomplished with pins, screws, wires, or tongs. Skeletal traction allows more prolonged traction with heavier weight than do the other two methods.

Are you familiar with traction equipment? If not, the illustrations on the following page will help you identify the various pieces used in traction therapy.

Traction

Learning about traction equipment

Your responsibility for obtaining and applying traction equipment depends on your hospital's policy. But, even if you won't be assembling traction setups, recognizing basic traction equipment and knowing how the components function together will help you monitor traction effectiveness.

Effective traction begins with a firm mattress. The preferred mattress is constructed with a solid base rather than springs. But, if this type isn't available, bed boards can be placed between the mattress and bed frame to provide additional support.

Traction frames, which extend from the head to the foot of the bed, are needed for almost all types of traction. Other equipment, such as pulleys and weights, hang from the frame to complete the traction assembly. Most frames are either steel or aluminum, but some combine both metals. Although steel frames are stronger, aluminum frames are more popular because they're lighter and easier to handle.

Note: Request a steel frame for a very tall, heavy, or restless patient.

Frame assembly varies according to the type of bed and the type of traction being applied. The upright poles supporting the overhead framework are either secured to the bed by clawlike attachments, or are inserted in I.V. holders located at each bed corner. The overhead framework usually consists of one or two bars suspended longitudinally across the bed.

The traction cord runs between the patient and the weight. The cord must be strong to avoid stretching or fraying. Cord thickness varies.

A trapeze is commonly added to the overhead framework. This piece of equipment (when indicated) provides the patient with a grasping device that promotes mobility and some independence, and enables you to expedite daily care.

The following set of illustrations shows you how to apply Russell traction, using a single overhead frame. As you can see, this particular traction involves many attachments. We've illustrated them individually as well as in position on the traction frame. This way, you'll understand how the pieces fit together.

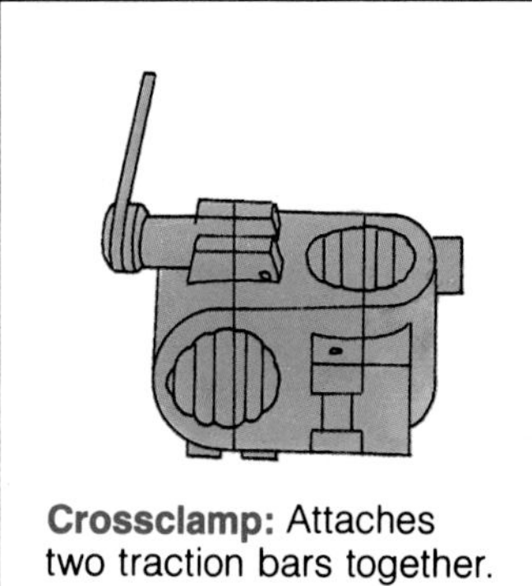

Crossclamp: Attaches two traction bars together.

Pulley: Holds the traction cord (which runs between the patient and weight), keeping the cord free of the bed; prevents cord erosion and allows patient movement; sizes vary according to traction cord thickness.

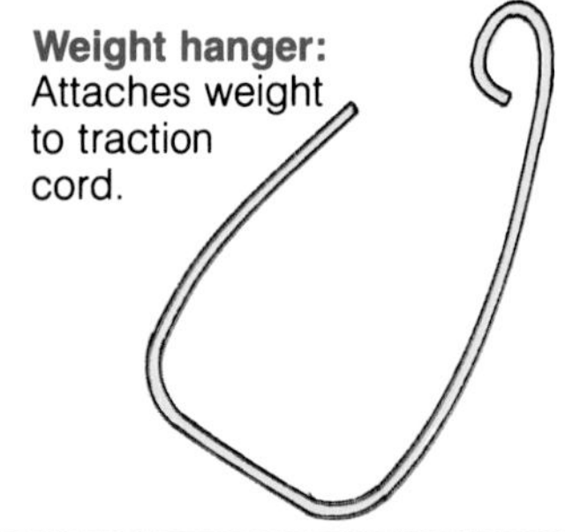

Weight hanger: Attaches weight to traction cord.

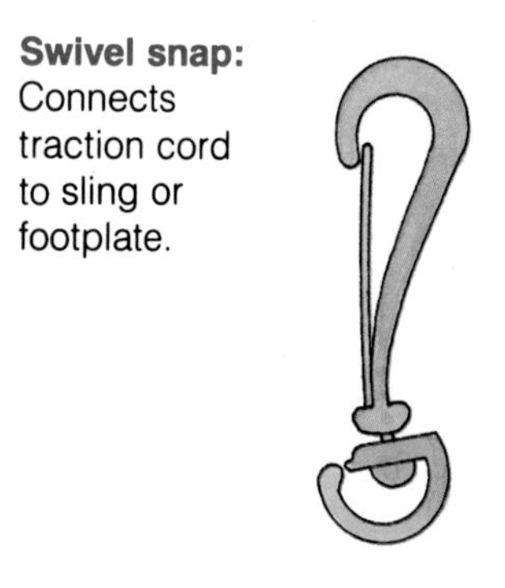

Swivel snap: Connects traction cord to sling or footplate.

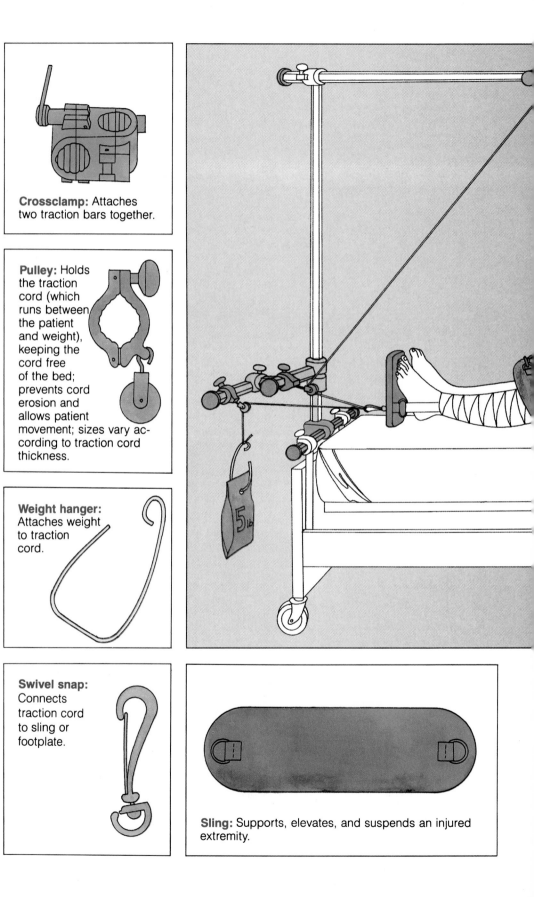

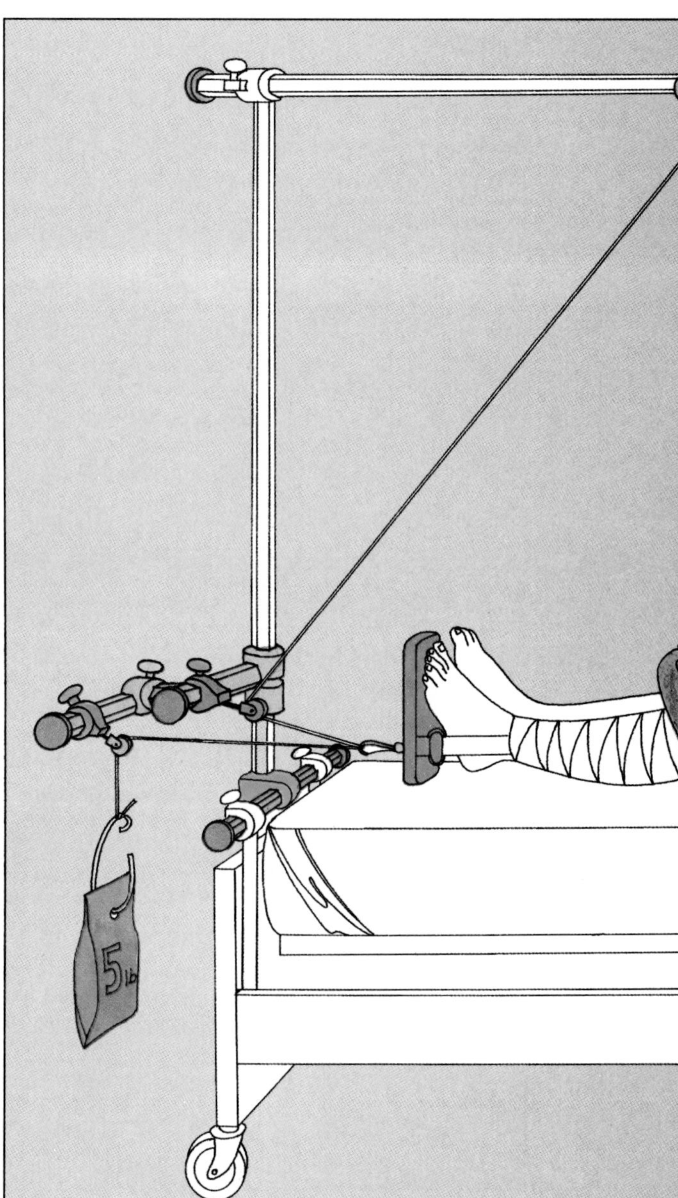

Sling: Supports, elevates, and suspends an injured extremity.

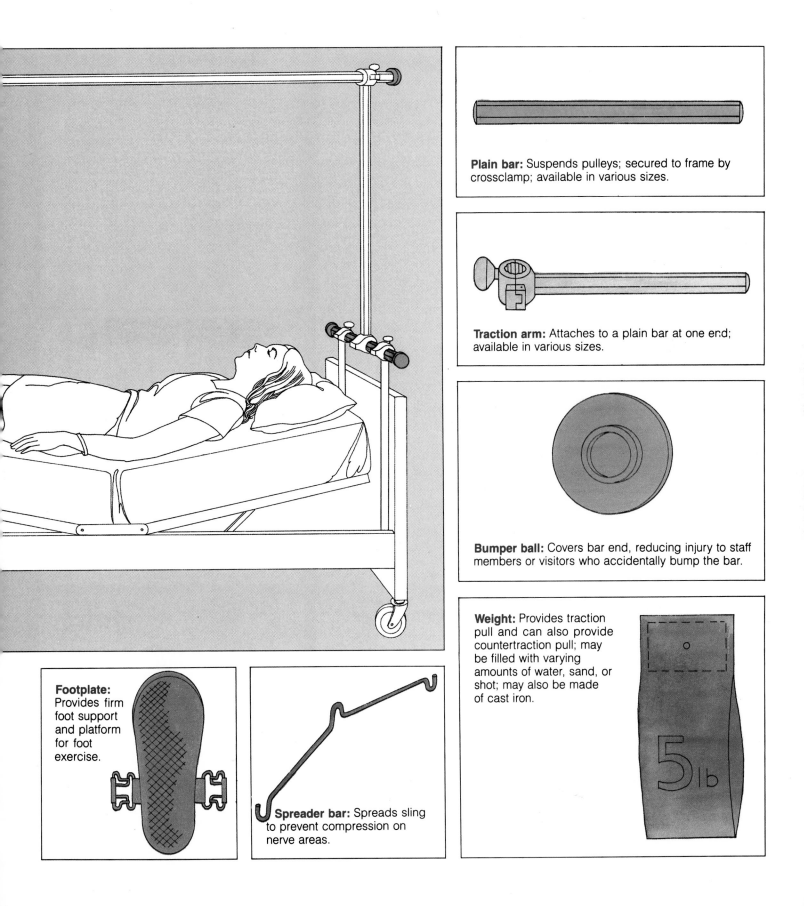

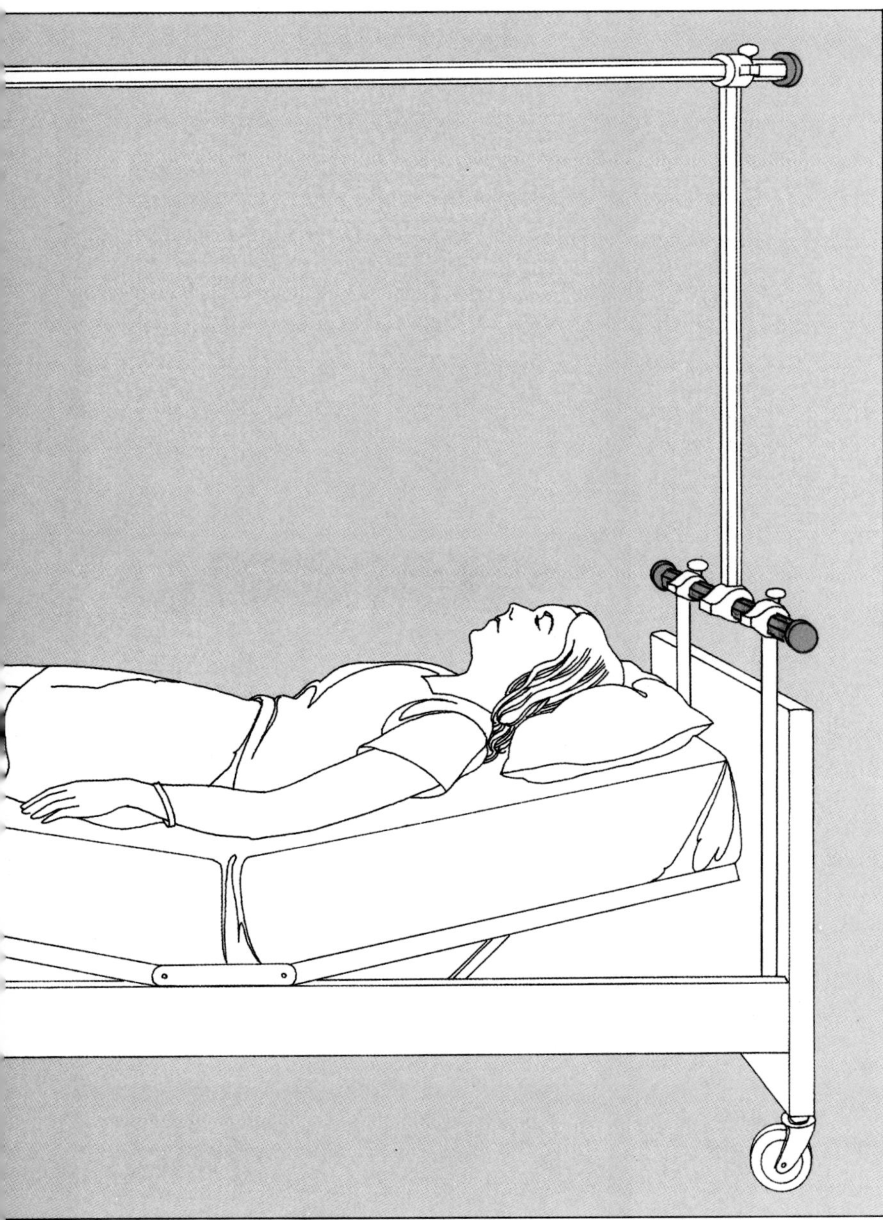

Plain bar: Suspends pulleys; secured to frame by crossclamp; available in various sizes.

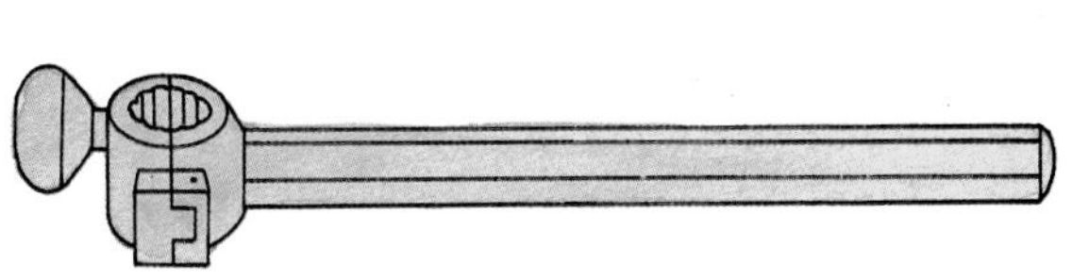

Traction arm: Attaches to a plain bar at one end; available in various sizes.

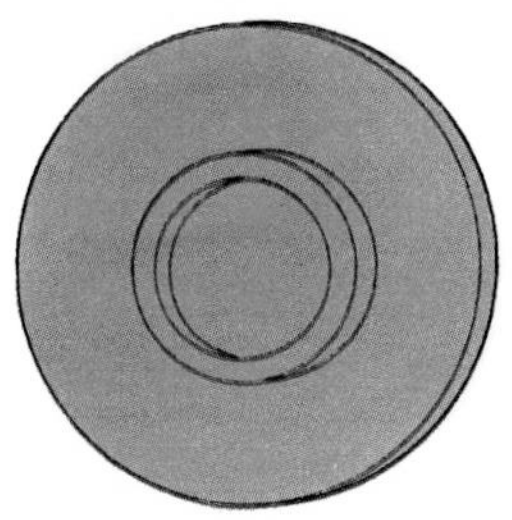

Bumper ball: Covers bar end, reducing injury to staff members or visitors who accidentally bump the bar.

Weight: Provides traction pull and can also provide countertraction pull; may be filled with varying amounts of water, sand, or shot; may also be made of cast iron.

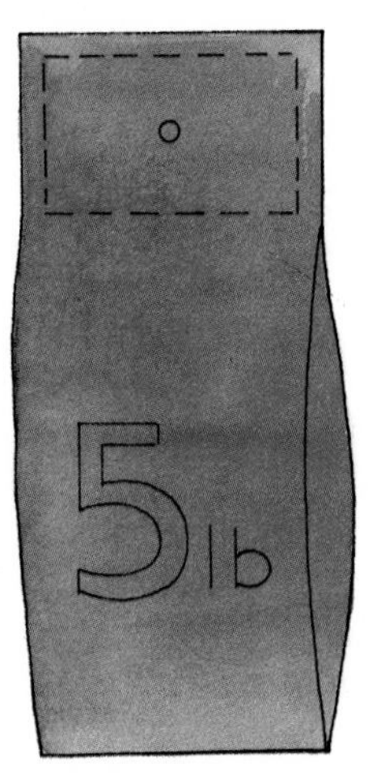

Footplate: Provides firm foot support and platform for foot exercise.

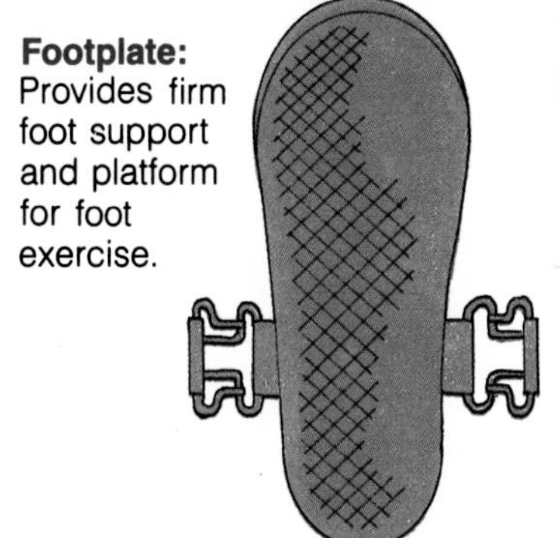

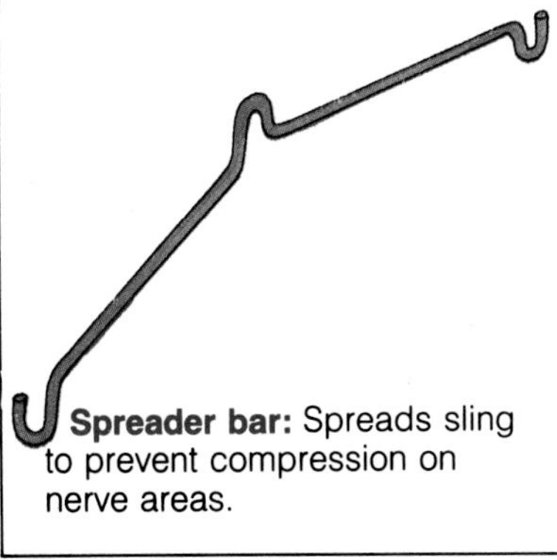

Spreader bar: Spreads sling to prevent compression on nerve areas.

Traction

Promoting traction effectiveness

Suppose your patient has been placed in traction. Whether he's in skin or skeletal traction, check the traction setup frequently to maintain its effectiveness. Do you know what to look for?

These guidelines should help you detect any problems. Always make sure that:

- the traction cords are aligned in each pulley's center track and hang free of the bed.
- the traction cords have not stretched excessively or frayed. *Note:* Never use the same traction cord for more than one patient. Dispose of the cord after the patient's traction is discontinued.
- the knots are tied tightly and hang no less than 1" (2.5 cm) *below* each pulley.
- the correct weight amounts have been hung on each hanger. Be sure this information is properly updated on the appropriate forms.
- the weights hang clear of the bed and floor.
- the spreaders, footplates, or splints don't touch the end of the bed.
- the bed linen doesn't interfere with traction pull.
- the line of traction pull hasn't been altered by movement of the extension bar, a pulley, or the patient's body.
- the patient's body is aligned correctly and the bed's positioned properly to maintain *counter*traction, if indicated.
- traction remains continuous, if ordered.

Tying a traction knot

1 *Do you know how to securely connect an S hook to traction cord? Several knot types may be used to link the two traction components. Just make sure you tie a secure knot that can safely bear traction weight. Important: For safety's sake, check all knots at least once every 8 hours.*

This photostory shows you how to tie a slipknot, a commonly used traction knot.

Remember, always obtain new cord when you put a patient in traction for the first time. Examine the cord for stretching or fraying. Then, if it appears sturdy, measure the length you'll need.

Nursing tip: Tape around the area you'll be cutting. After you cut through it, the cord end will remain taped to prevent fraying.

Now you're ready to tie the knot. You'll use one hand to tie the knot and the other to maintain tension on the cord. First, loop the cord under the S hook to form an S shape, as the nurse is doing here.

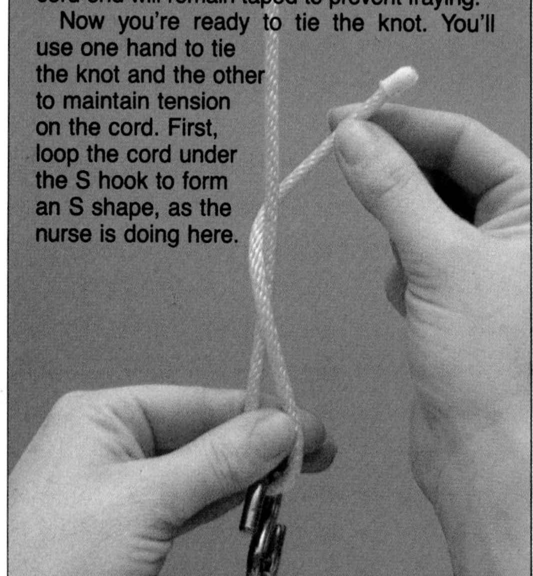

2 Next, pull the cord end down through the loop above the hook, and then through the loop you've just created, forming a pretzel shape.

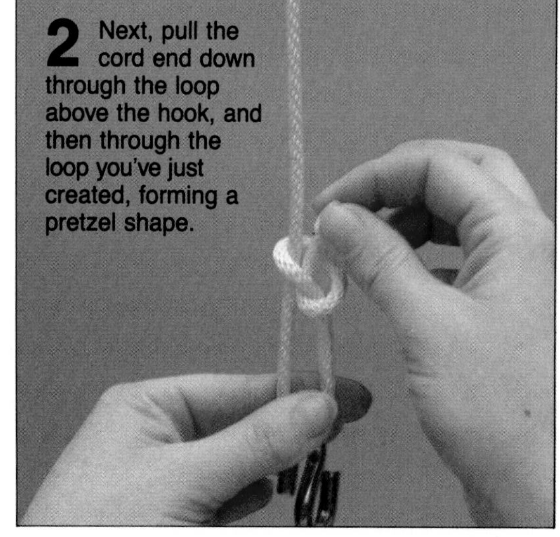

3 Then, tighten the knot.

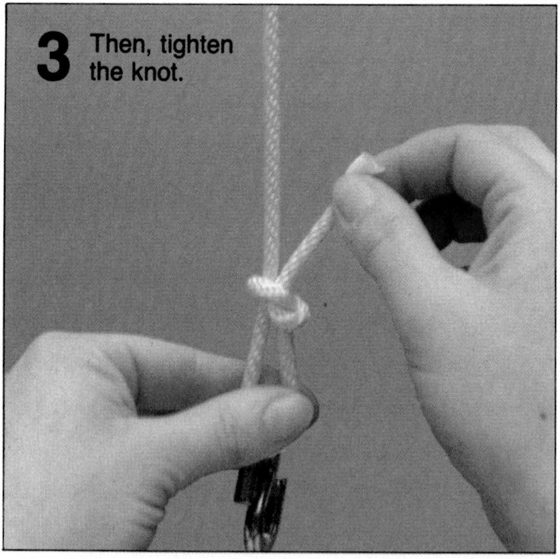

4 Now, slide the slipknot down against the S hook.

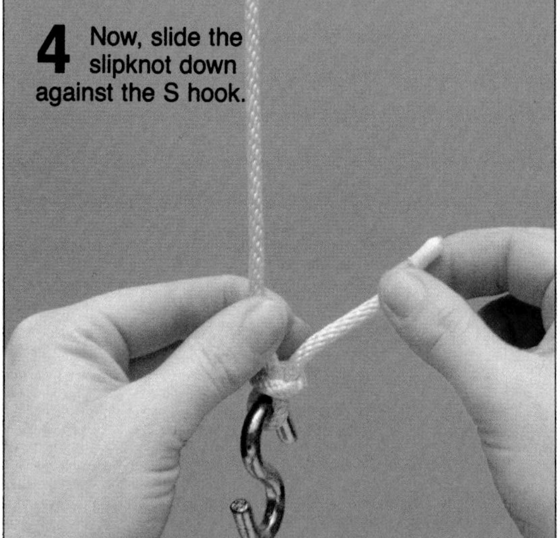

5 Secure the free cord end to the cord above the knot by wrapping it with adhesive tape. However, never cover the knot with tape.

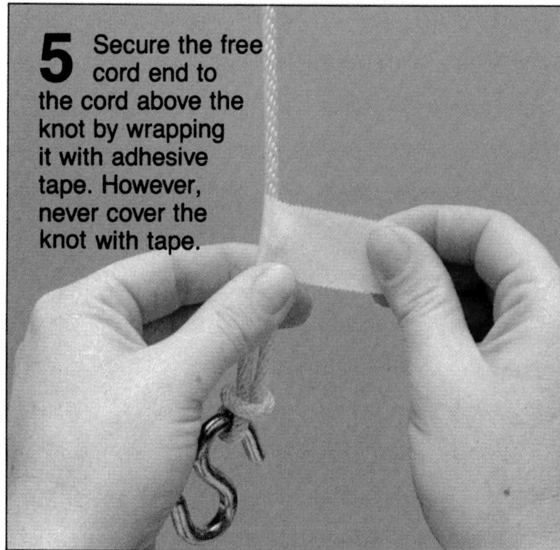

INDICATIONS/CONTRAINDICATIONS

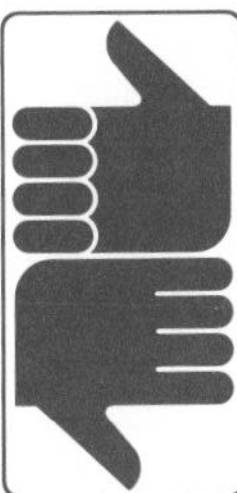

Does your patient need skin traction?

The doctor may order skin traction applied:
- to treat some stable fractures, particularly in the hip's subtrochanteric region.
- to treat fractures preoperatively; for example, before internal fixation of a fractured hip.
- to relieve muscle spasms.
- to correct deformities, such as flexion contractures of an arthritic patient's hip and knee.
- to reduce and treat dislocations.

However, the wraps and tape used with skin traction may cause skin irritation and breakdown from pressure. So, the doctor may decide to use another form of immobilization if the patient has any of the following conditions:
- an open, draining wound
- a dermatologic problem
- a preexisting disease, such as diabetes or a neurovascular disorder, which predisposes the patient to skin damage and poor healing.

Also, a patient with a fracture requiring prolonged traction or traction force beyond the 10 pound (4.5 kg) capacity of skin traction, will need skeletal traction. A patient with a joint disorder, where movement must be strictly controlled, will probably require a cast.

PATIENT PREPARATION

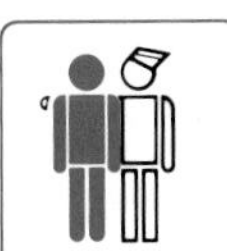

Preparing your patient for skin traction

Has the doctor ordered skin traction for your patient? If so, review the procedure before entering your patient's room. Then, you'll be prepared for any of your patient's questions.

In addition to answering his questions, emphasize these points:
- Name the various pieces of traction equipment and explain how each is used in the traction setup.
- Point out the need to keep the affected limb immobilized during traction, except for distal joint range-of-motion exercises.
- Discuss the general movements and positions he's allowed while in traction. Specify which activities he's permitted to perform.
- Instruct your patient to notify you immediately if any of his traction equipment becomes wet or soiled, so it can be changed promptly.
- Stress the importance of immediately reporting any of the following conditions in the affected extremity: pain or discomfort; change in skin color; coolness; decreased motion or loss of motion; decreased or unusual sensation, or complete loss of sensation.
- Notify the patient that you'll perform frequent neurovascular checks.
- Remind your patient not to readjust or remove his traction equipment unless the doctor has instructed him to do so. Tell him you'll check his traction equipment within 1 hour following application, and at least once every 8 hours after that. Also, instruct him to alert a nurse if any adjustments are needed; for example, if his traction tape has slipped, or if he needs to use a bedpan.

Preparing to apply skin traction

Skin traction's used primarily to maintain immobilization when light or noncontinuous pull is needed. It exerts pull directly on the skin and indirectly on the bone, using a weight-and-pulley system. But remember, anything stronger than the 5 to 10 pounds of weight recommended for this form of traction will produce extreme pressure on the patient's skin, leading to skin breakdown and further complications.

Depending on hospital policy, you may be responsible for applying and removing most types of skin traction. In addition, you'll need to monitor the effects of traction on your patient, to prevent nerve and blood vessel compression or skin breakdown.

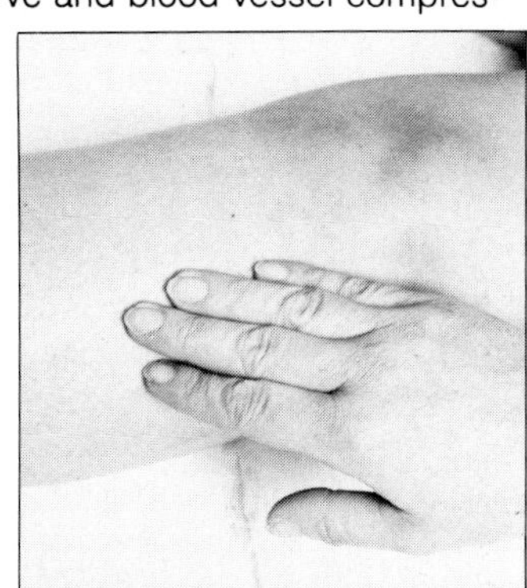

Has the doctor ordered skin traction for your patient? First, whether you're applying traction yourself, or assisting in traction application, take the following preliminary steps:
- Inspect your patient for circulatory problems, such as varicosities, or skin problems such as rashes, cuts, or ulcers.

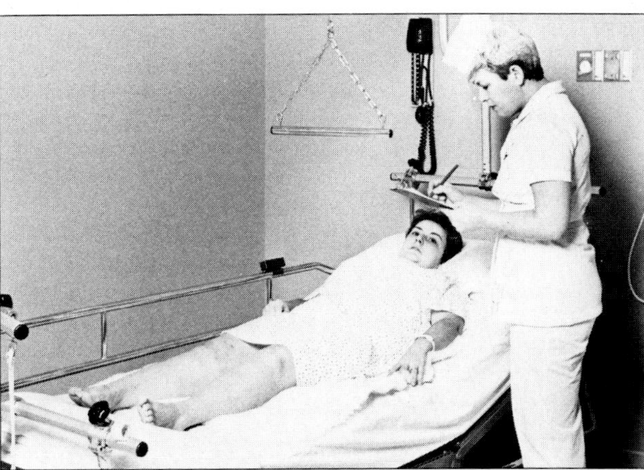

- Check your patient's history for any potential problems, such as diabetes or allergies. Make sure the doctor's aware of all pertinent information.
- Check skin preparation orders carefully. Is the affected area to be shaved? Avoid shaving unless you're applying adhesive strips. Then, only shave the area to be covered by strips. If shaving is ordered, avoid abrading or nicking your patient's skin.
- Skin surfaces must be clean and dry. Place padding over bony prominences, such as the malleoli, if you're applying adhesive tape and elastic bandages. This helps limit the chance of skin breakdown.
- Assess the neurovascular status of the affected and unaffected limbs to establish a baseline for comparison with subsequent assessments. (Remember, if you're putting a cervical halter on your patient, check the facial areas affected by the traction.) For information on neurovascular assessment, see page 24.

Traction

Applying Buck's extension using a skin traction boot

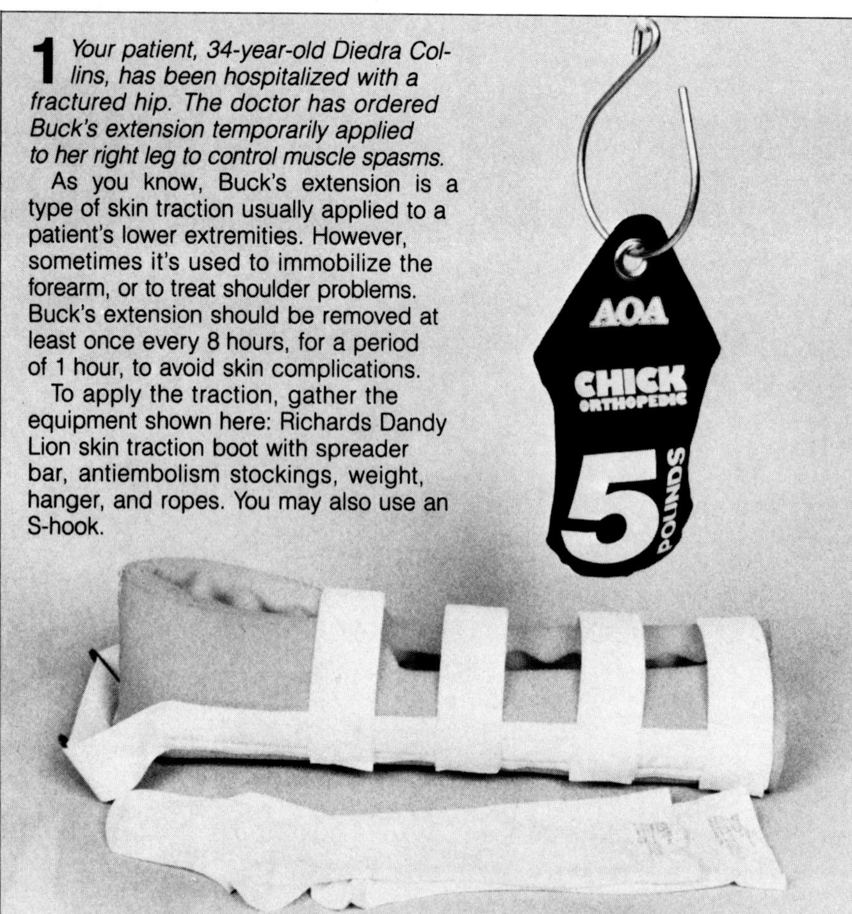

1 *Your patient, 34-year-old Diedra Collins, has been hospitalized with a fractured hip. The doctor has ordered Buck's extension temporarily applied to her right leg to control muscle spasms.*

As you know, Buck's extension is a type of skin traction usually applied to a patient's lower extremities. However, sometimes it's used to immobilize the forearm, or to treat shoulder problems. Buck's extension should be removed at least once every 8 hours, for a period of 1 hour, to avoid skin complications.

To apply the traction, gather the equipment shown here: Richards Dandy Lion skin traction boot with spreader bar, antiembolism stockings, weight, hanger, and ropes. You may also use an S-hook.

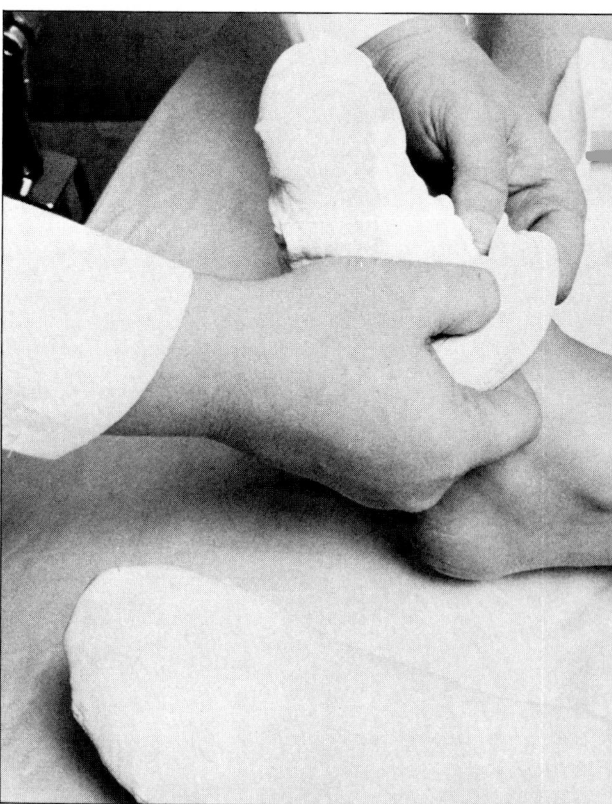

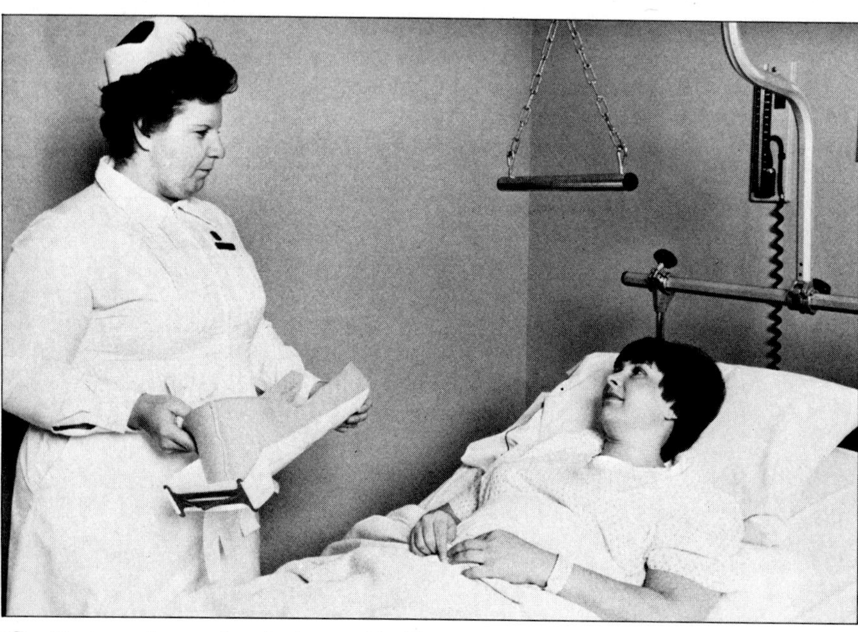

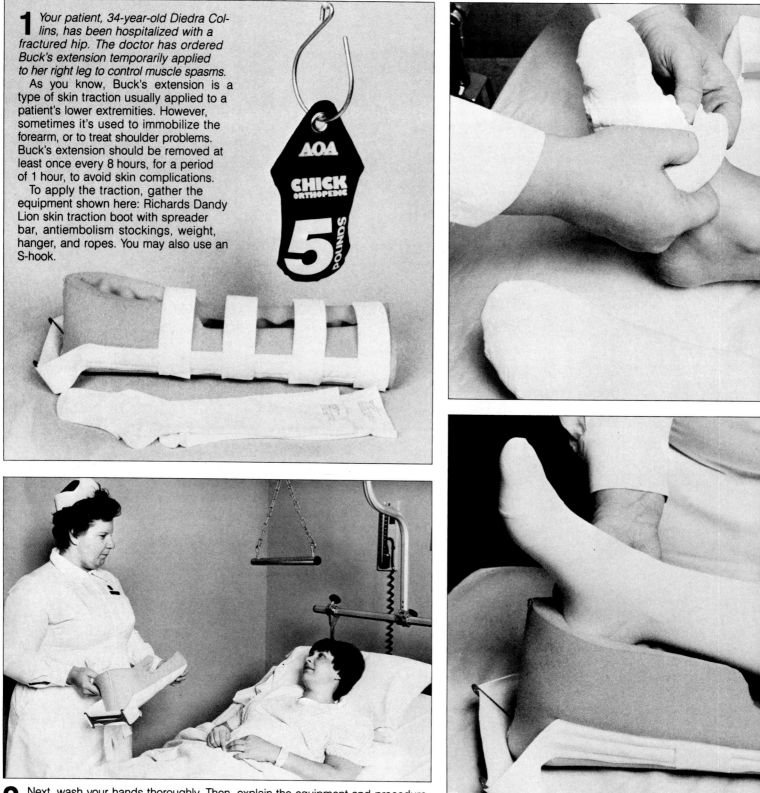

2 Next, wash your hands thoroughly. Then, explain the equipment and procedure to Mrs. Collins.

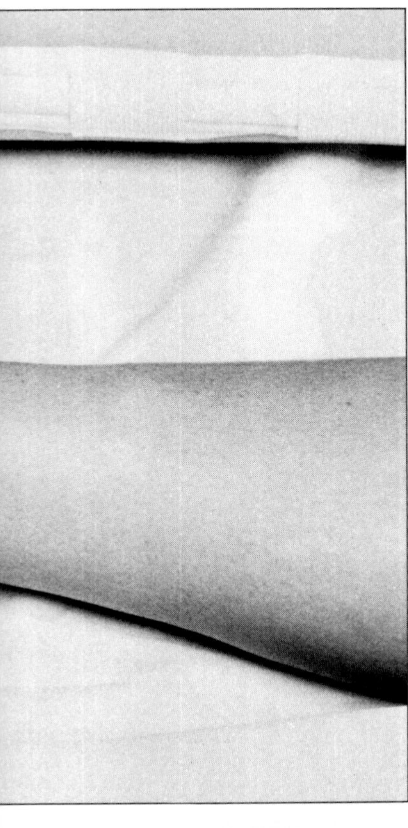

3 Apply antiembolism stockings to both of your patient's legs. These are used to decrease edema and promote venous blood return to the heart.

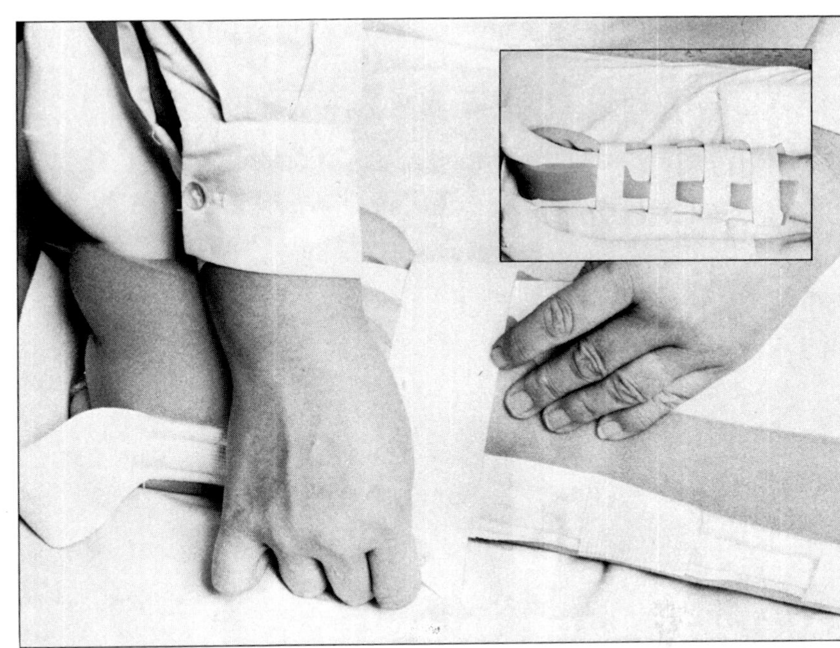

5 Now you're ready to fasten the boot. First, close the distal pressure occlusive strap, as shown. [Inset] Then, continue closing each strap, working toward the patient's knee. Don't tighten the straps too much as you proceed up her leg, or venous blood return from the foot could be impeded. Check for tightness by slipping your index finger under each strap. Loosen the strap if your finger won't fit under it.

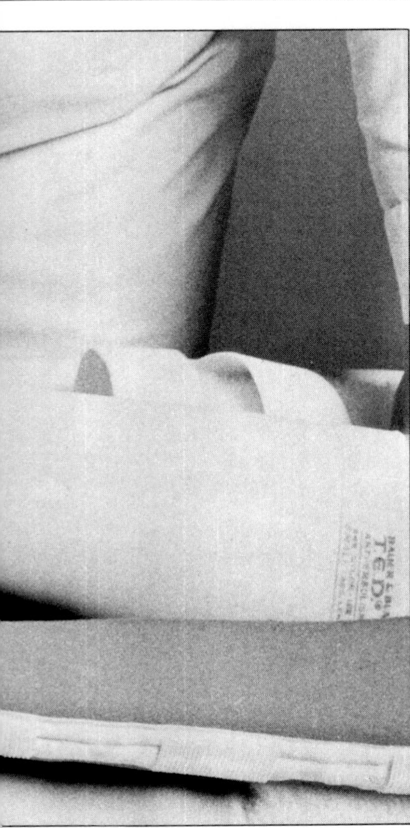

4 Next, position the boot on your patient's leg, as the nurse is doing here. Check the boot for correct fit, making sure the top of the boot doesn't cover the back of your patient's knee.

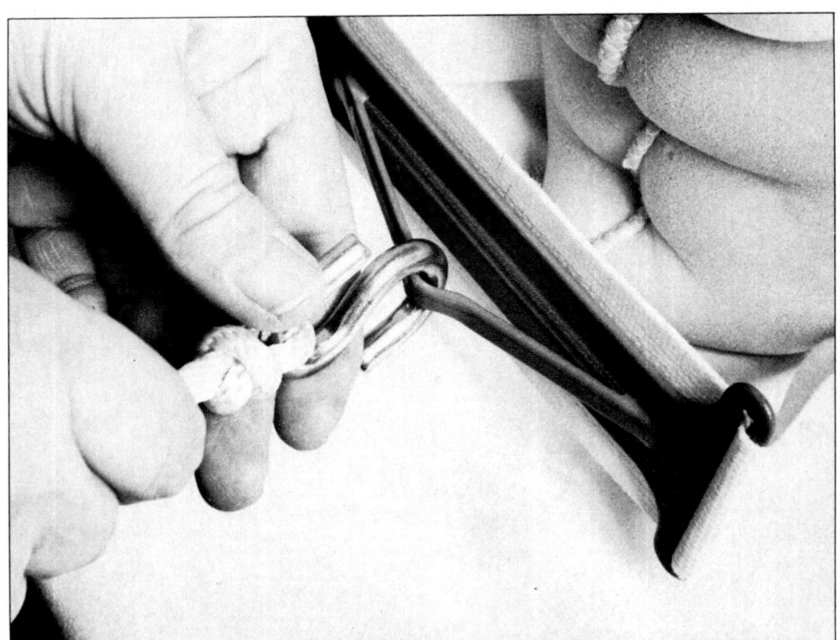

6 After fastening all the straps, secure the traction cord to the spreader bar. Then, apply the prescribed weight, making sure it clears the floor even when the bed's at its lowest position.

Now, after completing the setup, check the equipment for mechanical effectiveness. Then, document in your nurses' notes the procedure and the weight amount used.

Traction

Caring for a patient in skin traction

After skin traction's been applied, you'll need to closely monitor your patient's condition and provide the following general care. (Specific care guidelines for different types of skin traction are outlined on the following pages.)

• Perform neurovascular checks on the patient's affected and unaffected limbs. (If the patient's in cervical traction, also check the facial areas affected by the traction.)

• Closely monitor the patient for any edema at the injury site or distal to the injury. Measure the patient's limb every 8 hours. Check the equipment to see if it's too tight. Elevate the limb to reduce swelling. Notify the doctor if swelling doesn't decrease.

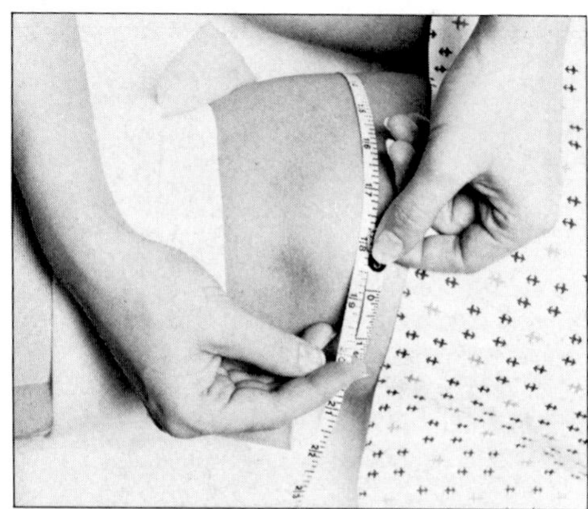

• Notify the doctor if the patient has increased pain or if his pain is unrelieved by medication.

• Frequently check the traction setup's mechanical effectiveness, as instructed on page 72.

• When you apply bandages, tape, or halters, make sure they aren't wrinkled or creased.

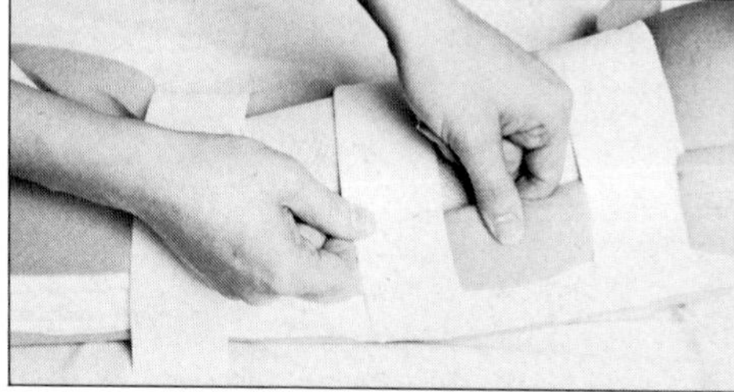

• Change your patient's position every 2 hours. Reposition her affected area, maintaining proper alignment and traction pull.

• At least once each day, remove skin traction (if not contraindicated). Inspect and massage bony prominences. If skin breakdown is severe, notify the doctor before reapplying traction.

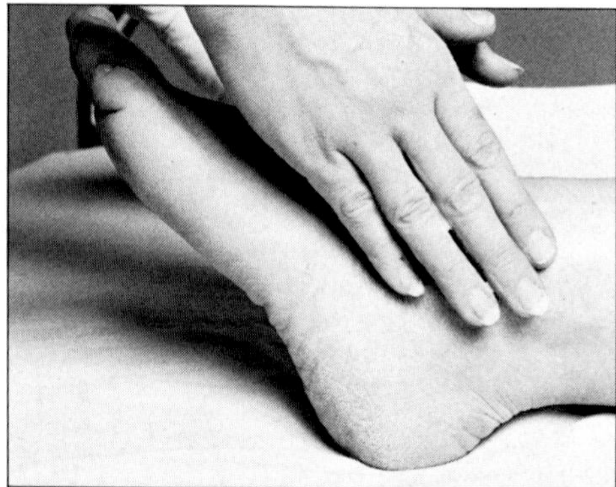

• Massage your patient's back every 3 to 4 hours. To do so, have her use the trapeze, or turn her 45° to either side, preferably *toward* the limb in traction. If the patient can't assist you, ask a co-worker to help.

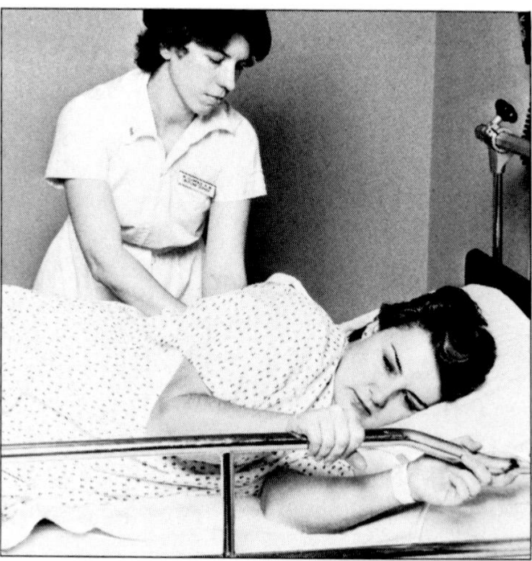

• To provide patient warmth and maintain privacy, cover her with a light blanket or sheet. Make sure the cover does not interfere with the traction.

Nursing tip: Put a sock or mitten on exposed toes or fingers for warmth.

• Encourage deep breathing and coughing to break up secretions in your patient's lungs and prevent respiratory complications.

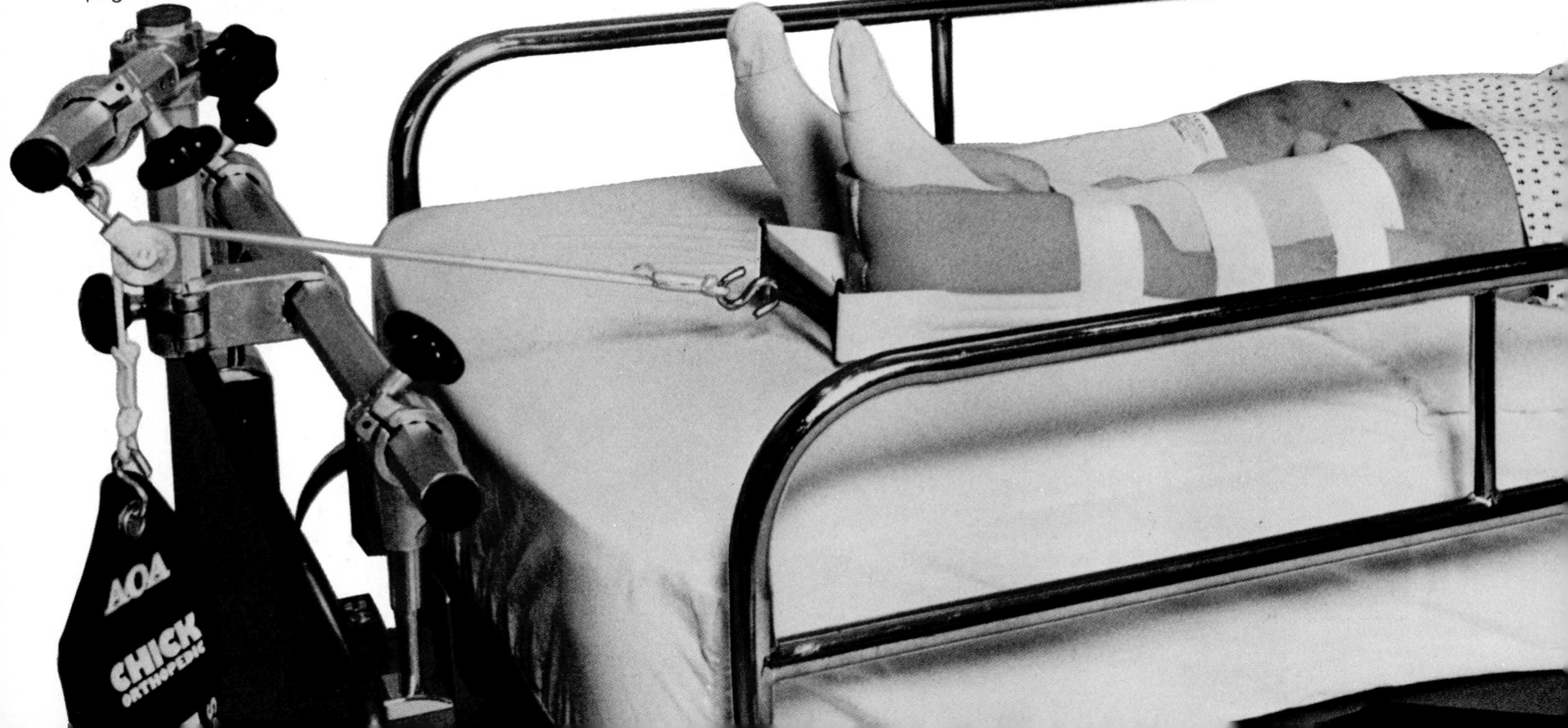

• Encourage exercise of all extremities (unless contraindicated) to prevent contractures, muscle atrophy, and venous stasis. Evaluate your patient's ability to exercise, according to her age and general condition. If she can't exercise, you must perform passive range-of-motion exercises.

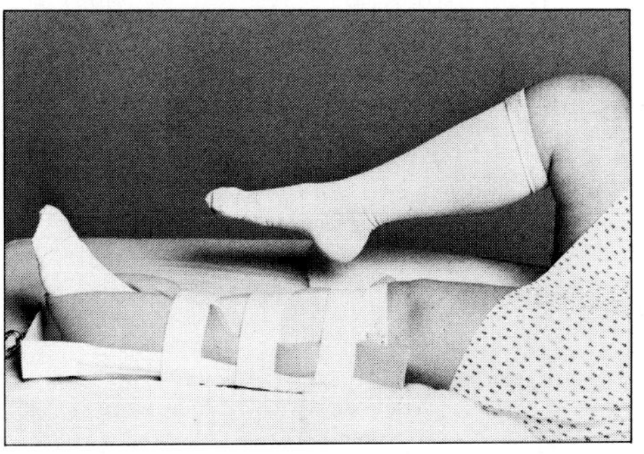

- Because your patient's mobility is limited, expect her appetite to diminish. To help provide adequate nutrition, give small frequent meals or supplemental nourishment between meals.
- Encourage increased fluid intake, as tolerated, to prevent urinary calculi and constipation.
- Take measures to avoid constipation by administering stool softeners, if ordered, or adjusting the patient's diet, as needed.
- Provide a fracture bedpan for comfort during elimination. Insert the fracture pan from her unaffected side. Seat the patient upright on the fracture pan, unless contraindicated.

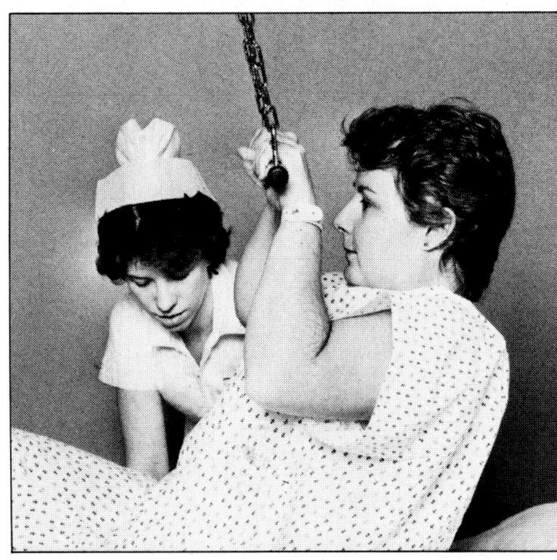

- Document all your findings in your nurses' notes.

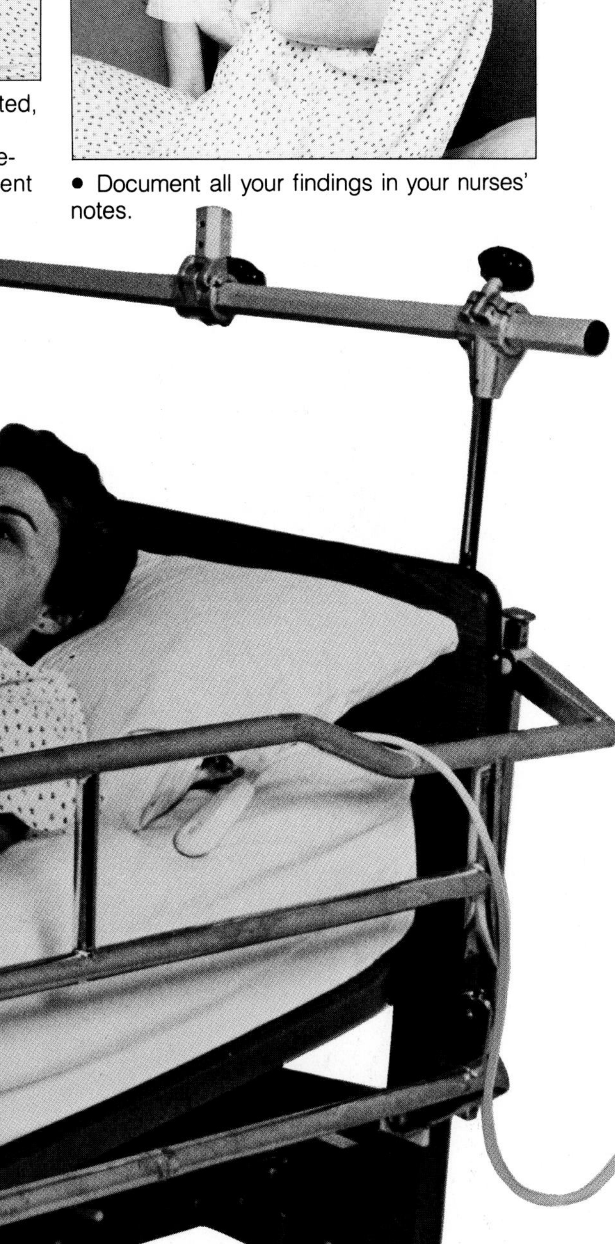

SPECIAL CONSIDERATIONS

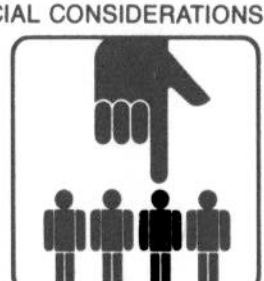

Using adhesive traction tape

Buck's extension is a common form of skin traction which can be applied in several different ways. One way is to first encase the patient's foot in a special boot, as shown on pages 74 and 75. Another way, which we will explain here, is to place strips of adhesive traction tape against both sides of the patient's leg.

To apply Buck's extension using this method, follow these guidelines:

- First, place your patient on a sheepskin, water-filled mattress, or an egg-crate mattress.
- Pad her malleoli, which will be covered by traction tape, to prevent skin breakdown.
- Alleviate foot edema by wrapping the patient's foot with an elastic bandage, starting above her toes. Then, hold the elastic bandage taut as you cover both sides of her leg with adhesive or foam traction tape strips. Start applying the adhesive or foam strips just above her malleoli, and end them just below her tibial crests. This way, you'll help prevent peroneal nerve damage.
- Now, continue to wrap the elastic bandage smoothly over the adhesive or foam strips, starting just above her malleoli. Avoid wrinkling or creasing the bandage, which could cause skin breakdown. Finish the wrap just below her tibial crests.
- Elevate your patient's *affected* heel by placing a folded bath blanket or towel under her leg from her calf to her ankle. Make sure the bath blanket doesn't put pressure on her Achilles tendon or popliteal space.
- Place the heel of her *unaffected* leg in a heel protector, to help prevent skin breakdown from pressure. However, continue to frequently check her heels for blisters.
- Prepare the traction setup carefully, gently attaching the rope, weight hanger, and weights.
- Remove Buck's extension at least once every 8 hours for skin inspection. Continuous Buck's extension can cause the patient's epidermis to be pulled away from her subcutaneous tissue.
- For further information, see the general care guidelines at left.

Traction

Applying a pelvic belt

1 *Tricia Squires, a 24-year-old secretary, has been admitted to your hospital with severe lower back pain. The doctor has ordered that Ms. Squires be placed in a pelvic belt for intermittent skin traction. Do you know how to apply the belt?*

Make sure you mentally review the procedure before entering her room, and be prepared for any questions she might ask. In some hospitals, an orderly gathers the equipment and assembles the frame. Otherwise, you'll have to complete the setup shown here. Then, assess your patient for traction application, as instructed on page 73.

Important: Some hospitals require that pelvic traction be applied directly on the skin. But, if you're applying the belt over pajama bottoms or underwear, make sure the clothing is cotton (for better traction) and wrinkle-free (to avoid excess pressure on the skin).

Be sure to wash your hands.

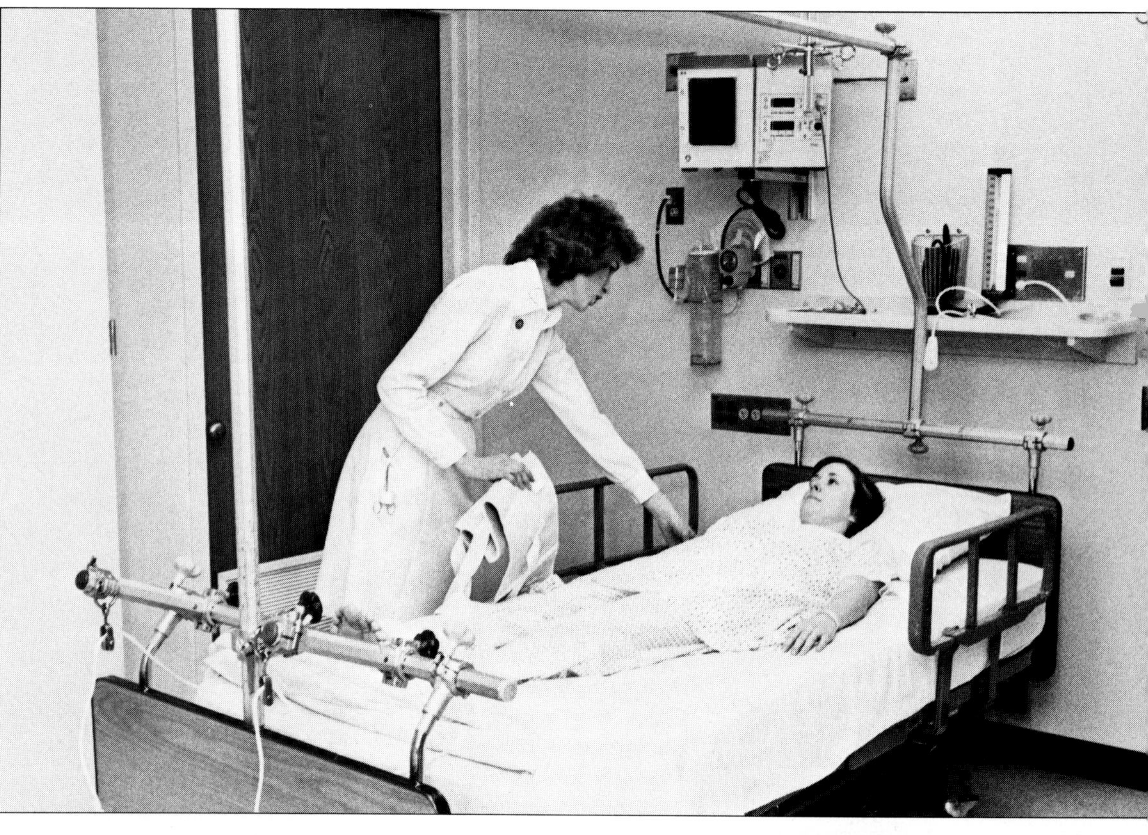

2 Now, carefully turn Ms. Squires away from you and fanfold half the belt, tucking it under her hip. Then, turn her toward you, as the nurse is doing here. Pull the fanfolded half of the belt from underneath her. She'll be lying on her side on the flat portion of the belt.

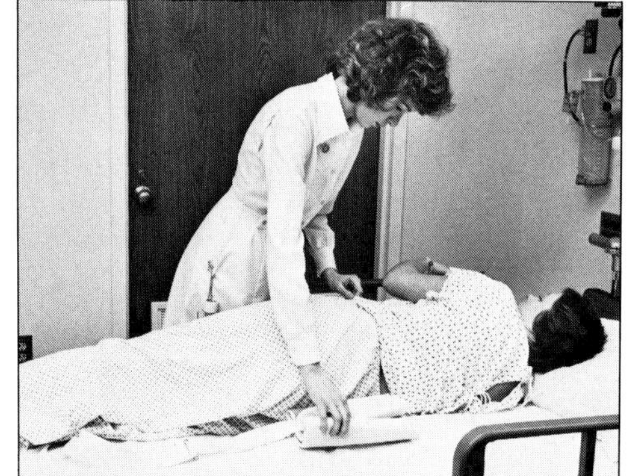

3 Now, return her to a supine position and pull the free ends of the belt around her hipbones, so her iliac crests are covered. Use both hands to tighten the belt, as shown, before pressing the Velcro ends together. Slip your finger beneath the belt's edges, and run it along the skin to check for proper fit. Readjust the belt, if necessary.

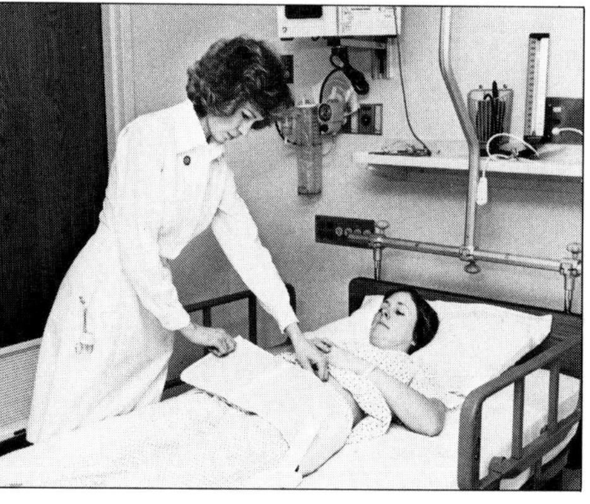

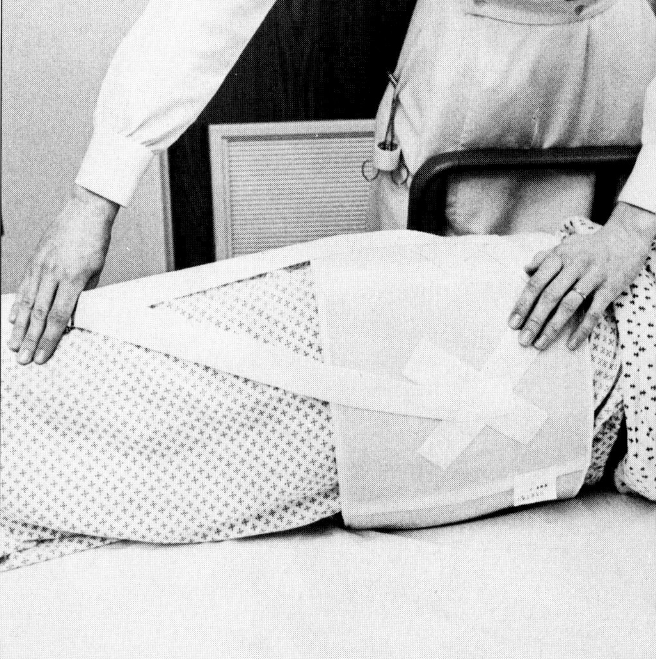

4 Next, correctly align the belt, positioning the strap sets over her hips. Make sure the straps will be parallel to each other and to Ms. Squires' thighs when attached to the traction cords.

5 Now, for each strap set, you have one loose strap and one strap attached to a triangular loop. Tie the loose strap end in a knot around the other strap end, just distal to the strap buckle, as shown here. Doing so will help prevent slippage.

Then, pull the knot taut. Make the same knot on the opposite strap set.

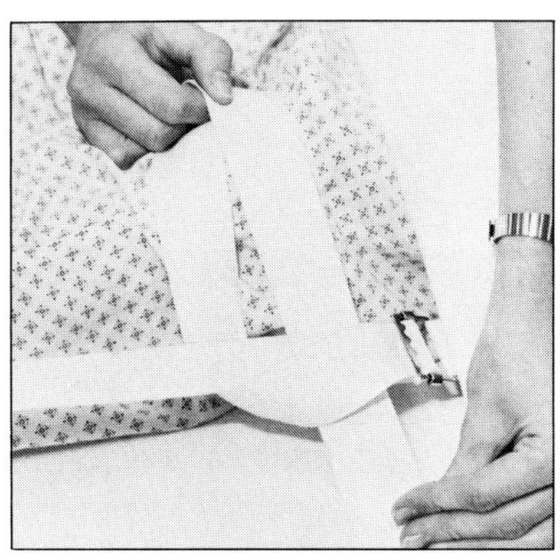

6 Place a traction cord through the pulley on the side of the frame you're working on. Attach one end of the cord to the triangular loop, tying it as the nurse is doing here. Then, repeat the procedure with the opposite cord and strap.

Using a weight carrier, simultaneously attach the ordered weights on the end of each cord. Make sure you're placing the same amount of weight on each side.

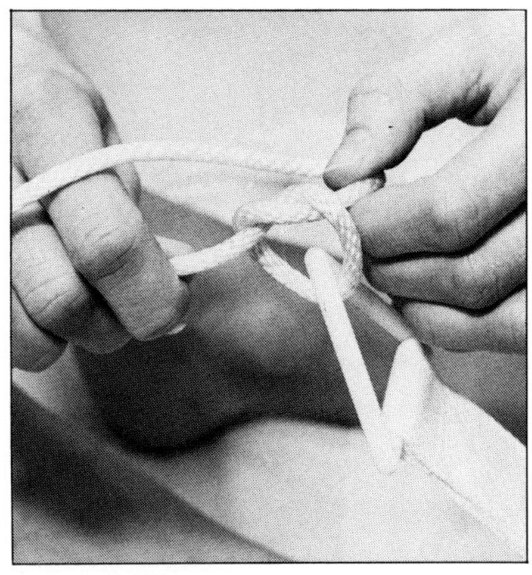

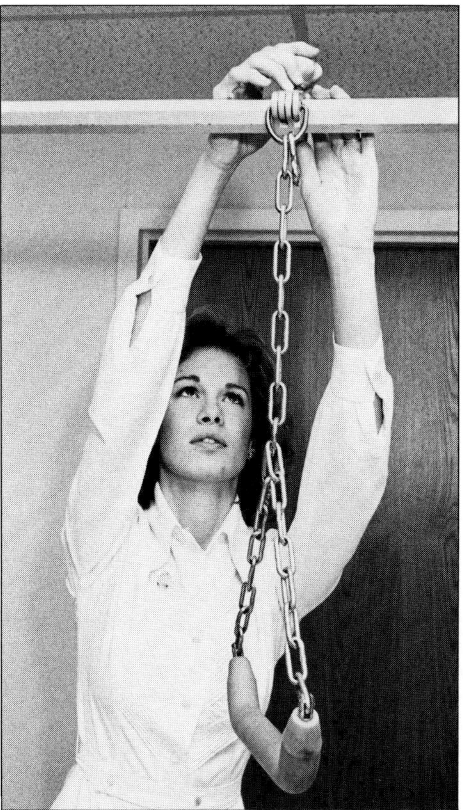

8 Hang a trapeze on the overhead frame, unless contraindicated. The trapeze will enable Ms. Squires to exercise to reduce immobility complications. Encourage her to use it.

Finally, assure your patient that someone will return within an hour to check on her and that she should use her call bell if she needs help.

Document the traction setup and weight amount on your patient's chart.

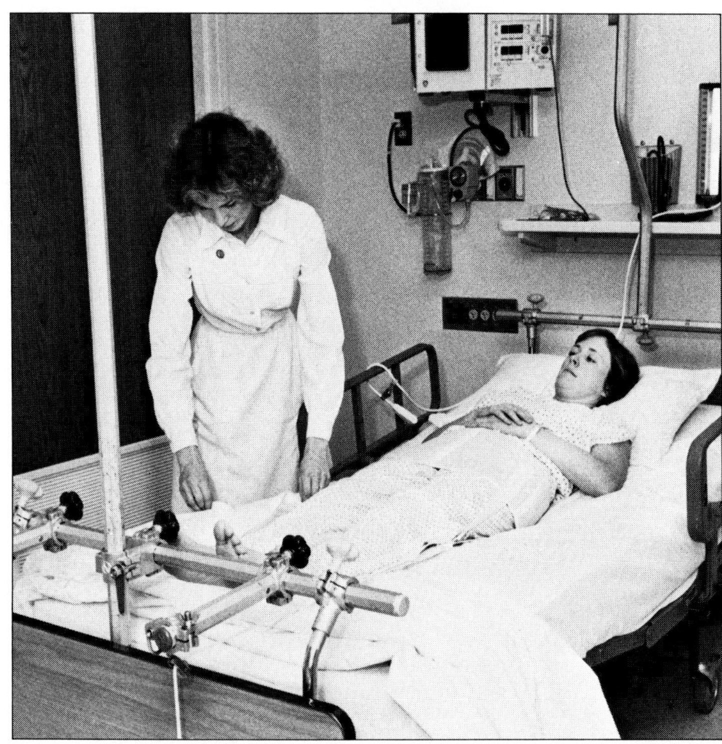

7 Now, you've completed the traction assembly. Check the knots, traction cord, and pulleys for proper alignment.

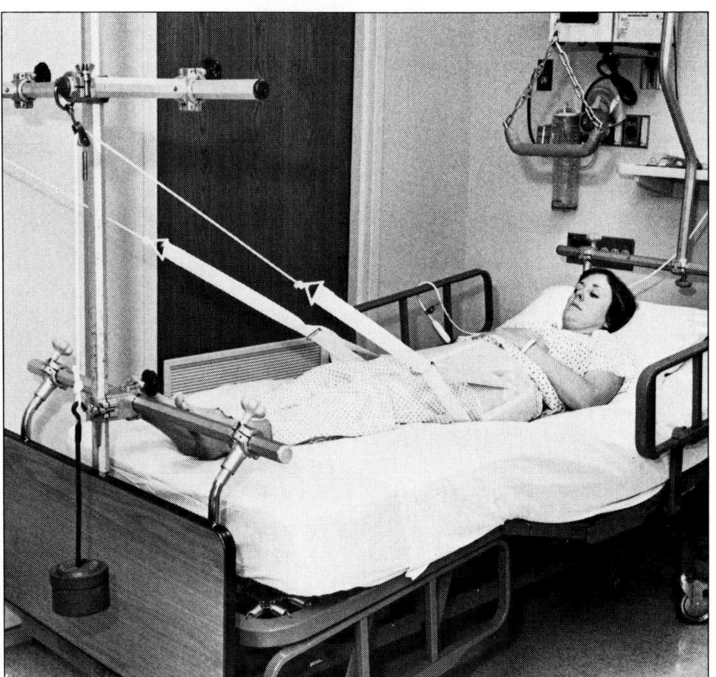

9 Pelvic belt setups can differ, according to doctor's orders. In this alternative setup, the traction bar holding the pulleys is positioned higher, creating a greater upward pull on your patient's lower back.

Traction

Caring for a patient in a pelvic belt

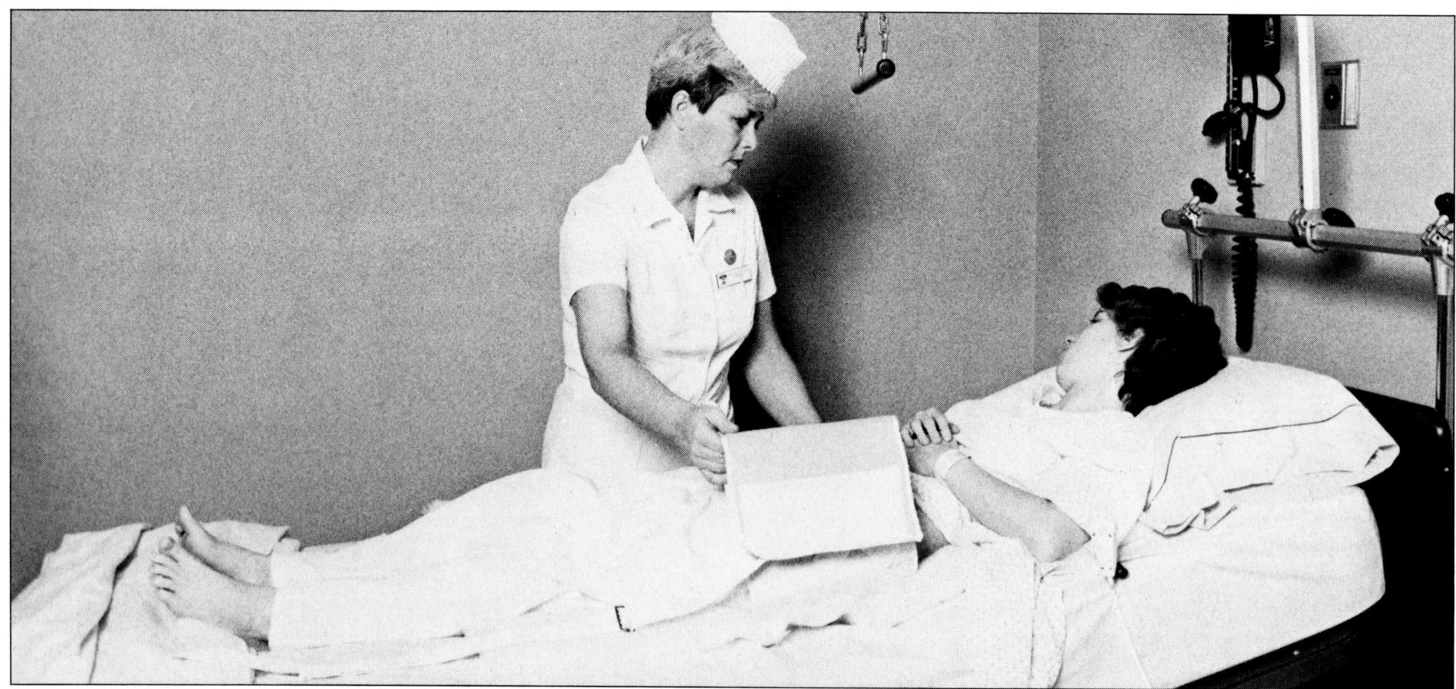

The doctor may order pelvic belt application for a patient with lower back pain; for example, pain caused by a suspected lumbar disc herniation. Most pelvic belts are adjustable, with Velcro closures.

Provide the following daily care for your patient:

- Place your patient in Williams position, with her hips flexed 30° and her knees flexed 30° (or the foot of the bed elevated 30°). Encourage her to keep her back flat against the mattress during traction, as shown above. Instruct her to lie prone or on her side with the bed flat when she's not in traction.
- Periodically, check the belt's location. Make sure it's securely applied around the pelvis, but doesn't squeeze the area above the iliac crests. Also check that pelvic belt straps are parallel to each other, as shown at left. If the belt's applied over your patient's pajama bottoms, make sure the pajama bottoms don't wrinkle under the belt.

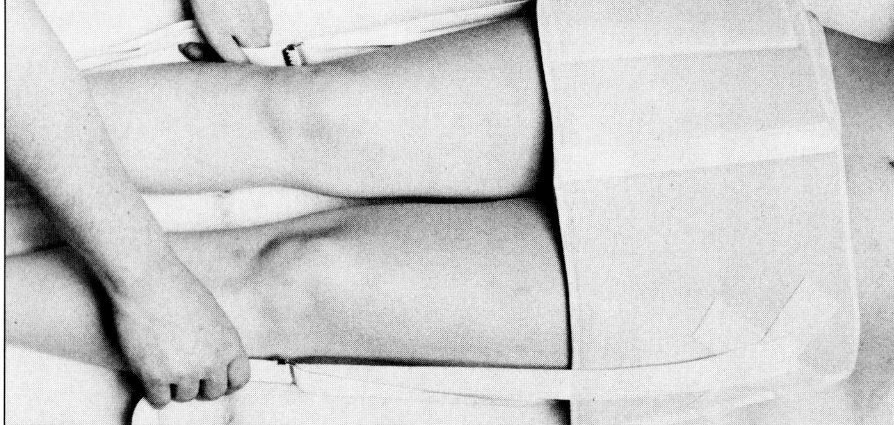

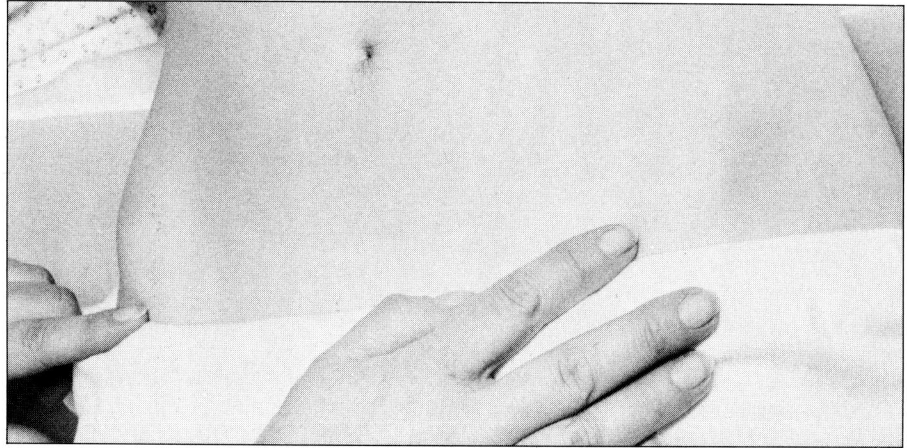

- Frequently assess your patient for any signs of sciatic nerve pathway constriction from poor positioning or a misplaced belt. This problem is indicated by increasing numbness or tingling in her legs or feet (particularly in the medial and lateral areas just above her knee and ankle). Relieve constriction with position changes and massage.
- Inspect your patient every 2 hours for skin irritation, particularly her elbows, coccyx, and iliac crests (see photo at left). Massage these areas after each inspection. Pay special attention to skin care if the belt's been applied directly on the skin.

Applying a cervical halter

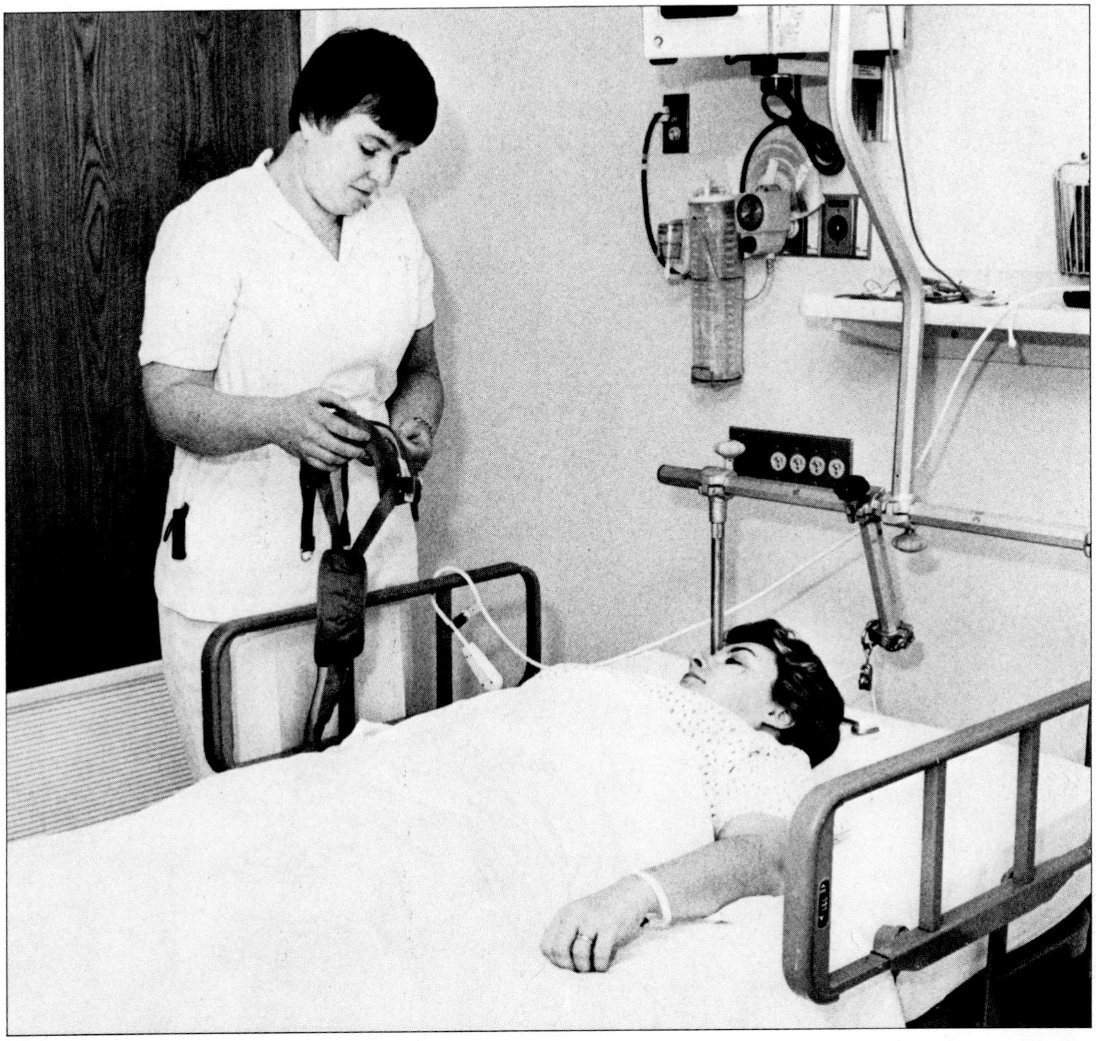

1 *Your patient, 34-year-old Andrea Sims, has been hospitalized with neck pain after falling off a horse. The doctor has ordered skin traction applied, using a cervical halter. Keep in mind that the cervical halter can cause skin irritation and patient discomfort, which contraindicates its use for extended periods.*

Mentally review the traction application procedure before entering Ms. Sims' room, so you can answer any questions she might have about the traction. Then, make sure you have the components needed to assemble cervical traction: traction cord, weights and weight carriers, clamps, bars, pulleys, spreader bar, and cervical halter. Next, remove the bed's headboard.

Make sure your patient's comfortable, her body properly aligned, her shoulders level and relaxed, and her back flat against the mattress. Leave room for a spreader bar and traction cord to fit between her head and the head of the bed.

Explain to your patient what you'll be doing. Then, prepare the head halter for application, as the nurse is doing here, making sure the label faces the patient's bed, not the back of her neck.

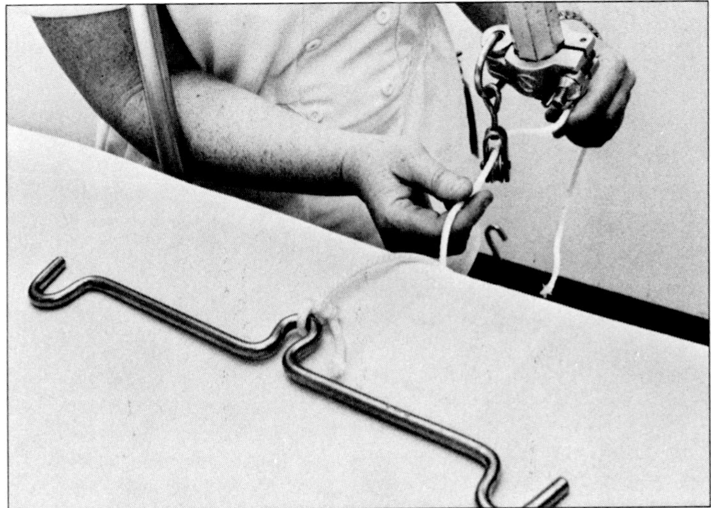

2 Next, attach the traction cord to the spreader bar. Thread the cord through the pulley at the head of the bed.

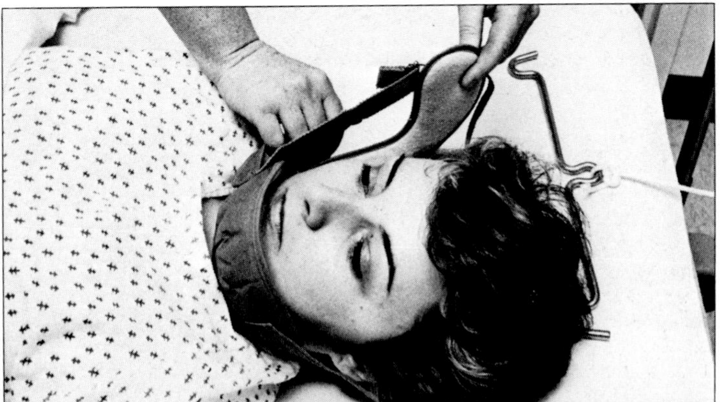

3 Now, place your patient in the cervical halter, positioning the back of the halter beneath her head and aligning the sides so they don't cover Ms. Sims' ears. The chin and front straps should be fastened (or unfastened) on the right side, as shown in the photo.

Note: Make sure all straps are straight before proceeding.

Traction

Applying a cervical halter *continued*

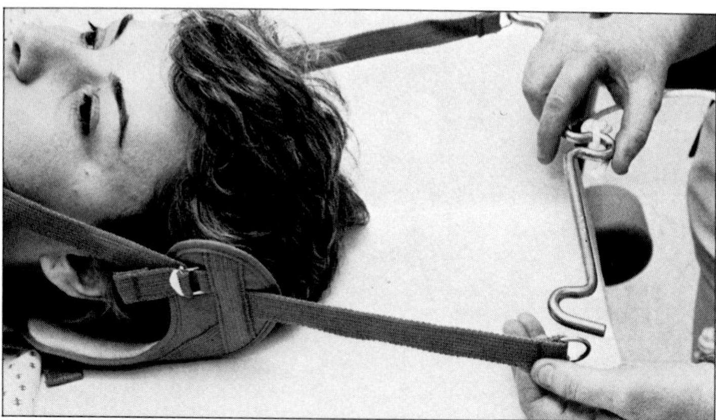

4 After the halter is fitted on your patient's head, place the ends of the spreader bar through the metal loops located on the ends of the cervical halter strap. Then, attach the weight to the traction cord.

Note: Make sure the weights don't touch the floor.

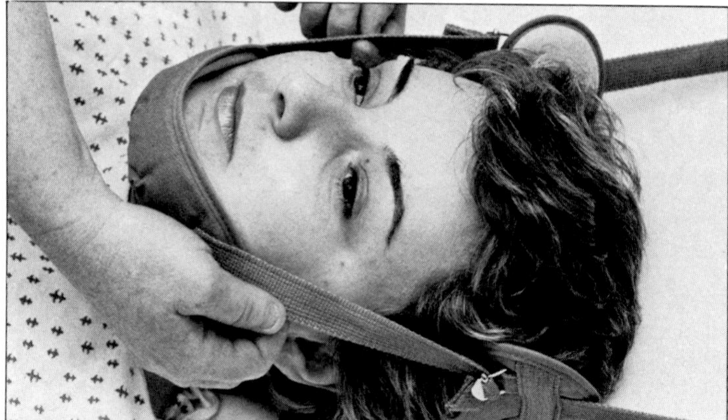

5 Next, align the halter on your patient's head, so that equal pull is exerted on both sides. The straps leading to the sidepieces should be loose over the patient's cheeks, to avoid zygomatic nerve damage.

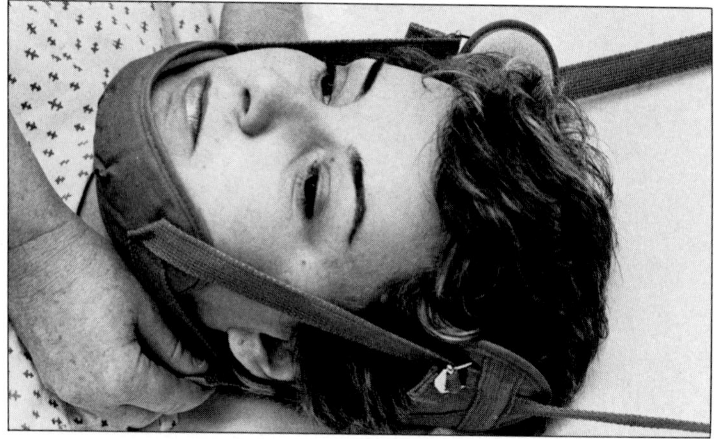

6 If any adjustment on the posterior strap is necessary, make it first, as shown. Then, adjust the front straps, if necessary.

7 Adjust the chin piece for patient comfort, as the nurse is doing here. Make sure it's not positioned over your patient's throat.

Note: Don't put additional padding under your patient's chin. This increases traction pull.

Now, give the halter a final check to make sure pull is equal on both sides of the patient's face.

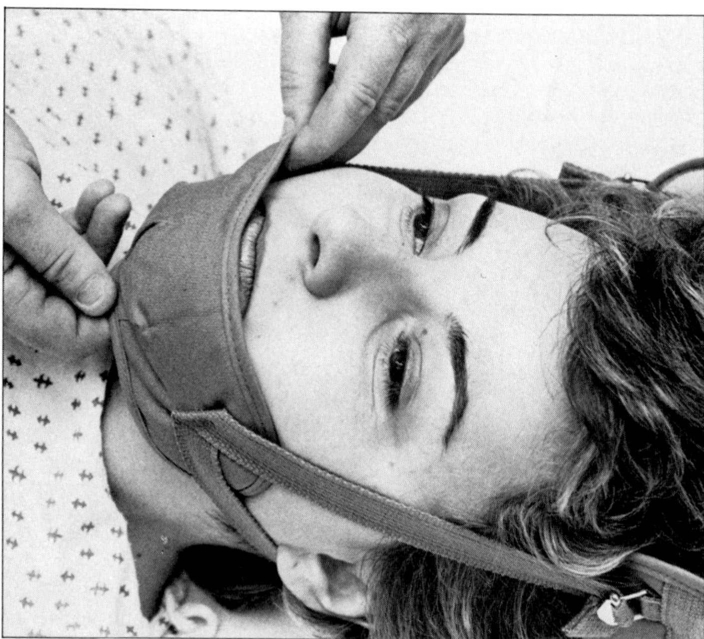

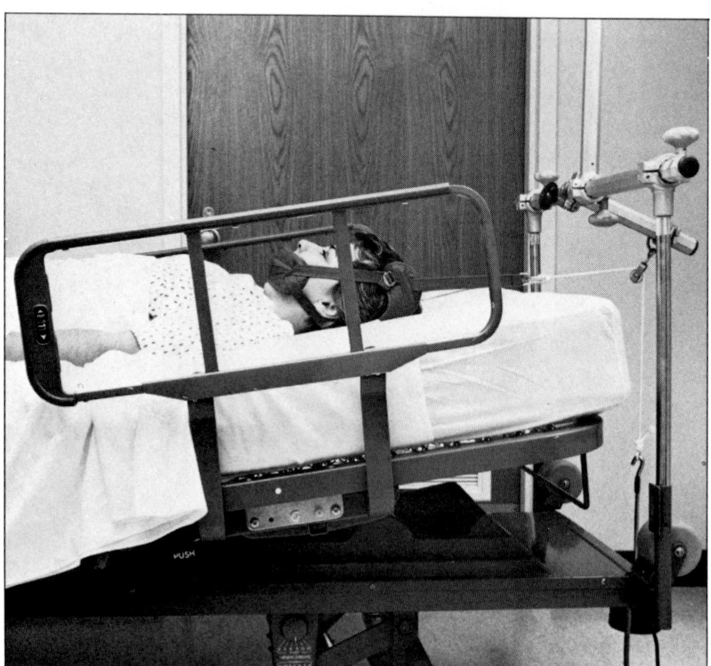

8 The doctor may want the head of the bed elevated. This photo shows cervical traction with the head of the bed elevated 20° for patient comfort.

Document in your nurses' notes the halter application procedure and any special positioning.

Caring for a patient in a cervical halter

The doctor may order a cervical halter to relieve muscle spasms from cervical sprains or strains (for example, in whiplash injury). The halter may also be used to relieve cervical pain caused by nerve root compression secondary to degenerative joint disease.

This form of traction can only be applied intermittently, as continuous application will lead to patient discomfort and skin breakdown. Never apply cervical traction with the patient in a sitting position. The bed should be flat, unless the doctor specifically prescribes that the head be elevated.

Provide the following special care after you've applied cervical halter traction:

- Instruct your patient how to unfasten his halter in case of emergency, such as nausea, vomiting, or choking. But, remind him never to remove his halter or weights *unless* an emergency develops. If any of these emergencies occurs, he should remove the cervical halter, roll on his side, and use the call bell to immediately notify the nurse. Make sure the call bell is fastened to his bed, close to his hand.
- Remove the halter for skin care, meals, and medication. Remember, your patient should be fed at least 1 hour before the traction's reapplied.
- Place your patient on a sheepskin, water-filled mattress, or egg-crate mattress for his comfort.
- Give thorough back rubs every 2 hours during traction. Teach your patient leg exercises and other range-of-motion exercises he can perform to help prevent immobility complications.
- Encourage prone or side-lying positions, as well as ambulation, while the patient's out of traction. This way, you'll reduce the number of hours he must remain supine.
- Frequently check to make sure equal pull is exerted on both halter strap ends.
- If your patient complains of severe discomfort, remove the halter and notify the doctor immediately. He may want to decrease the amount of weight or discontinue the traction altogether.
- Discourage your male patient from shaving. Doing so could cause skin irritation.
- Inspect skin areas along the jaw and sides of your patient's face for pressure areas and abrasions. Also, check your patient's elbows, heels, and coccygeal area for skin breakdown.
- Make sure the front straps fit loosely over your patient's cheeks, to avoid zygomatic nerve damage.

Understanding skeletal traction

When your patient has skeletal traction applied, force is exerted directly on one or more of his bones, using pins, wires, or tongs. This type of traction is usually employed for extended periods. It accommodates large amounts of weight, allowing very strong traction pull. Direct pull on the bone lessens the chance of secondary injuries at the fracture site, by stabilizing the bone fragments in correct alignment, decreasing muscle spasms, and reducing internal inflammation (through strict immobilization). The pins may be introduced in surgery, or under local anesthesia (in the emergency department or patient's room), using strict aseptic technique.

Since this form of traction communicates directly with the skeletal system, infection control is mandatory. Meticulous care around the pin entry and exit sites is important to prevent any complications, such as osteomyelitis.

Pins and wires used in skeletal traction may be smooth, but threaded varieties are used more commonly to reduce slippage. The pin or wire used in skeletal traction connects to a U-shaped bow or caliper, which attaches to a weighted rope carried by a pulley system.

Skull tongs are used for a patient who requires long-term cervical traction for a cervical or thoracic fracture, or for a critical dislocation or subluxation. The tongs are often used with a specially designed turning frame, such as a Stryker® frame. For more information on special beds, refer to the last section of the book.

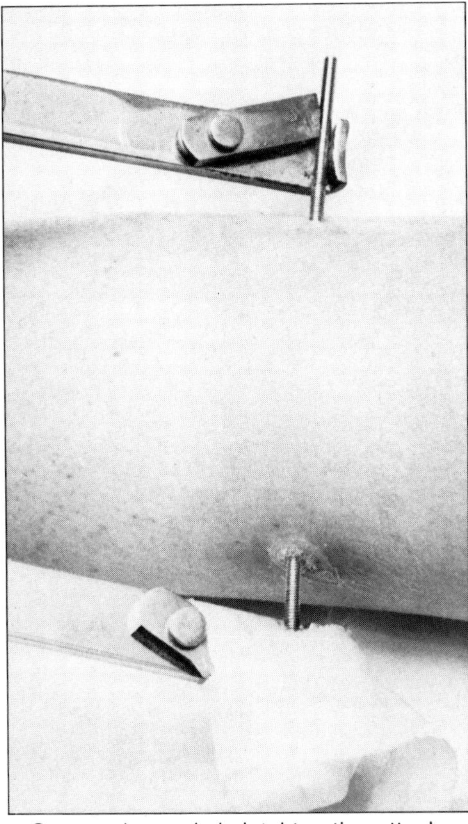

Commonly used skeletal traction attachments include Steinmann's pin, the Kirschner wire, and Gardner-Wells tongs.

You'll be responsible for providing your patient's care while he's in skeletal traction. Follow these general guidelines:

- Check the weights when your patient's moved or his body position is changed, making sure they continue to hang freely. Also, frequently check the mechanical effectiveness of the setup.
- Avoid removing or lifting the weights during any procedures. Lifting the weights releases traction, and could cause violent muscle contractions, leading to further damage or disruption of the fractured bone fragments.
- Avoid bumping the weights attached to the U bow. Doing so could move the traction cord and cause pain at the pin site.
- Cover the traction pin or wire ends with cork or adhesive tape to protect you and your patient from accidental injuries.
- Check the skin around the pin or wire for skin tears at the entry or exit sites, and report any to the doctor.
- Observe the pin or wire entry and exit sites for any signs of bright red bleeding or purulent drainage. Notify the doctor immediately.
- Assess your patient for secondary complications of immobility, such as phlebothrombosis or atelectasis.
- Perform meticulous skin care at least once every 8 hours, following the instructions on page 55. Give particular attention to bony prominences.
- Instruct your patient to perform range-of-motion exercises.
- Provide emotional comfort (see page 89). For example, find out your patient's needs by talking with him. Then, resolve as many as possible.

Traction

Performing pin care

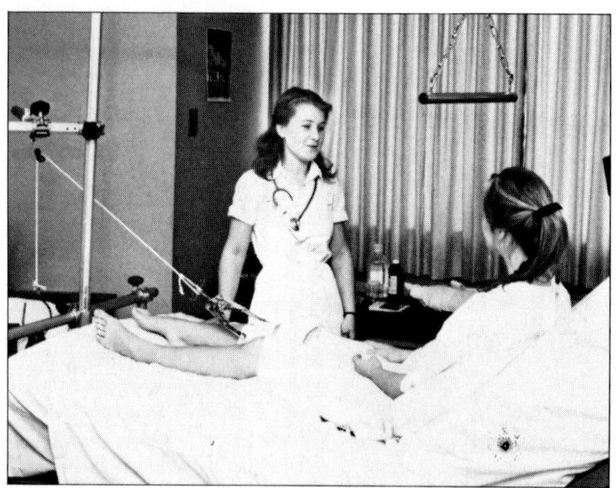

1 *Leslie Swope, a 25-year-old chef's assistant, fractured her right tibia in a skiing accident. Her leg is being immobilized in skeletal traction, and you've been ordered by the doctor to perform pin care to prevent infection.*

Caution: Pin care may vary according to the doctor's preference and hospital policy. Make sure you receive a specific order before initiating pin care.

First, gather the following sterile supplies: several packages of 4"x4" gauze pads, a bowl, applicator sticks, gloves (optional), normal saline solution, and a suture set. You'll also need a spray container of povidone iodine, a bottle of hydrogen peroxide, and a plastic bag for disposal of used pads.

Note: Make sure you use the bottles of solution individually marked for your patient.

Remember to explain the procedure and its purpose to your patient.

Now, wash and dry your hands thoroughly. Then, prepare your supplies, using aseptic technique. Open four gauze pad packets and slit them with your suture set scissors, unless the pads are preslit. Pour equal amounts of hydrogen peroxide and normal saline solution into the bowl.

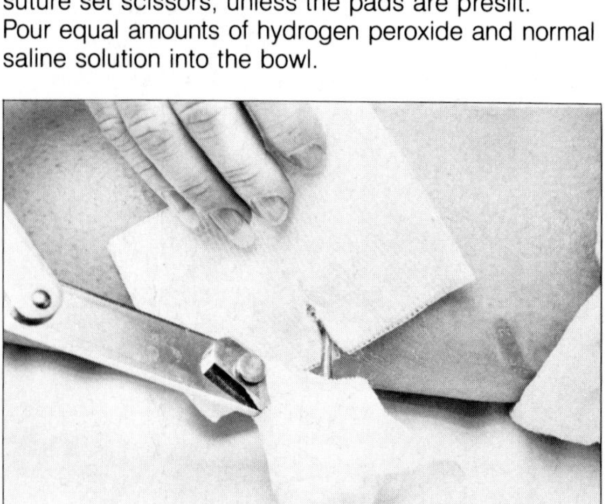

2 Then, remove the old dressing, as the nurse is doing here. Dispose of the soiled dressing in the plastic bag. Repeat the procedure on the patient's opposite side. Wash your hands again.

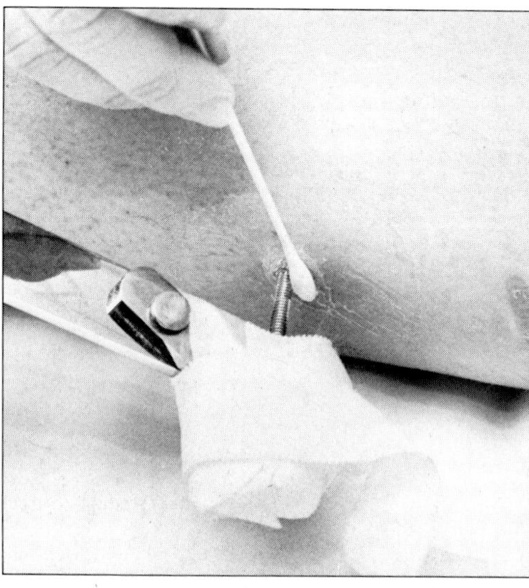

3 Next, insert an applicator into the hydrogen-peroxide/normal saline solution mixture. Then, cleanse the pin site, as shown.

Note: Make sure you use a new applicator for each pin site. After an applicator is used, place it in the plastic bag.

After cleansing each pin site, use a dry applicator around the site to absorb any excess solution. Then, with the gauze pads removed and the area cleaned, visually inspect each pin site for reddened skin, purulent drainage, or edema. Notify the doctor if you notice any of these signs.

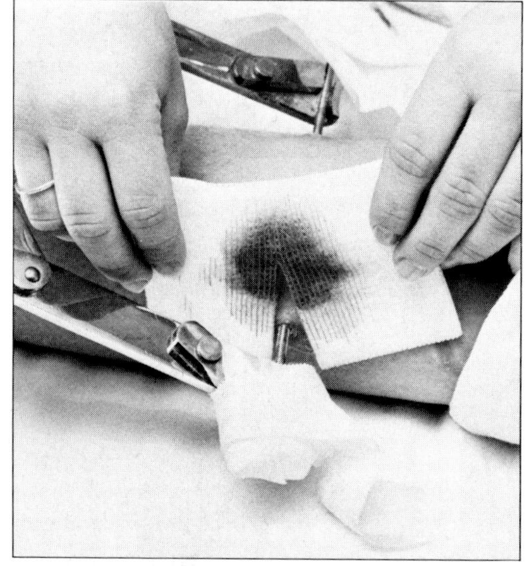

4 Now, spray each gauze pad with povidone iodine, directing the spray at the area around the top of the slit. Then, place a pad at the pin site, sliding the slit over the pin, as shown.

Note: Discontinue povidone-iodine applications if they irritate the patient's granular tissue or when the pin site has healed.

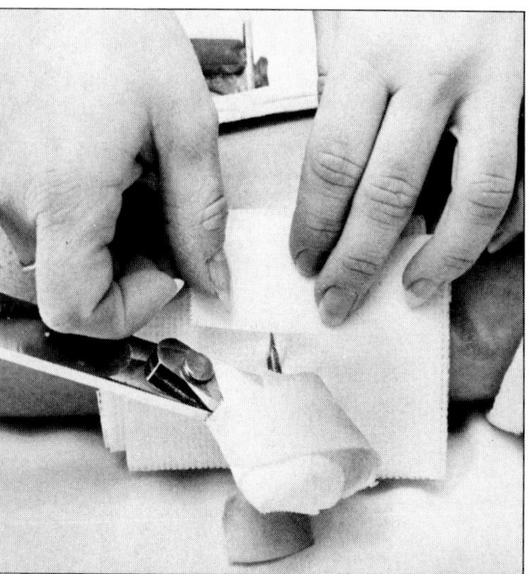

5 Next, place a dry gauze pad at the pin site, positioning it over the pad saturated with povidone iodine. Slide it over the pin in the direction opposite to the saturated pad. Then, place a strip of nonallergenic tape at the common borders of the pads to secure them, as the nurse is doing here.

Caution: Don't attach the tape to your patient's skin.

When you've completed the procedure, place your gloves and suture set in the plastic bag. Dispose of the plastic bag, according to hospital policy. Wash your hands. Remember to document the procedure.

Providing care for a patient in halo skeletal traction

Do you understand halo skeletal traction? The halo head attachment and accompanying torso vest are applied by the doctor to reduce or immobilize stable cervical fractures or dislocations. Permitting mobility is halo traction's primary advantage over other forms of skeletal traction. It allows the patient to sit, stand, and walk. Giving the patient freedom from strict bed confinement reduces the risk of respiratory and circulatory problems, as well as muscle atrophy.

The halo's a metal ring that's secured around the patient's head by four pins, two anterior and two posterior (see illustration). These pins penetrate the skull about ⅛", and don't require skin incisions and drill holes needed for some cervical spine traction. This reduces infection risk as well as patient discomfort. The headpiece attaches to a plaster or plastic vest. The latter is lined with sheepskin for patient comfort and to help reduce skin breakdown.

Note: You should know how to remove the vest quickly in an emergency; for example, when the patient's vomiting or choking. Tape the traction adjustment wrench to the front of your patient's vest. Also, place the toolbox containing other adjustment tools (with its contents correctly labeled on the outside of the box) in full view near his bed.

To provide the best care for your patient, follow these guidelines:

- Assess your patient's neurovascular status at least every 8 hours, and notify the doctor immediately if you note any sensation or motor loss, or muscle power loss. These are the major signs of spinal cord trauma.
- Show your patient how to change his body position every 2 hours to prevent nerve and vascular constriction. Assist him with the position changes only if he's lost sensory or motor function.
- Encourage use of an incentive spirometer once an hour while your patient's awake. Auscultate for rales or rhonchi every 4 hours to make sure the vest isn't impeding his breathing.
- Specially trained personnel should remove the vest daily to perform complete skin care and inspection (see page 55). Check in particular the skin areas where the vest's edges rest, for signs of pressure.
- If you suspect the vest is fitted improperly, have it adjusted by trained personnel. Temporarily pad the areas of improper fit, *not* the areas showing signs of pressure.
- Keep the vest's inner padding clean and dry. Replace the padding, as necessary.
- Teach him range-of-motion exercises to prevent muscle atrophy. Encourage your patient to walk, unless contraindicated. To prevent a fall, assist him when he first tries to walk.
- Twice each day, provide pin care (if ordered), following your hospital's policy. Notify the doctor if the areas around the pin entry sites become infected. He may want to either increase the frequency of pin care or discontinue the care (see the previous page).

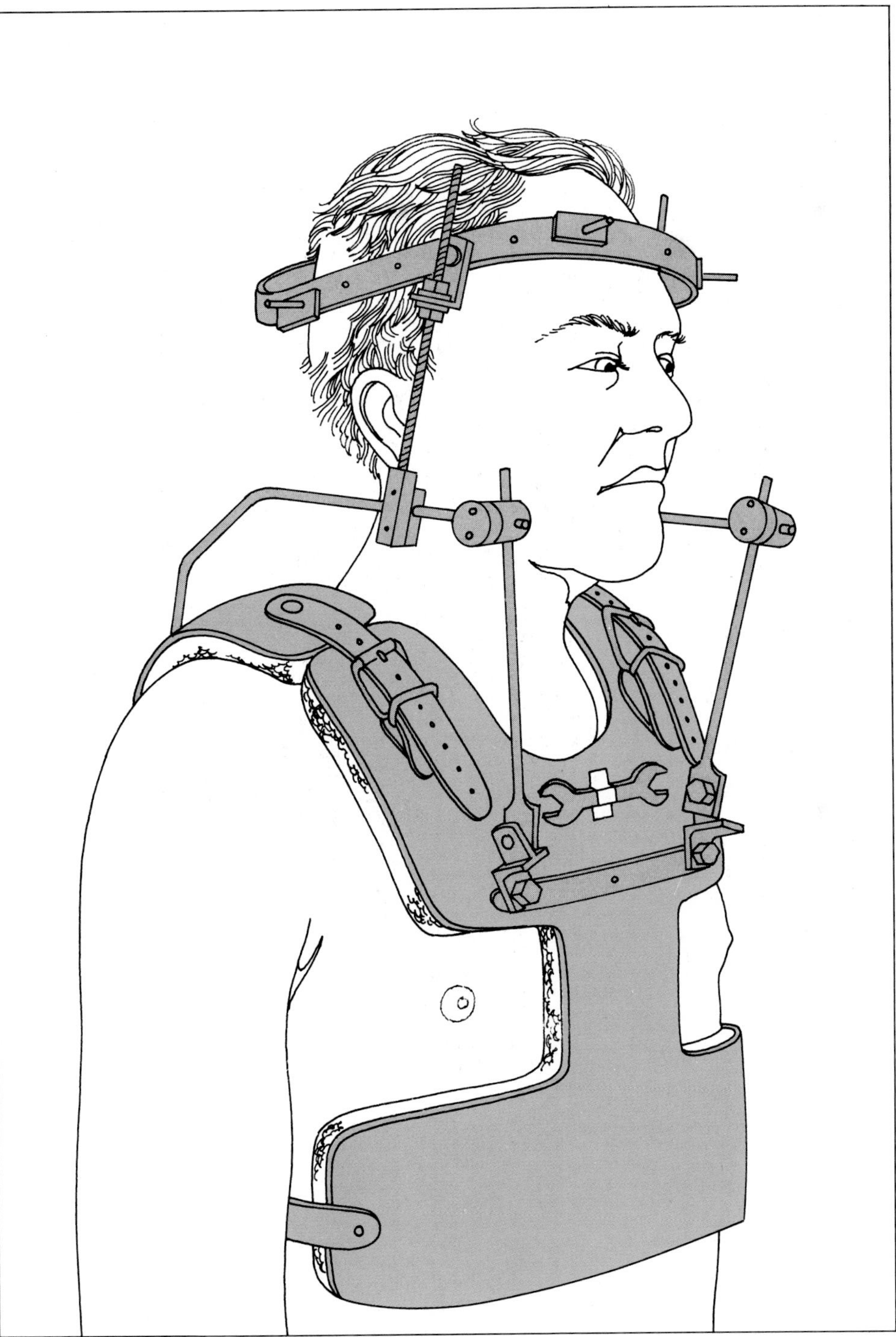

Traction

Caring for a patient in cervical traction

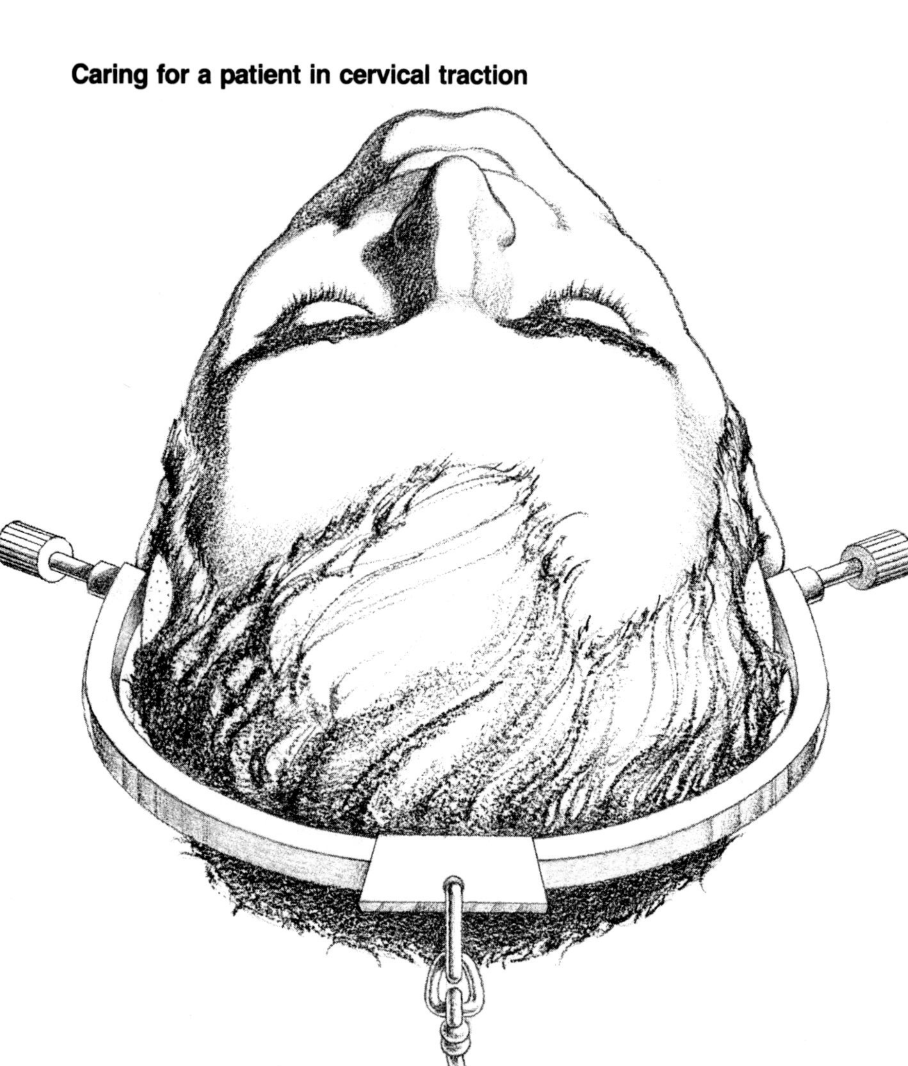

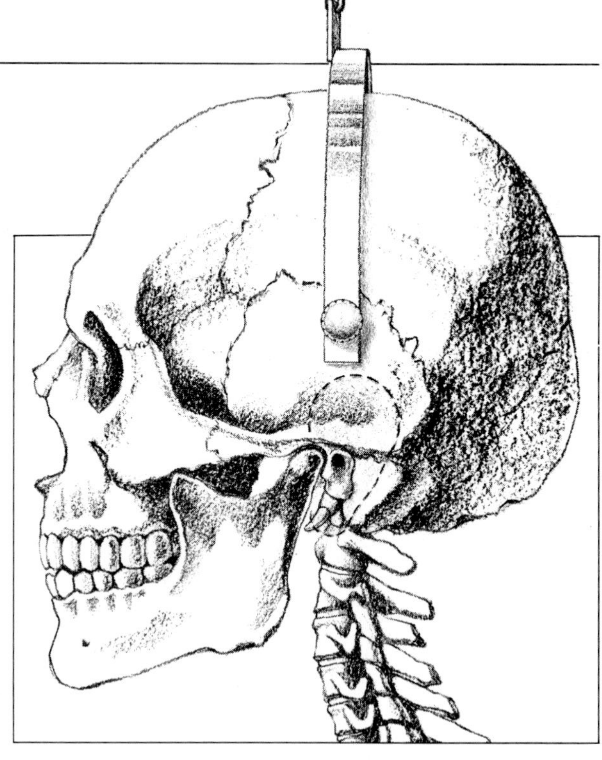

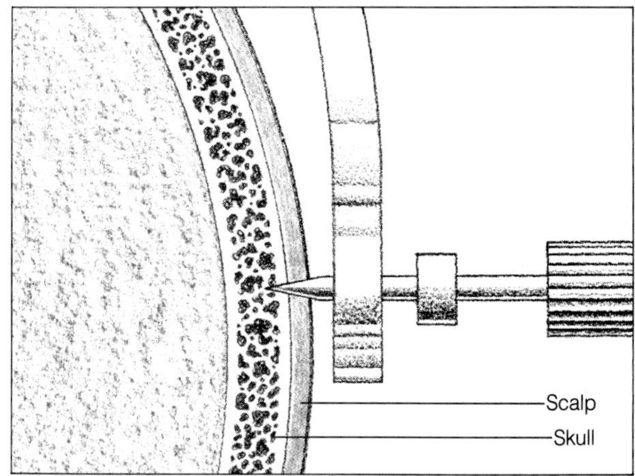

Cervical traction is applied following fractures or dislocations of the cervical or high thoracic vertebrae. Tongs attached to the patient's skull are used with a weight-and-pulley system to exert pull along the axis of the spine. This arrangement promotes vertebral alignment and decreases the possibility of inadvertent movement and further injury. However, it does carry the risk of spinal cord injury from excessive manipulation of the patient's head and cervical vertebrae during traction application.

Three types of tongs are used in cervical spine traction: Gardner-Wells (see illustration), Crutchfield, and Vinke. Gardner-Wells tongs are considered the least likely of the three to slip and tear the skin from prolonged use, or use with excessive amounts of weight.

If you're caring for a patient in cervical traction, provide the following special care:

- Turn your patient as soon as possible after the skull tongs are applied and the desired vertebral alignment has been confirmed by an X-ray. Use a special bed or frame, such as the Circle® bed or Stryker frame, so you can turn your patient without disrupting vertebral alignment.
- Monitor your patient's blood pressure, pulse, respiratory rate, and temperature every hour until stable, and then every 2 to 4 hours thereafter. Remember, low systolic blood pressure (90 mmHg and below) is one indication of spinal cord trauma. Also, respiratory complications are more common with high cervical injury.
- Note the degree and location of pain, paresthesia, paralysis, or loss of muscle power, before tong application, and hourly for the first 24 hours following tong application. Continue assessment thereafter according to doctor's orders.
- Check the tongs often for correct placement.
- Perform pin care at the tong insertion sites, depending on hospital policy or doctor's orders. Expect only minimal bleeding at these sites following application, since the anesthetic of choice contains epinephrine. Notify the doctor if bleeding persists.
- Observe and frequently assess all bony prominences, including the heels, elbows, and occipital area.
- Provide meticulous skin care and position changes every 2 hours, unless contraindicated, especially if your patient has any sensory or motor function loss.
- If ordered by the doctor, provide padding or support under your patient's head, neck, or shoulders.
- Encourage your patient to feed himself, if possible. Turn him on his side for feeding. Supply a high-protein and high-caloric diet, or a soft diet if it's painful for your patient to chew.
- Provide rectal stimulation, as ordered, for bowel function.
- Provide emotional and moral support for your patient and his family. They'll probably be particularly anxious, considering the implications of spinal cord injury.
- Document all your care in your nurses' notes.

Learning about balanced suspension traction

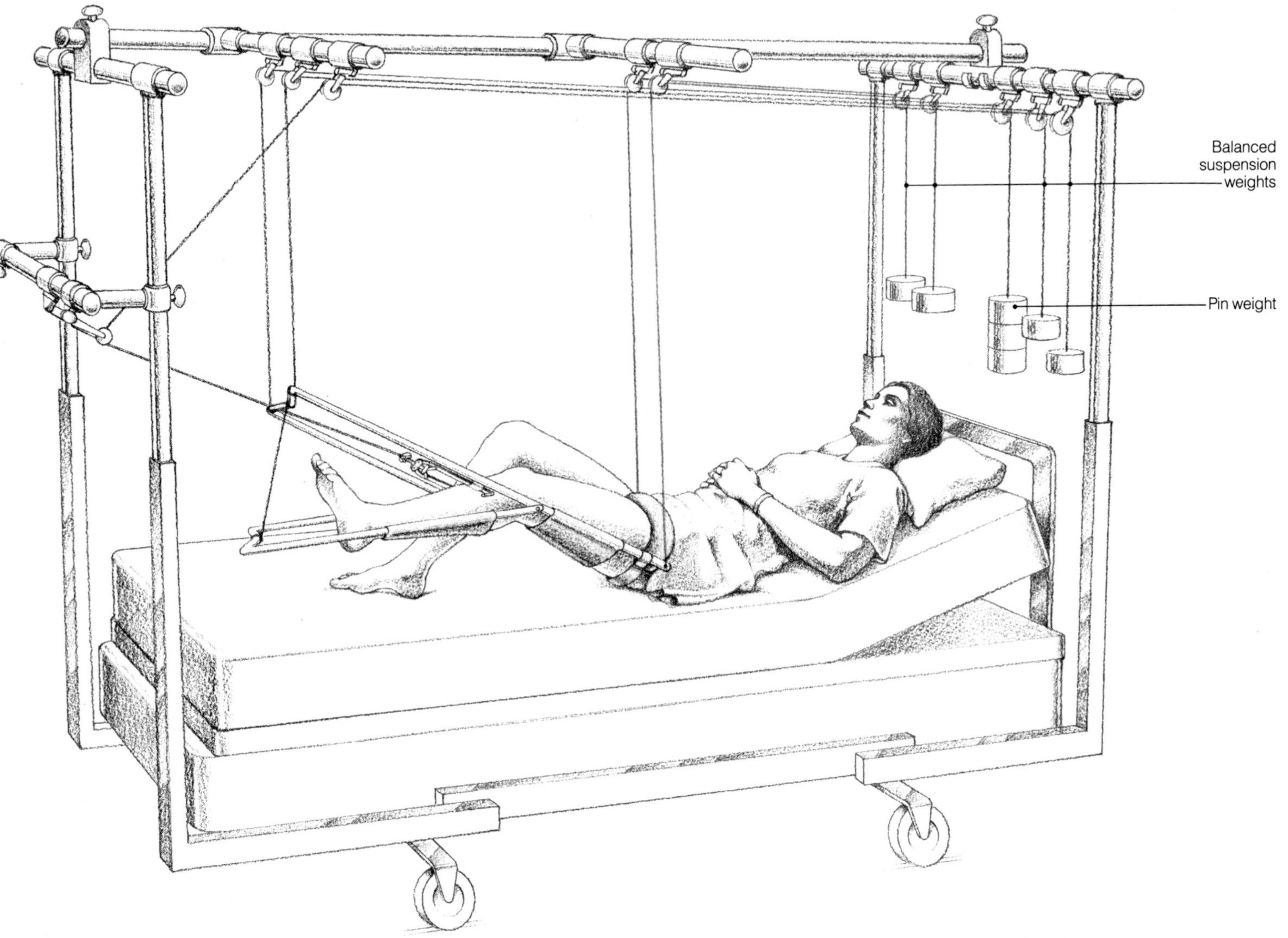

Have you ever cared for a patient in balanced suspension traction? As you know, this form of suspension is most commonly used with skeletal traction. A hammock or splint, such as a Thomas' splint with Pearson attachment, provides leg support. Balanced suspension is most commonly used to support leg injuries such as femoral fractures with displacement, and nonaligned bone fragments.

In balanced suspension, the weight that suspends the affected extremity equals the weight of the countertraction being applied. In other words, the suspension weight of the affected extremity, splint and attachment are countered through the backward pull of ropes and weights attached to the groin end of the splint. This assembly promotes neurovascular integrity by decreasing prolonged pressure on the back of the patient's leg. It also allows more range of motion than other forms of traction, without affecting the line of traction pull.

Caring for a patient in skeletal balanced suspension traction should include the following nursing considerations:

- Perform hourly neurovascular assessments during the first 48 to 72 hours after initial application. Then, continue assessing your patient at frequent intervals, taking care to note (and correct) any circulatory impairment from equipment.
- Prevent any pressure on the peroneal, femoral, popliteal, and sural nerves. Increased numbness or pain in the affected extremity could indicate nerve constriction.
- Check peripheral nerve function by having your patient perform flexion, extension, and hyperflexion of the affected extremity. Nerve pressure or disruption may be indicated by a slowness or inability to perform these movements.
- Frequently inspect your patient's skin, especially over her bony prominences. Closely inspect your patient's buttocks and back. Provide the skin care described on page 55.
- Observe the pin entry and exit sites for drainage, swelling, pain, redness, or skin warmth, all indications of possible infection. Notify the doctor if you note any of these signs. Perform pin care, as ordered by the doctor, or according to hospital policy.
- Instruct and assist your patient in exercising her suspended limb and maintaining range of motion in her other extremities.

Traction

Caring for a patient in a Thomas' splint with Pearson attachment

Has your patient fractured his femur? Skeletal traction will provide fracture alignment and stabilization. Also, the doctor may order a Thomas' splint with Pearson attachment to support the distal limb. The Thomas' splint fits around the patient's thigh. The distal end is attached to a weight for suspension. The Pearson attachment is a frame that supports the patient's lower leg or calf area, allowing knee flexion and lower leg movement, as shown in the illustration.

Nursing care for a patient in a Thomas' splint and Pearson attachment includes the following:

- Make sure the ring of the Thomas' splint is correctly positioned around the upper thigh, without constricting his groin area. Check splint fit often; eliminate any pressure on the groin.
- Also, keep the Pearson frame from pressing against the lateral side of your patient's knee.
- Attach footplates to the Pearson frame to prevent footdrop. These can be moved to facilitate foot exercises.
- Reduce the risk of hip flexion contractures from prolonged semi-Fowler's position, by scheduling periods of hip extension every 8 hours. Position the bed flat for each session.
- Encourage frequent lower leg exercise.
- Perform the general care listed on pages 83 and 87.

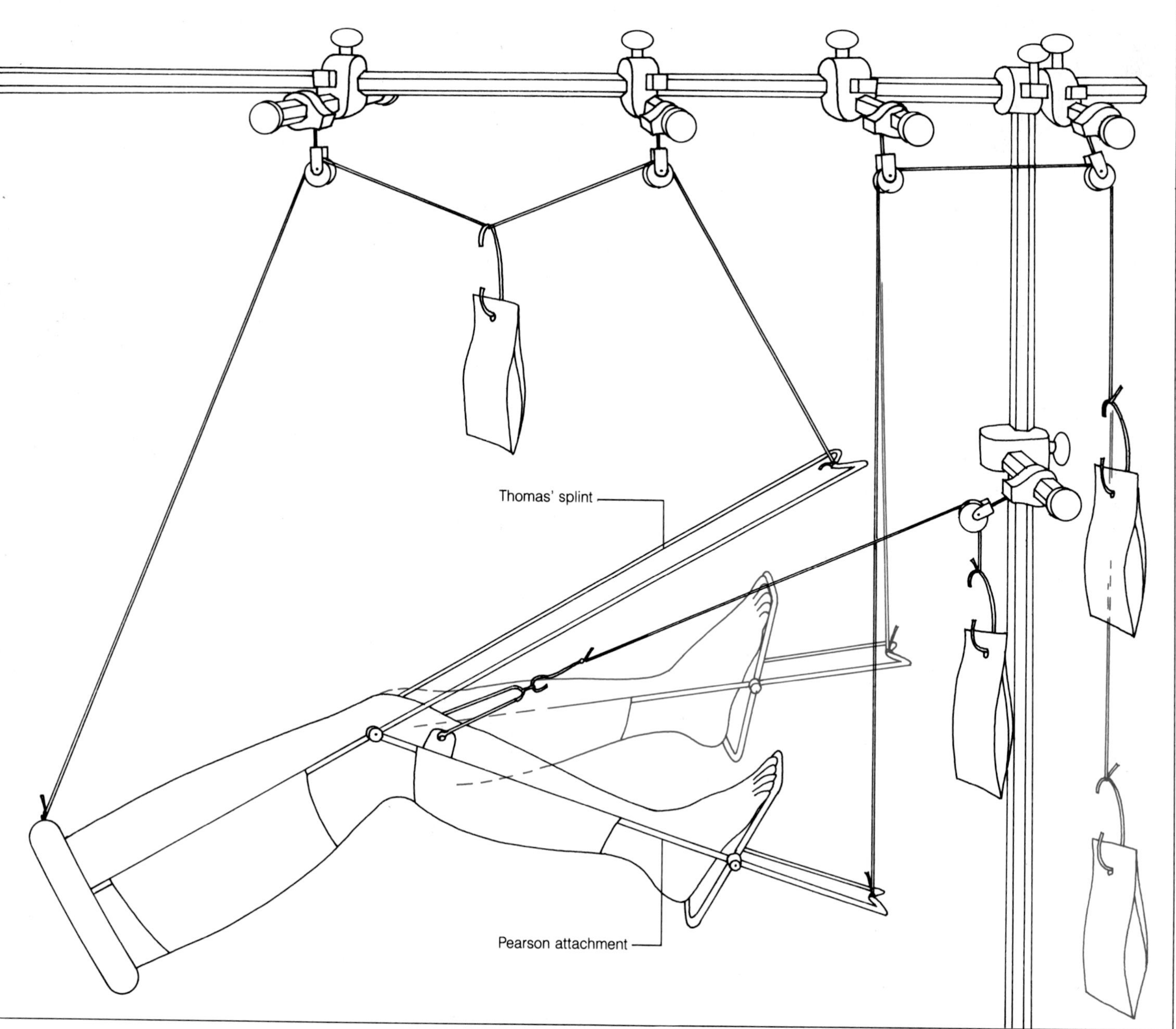

Providing emotional and psychological support

Often, the frustration and boredom caused by an extended period of immobilization creates more problems than the injury that led to traction application. You must be sensitive to your patient's need for emotional support as well as physical care. Of course, the psychological support each patient needs will differ, depending on age, level of consciousness, and lifestyle before he was placed in traction.

Never be timid about making practical suggestions to the doctor regarding your patient, such as increasing his mobility by adjusting the traction setup. Remember, you spend more time with the patient, so you best know his needs.

Allow your patient as much control as possible over his environment. Give him some choice over the times of his care.

Try to maintain his orientation, and provide diversion. Enlist others, such as physical and occupational therapists, clergymen, and volunteer aides to supplement your efforts. Perhaps the patient's family could occasionally bring in meals and eat with him. Make sure the patient receives a daily newspaper, and that a transistor radio, TV, and phone are readily accessible. Spend a few minutes with your patient whenever possible, and listen attentively to what he says. If you can, put patients of the same age and interests together in the same room. Remember, the personal care you provide helps your patient cope with his strange new environment, and ultimately speeds his recovery.

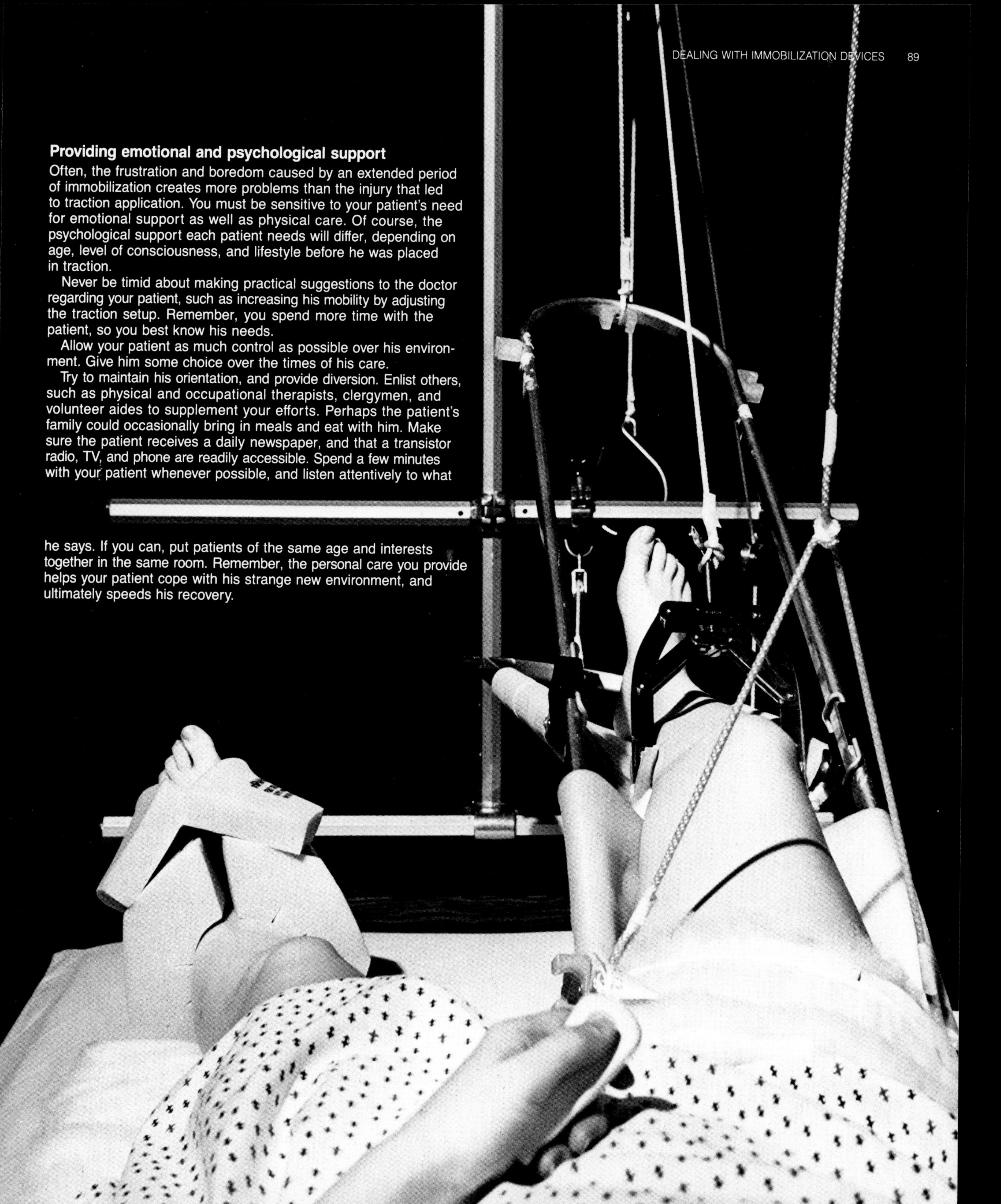

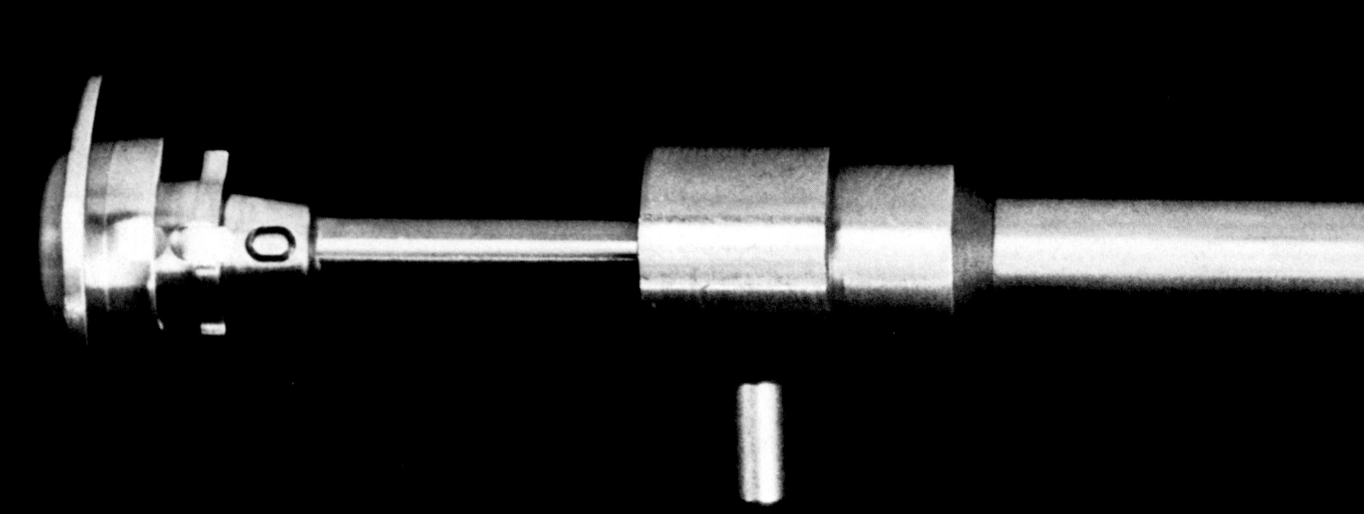

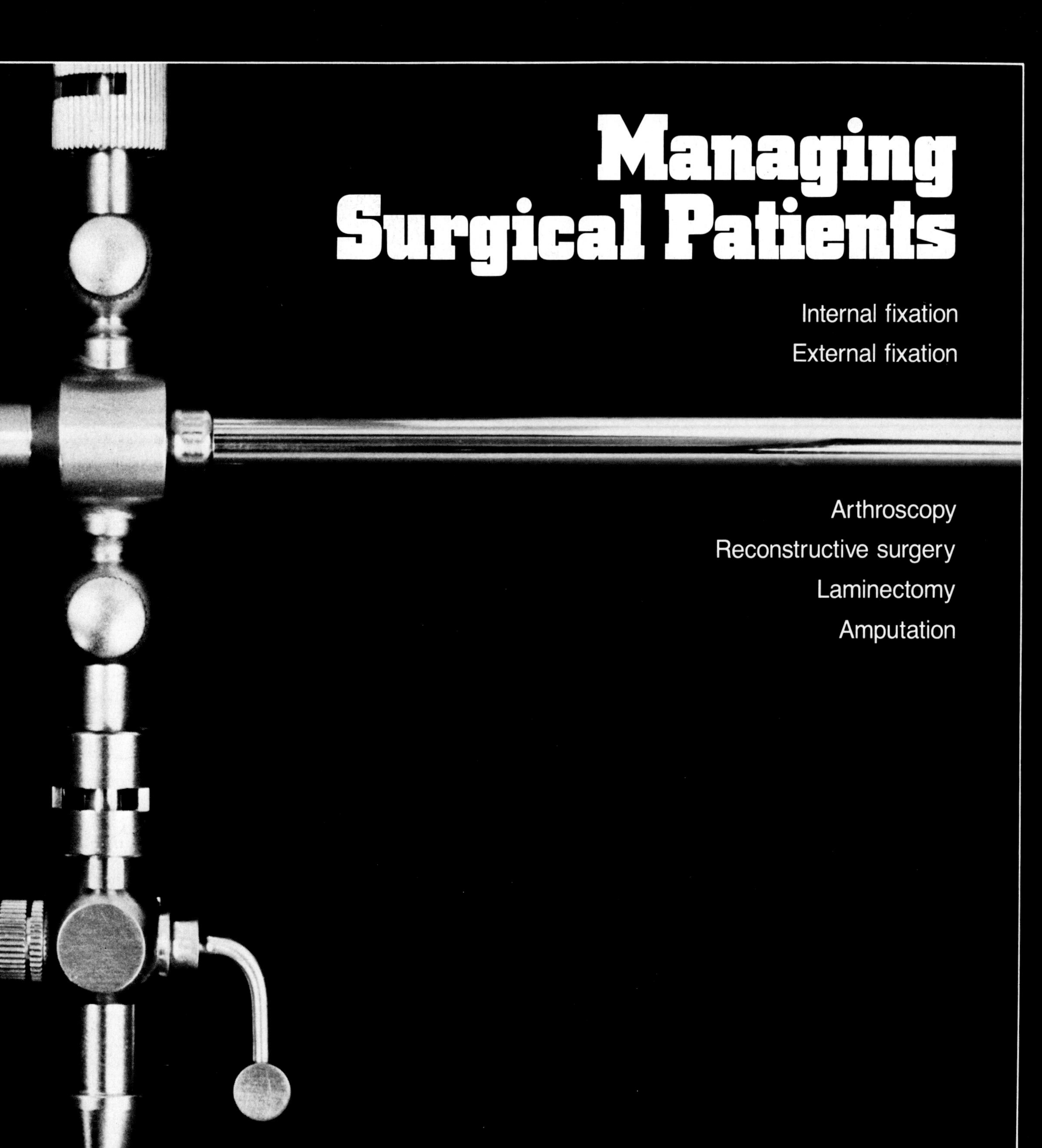

Managing Surgical Patients

Internal fixation

External fixation

Arthroscopy

Reconstructive surgery

Laminectomy

Amputation

Internal fixation

What does internal fixation mean to you? Did you realize that a pin, screw, nail, or plate is actually inserted in your patient's bone, to hold bone fragments together during healing? With one or more of these devices securely fixating his fracture, your patient can begin weight-bearing ambulation relatively early.

One common form of internal fixation is hip pinning. Caring for a patient who has a hip pin in place requires specific turning, positioning, and early-ambulation procedures.

Read the following pages for all the details you need to help your patient successfully recover from hip-pinning surgery.

Learning about internal fixation

Internal fixation is a way of immobilizing fractures. It involves the surgical insertion of a metal nail, pin, or screws, sometimes in conjunction with a plate, to bind the fractured bone fragments together. After the bone heals, the device may be removed. To find out when internal fixation's indicated, see the box at right.

Suppose your patient has a hip fracture, and the doctor decides to perform internal fixation. How does he choose the proper fixation device? First, he considers the angle and location of the fracture line. Then, he selects a device that will bind the fractured fragments securely, yet cause the least bone disruption during insertion. See the chart at right for information on fracture types and the internal fixation devices indicated for each.

As you can see in the chart, a pin and plate are commonly used to treat trochanteric fractures (a type of hip fracture). How does the doctor insert them? First, he surgically opens the area for better visualization during reduction. Then, if internal fixation's indicated, he'll insert the threaded pin through the femur neck into the femur head. He'll attach the plate, which anchors the pin, to the femur's outer side (see illustration). To complete the pinning, he applies compression to the fracture line by inserting a small bolt up through the plate.

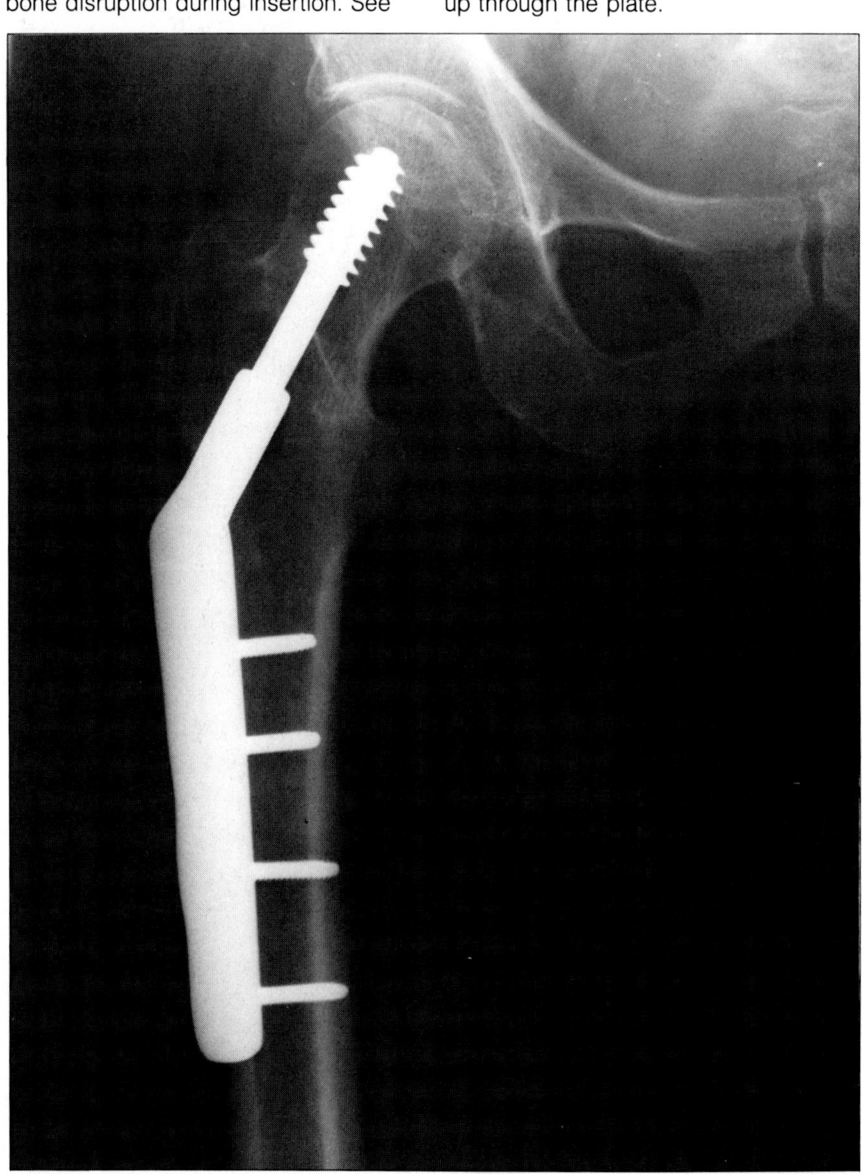

Does your patient need internal fixation?

The doctor may perform internal fixation for a patient with:

- an intra-articular fracture.
- a fracture with associated vascular injury.
- an open fracture following multiple trauma.
- a severely displaced long-bone fracture.
- a femoral neck fracture in an older patient.

The doctor probably won't perform internal fixation for a patient with:

- a severely comminuted fracture, which provides too little firm bone for good fixation, and which requires an amount of surgical dissection that disrupts blood supply to the injury site.
- a fracture in a bone seriously weakened by osteoporosis, which won't provide a firm anchor for the internal fixation device.

Internal fixation devices by fracture type

Fracture type
Trochanteric (femoral)
Internal fixation device
Hip pin or nail (with or without plate), or screwplate. Choice of pin, pin with plate, or screwplate depends on specific fracture type and configuration.

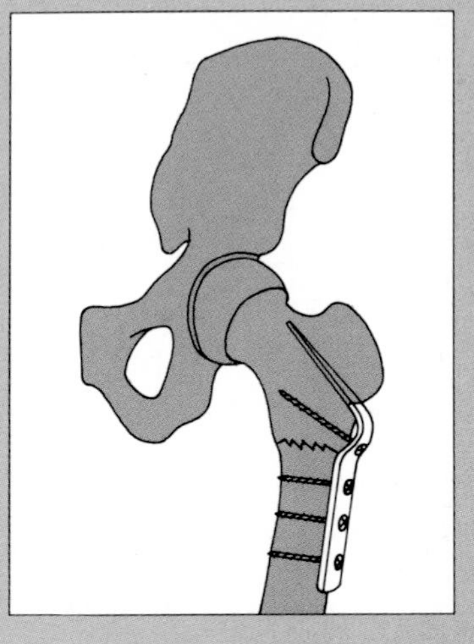

Fracture type
Supracondylar and condylar femoral fractures
Internal fixation device
Rod, nail, plate, or screws. Traction is treatment of choice, because internal fixation carries risk of damage to the sciatic nerve or popliteal artery. However, for transverse or oblique fractures, and other fractures that aren't complex, internal fixation may be used.

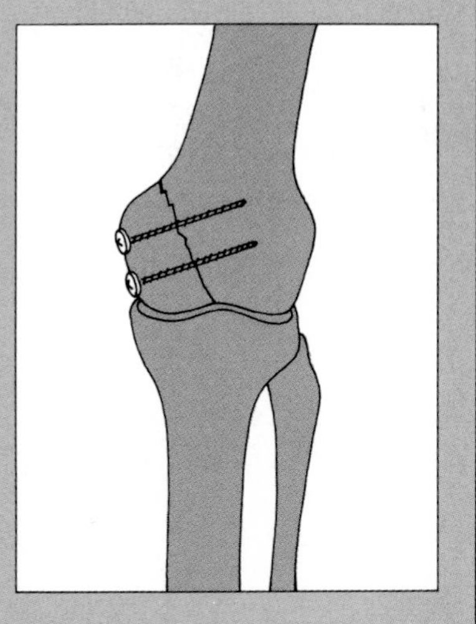

Fracture type
Subtrochanteric (femoral)
Internal fixation device
Hip pin or nail (with or without plate), or screwplate. Because of the great stresses imposed on this area by weight bearing, strong control of both proximal and distal bone fragments is required. Pin and plate with extra nails stabilize the fracture by impacting the bone ends at the fracture site.

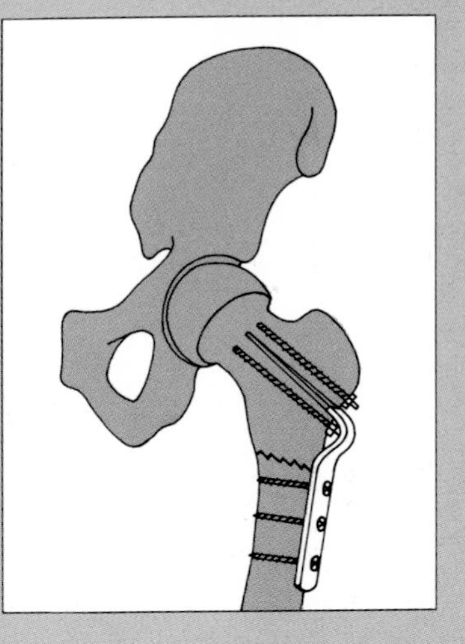

Fracture type
Tibia fracture
Internal fixation device
Intramedullary rod or screwplate. Intramedullary rod may be used for a severely displaced fracture. Screwplate may be used for a comminuted fracture.

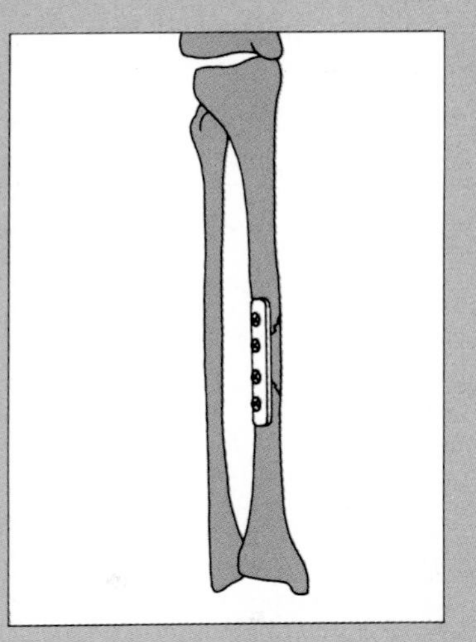

Fracture type
Femoral shaft
Internal fixation device
Intramedullary rod. If fracture's not complex, and the patient is healthy, with no soft tissue damage, open reduction with insertion of an intramedullary rod is indicated. This procedure permits early ambulation with partial weight bearing.

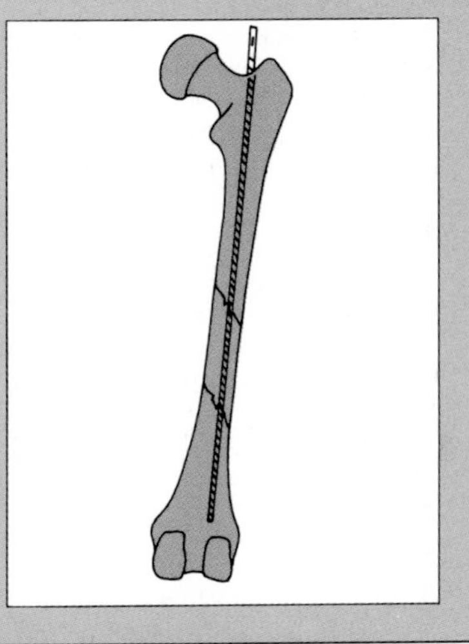

Fracture type
Upper extremity fracture
Internal fixation device
Plate, rod, or nail. Good circulation and soft tissue coverage of the upper extremity mean fewer complications from internal fixation. Most radius and ulna fractures may be fixed with plates. Humerus fractures may be fixed with rods. Because of the elbow joint's complexity, elbow fractures almost always require internal fixation.

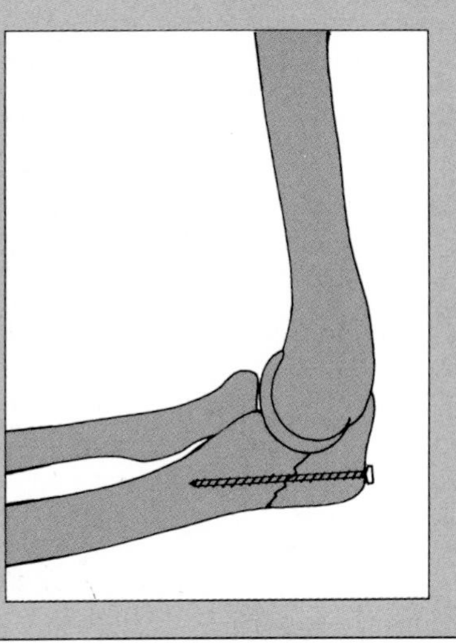

Internal fixation

PATIENT PREPARATION

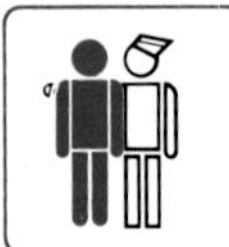

Hip internal fixation: Before the procedure

Hip fractures usually require prompt repair, so lengthy preoperative patient preparation probably won't be feasible.

In many cases, your hip fracture patient will be an older woman. Briefly explain the procedure to her. Help her understand that after surgery she'll have a hip pin or other device in place for an extended period. Tell her the device may be removed after her hip has completely healed. The pin will allow weight-bearing ambulation much sooner than a cast or traction would.

Prior to surgery, assess your patient carefully to establish a baseline for postoperative evaluation. Begin by taking a general surgical history. To do so, follow the guidelines we give in the NURSING PHOTOBOOK CARING FOR SURGICAL PATIENTS. Then, perform a complete physical assessment, including a detailed orthopedic assessment (see pages 34 to 39).

In performing your assessment, you may note that your patient has the following signs and symptoms:

- hip pain which increases during movement
- slightly shortened affected leg
- externally rotated affected leg.

If your patient's elderly, pay special attention to any problems associated with aging such as nutritional deficiency, skin conditions, or osteoporosis, and any chronic diseases such as coronary artery disease, diabetes, or organic brain syndrome.

Suppose your assessment indicates a condition requiring treatment before surgery; for example, recent myocardial infarction. The doctor may delay surgery for 24 to 48 hours while the patient's condition stabilizes. If surgery's delayed, the doctor may order that your patient's injured leg be immobilized in Buck's extension. Doing so will relieve muscle spasms and prevent further soft tissue damage.

For specific guidelines on Buck's extension application and care of a patient in Buck's extension, see pages 74 and 75.

Internal fixation: Providing postop care

Clara Bruno, a 50-year-old elementary school teacher, has just returned from surgery. You must monitor her vital signs frequently, encourage deep breathing and coughing, and turn Ms. Bruno every 2 hours. Check dressings and linens frequently for drainage and bleeding. Your patient may have a surgical wound evacuator (for example, a Hemovac™) in place to prevent drainage accumulation inside the wound. If so, provide appropriate care, using meticulous aseptic technique.

To prevent thrombophlebitis, use elastic antiembolism stockings, as ordered. Remove the stockings every 8 hours for 1 hour. Wash and dry her legs completely before reapplying the stockings.

To prevent dehydration, provide adequate fluids, either parentally or orally, as ordered. Encourage oral fluids as soon as possible. Administer antibiotics and pain medications as ordered, and observe and document their effects.

Throughout the postoperative period, monitor your patient closely for indications of shock, hemorrhage, infection, paralytic ileus, thrombosis, and pressure sores. See the box at right for more information on specific complications of internal fixation.

Don't neglect Ms. Bruno's nutritional needs. (For information on nutrition, see page 111.) She'll require adequate proteins, vitamins, and calcium for proper bone healing. Have the dietition visit Ms. Bruno to assess her nutritional status. Because her appetite may be depressed from limited mobility, try feeding her small frequent meals. Or, give supplemental feedings between her regular meals.

Use a fracture bedpan to help reduce discomfort during elimination. Provide stool softeners, as ordered.

Because a patient with a fractured hip may have overflow urinary incontinence, provide a bedpan at frequent intervals.

Note: Indwelling catheterization should be avoided, to help prevent urinary tract infection.

For more details on providing postop patient care, see the NURSING PHOTOBOOK CARING FOR SURGICAL PATIENTS.

Remember to document all care in your nurse's notes.

COMPLICATIONS

Internal fixation complications

Complications associated with internal fixation include nonunion and avascular necrosis. Nonunion is the failure of the bone to heal completely. Although the fracture undergoes preliminary bone-healing stages, the wound repair tissue isn't converted into bone. Motion at the fracture site may indicate nonunion. Treatment may include a bone graft, femoral prosthesis insertion, or electrical stimulation of the bone fragments (see page 98). The fixation device may or may not require removal.

Avascular necrosis is caused by interruption of the blood supply at the fracture site, destroying bone tissue. Signs and symptoms include pain, muscle spasm, and limping during weight-bearing ambulation. Weight bearing may further erode bone tissue. Although these signs and symptoms are to be expected early in the bone-healing period, suspect necrosis if they're prolonged. If the bone is to be salvaged, nonunion and necrosis must receive early treatment.

Another internal fixation complication includes weakening or breaking of the fixation device, causing soft tissue damage. If postoperative pain, swelling, or tenderness are prolonged, or if the patient loses motion in his leg, notify the doctor. Replacing the internal fixation device with a prosthesis may be necessary.

Positioning your patient

If you're caring for a patient after internal fixation of the hip, you must pay special attention to positioning.

Teach the patient which activities and positions are allowed and which are contraindicated. For example, don't allow adduction, external rotation, or acute flexion of the patient's hip, because these positions will increase her pain and put undue strain on the fracture site. Until your patient's ambulatory, you must maintain her leg in strict *abduction.*

To help maintain abduction, position your patient supine, and place a pillow between her legs. This will keep her affected leg to one side of her midline. Or, use an abductor triangle, if one's available (see upper photo). Important: Warn your patient *never* to cross her legs.

To avoid extreme external rotation, use a trochanter roll or properly placed sandbags beside her thigh. Use the sandbags if your patient is restless and needs strong support. Otherwise, you may use the trochanter roll. Here's how: First, place the patient on her side. Then, position a bath blanket, folded into a 2'x2' square, so that its far edge is well under her buttocks. Place the patient on her back again. Roll the blanket up tightly against her pelvis and thigh, with the roll facing down (see middle photo). Or, roll up the bath blanket. Securely tape the roll to maintain its shape. Place it against her hip (see inset).

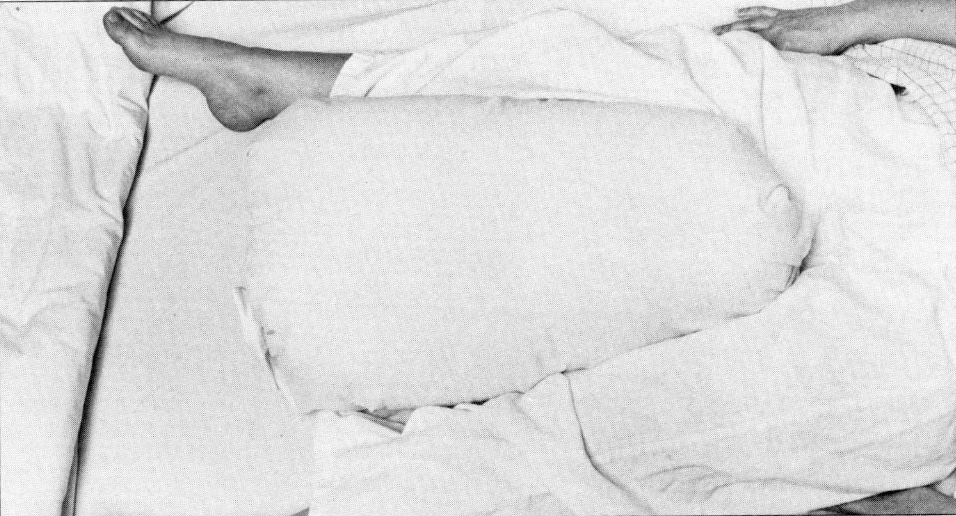

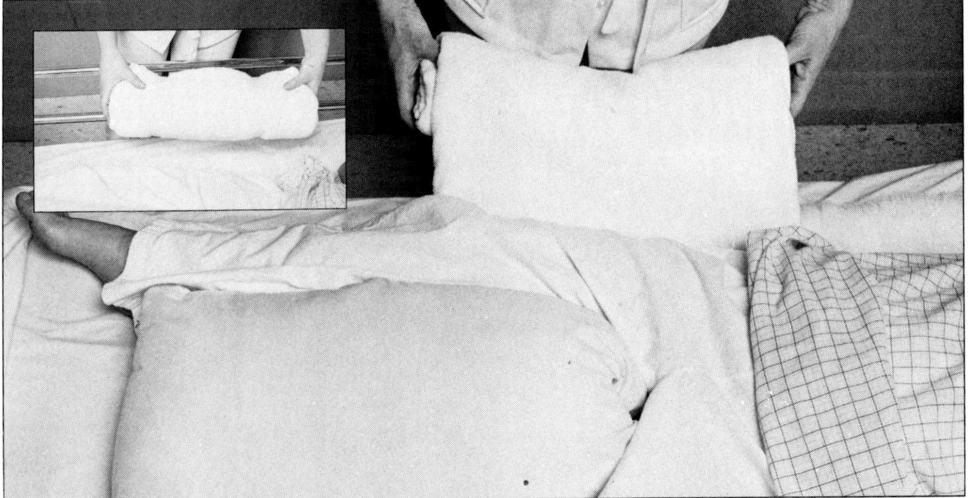

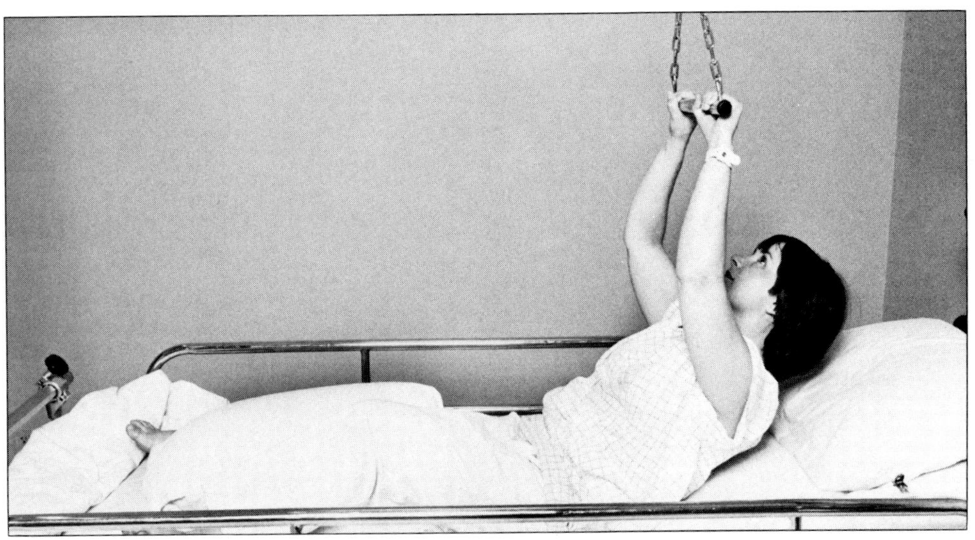

Check with the doctor to determine whether the head of the bed can be elevated. Usually, the doctor will order it elevated 30° to 40°. Tell your patient not to lean forward any further, which would increase hip flexion. If your patient's confused or restless, apply a jacket restraint. *Note:* Keep everything your patient needs, such as the call bell, within her reach.

Check your patient often to make sure her hip, leg, and foot are in proper alignment.

Finally, provide a trapeze for your patient's exercise. Hang the trapeze on an overhead bar. As ordered, teach your patient how to use it to help reposition herself and perform arm-strengthening exercises.

Change your patient's position every 2 hours. When you do so, provide skin care and massage bony prominences. For the proper turning procedure, see the following photostory.

Internal fixation

Turning your patient

Is it time to turn your patient? You may turn her on either side, providing you keep her affected leg abducted with pillows. Alternating from side to side will help promote good circulation. However, your patient may prefer to turn on her unaffected side, because it's less painful.

Note: Anytime you turn your patient on her affected side, make sure she receives pain medication 15 to 20 minutes before turning.

To turn your patient on her side, have an assistant stand on the side of the bed you'll turn the patient toward. If you're turning your patient on her *affected* side, the assistant should position her hands on the patient's shoulder and hip.

If you're turning her on her *unaffected* side, so that her affected leg is uppermost, your assistant should grasp her hip *above the incision site.*

Encourage the patient to help by holding onto the bedrail as your assistant pulls her toward her. As the patient turns, support her affected leg in abduction (see upper photo). Once she's repositioned, keep her hip and knee elevated on pillows, in the same plane as her other leg (see lower photo). Also, place a pillow behind her back.

Document what you've done in your nurses' notes.

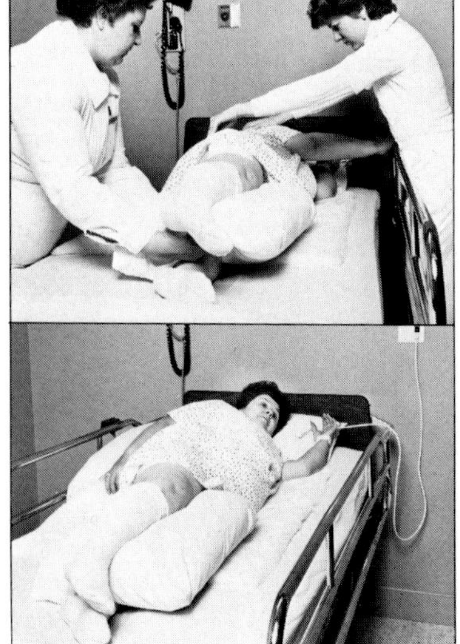

Early ambulation after hip fixation

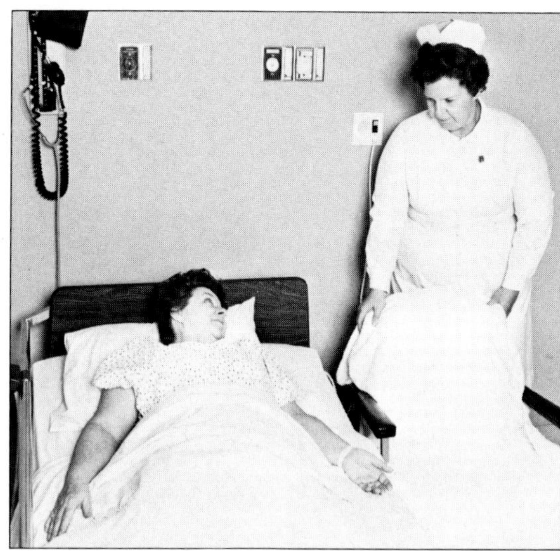

1 *Suppose your patient's surgery is uncomplicated. The doctor will probably order that you help your patient sit in a chair the morning after surgery. However, the patient must do this without putting weight on her* affected *leg. How can she do so? With your help, she'll stand on her unaffected leg and pivot into a chair.*

To avoid injury to either yourself or your patient, perform the task slowly and deliberately. Although this situation presents an opportunity for your patient to gain self-confidence after surgery, she'll probably be quite apprehensive. Explain very clearly what you're going to do and encourage her active cooperation.

Take these preliminary steps: Obtain a straight-backed, relatively high chair with arms. Place it close to the bed, on your patient's *unaffected* side.

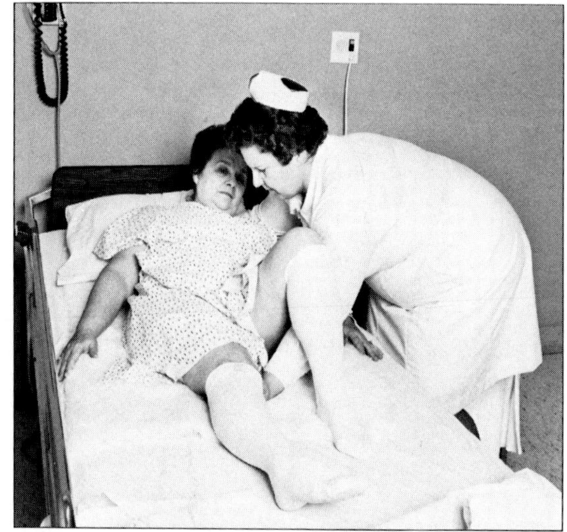

2 To bring your patient to a sitting position on the bed, first raise the head of the bed to 30°. Then, have her flex her unaffected leg at a right angle. Also, ask her to partially flex her affected leg. But, don't permit her to do so if it causes pain. Next, have her push herself up by placing her palms against the mattress.

Then, place one arm behind her back at shoulder level and the other under her knees.

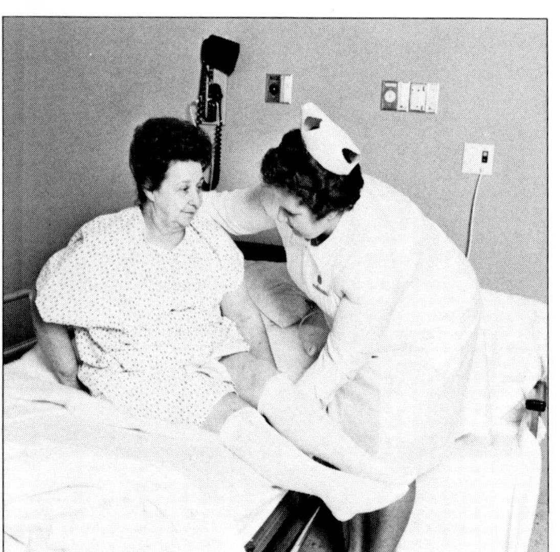

3 Using good body mechanics, gently swivel her into a sitting position on the side of the bed. Have the patient keep her affected leg straight, with her hip slightly flexed.

Permit her to rest in this position for several minutes.

Now, place a shoe with a nonskid sole on the foot of her unaffected leg.

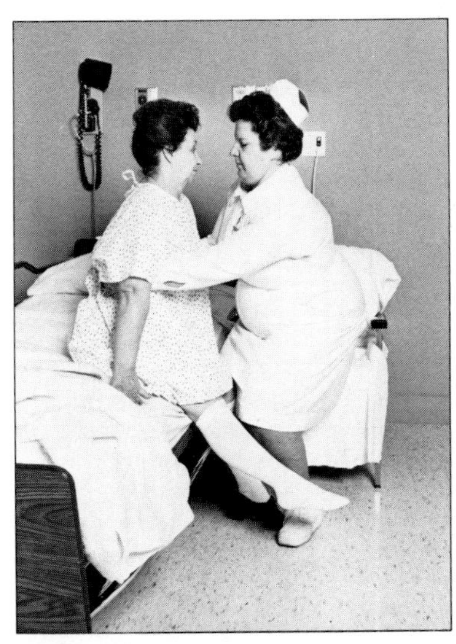

4 If she can continue, move in close to her and grasp her under her arms.

Important: Never allow her to hold you around your neck.

Stabilize her by bracing one of your legs against her unaffected leg.

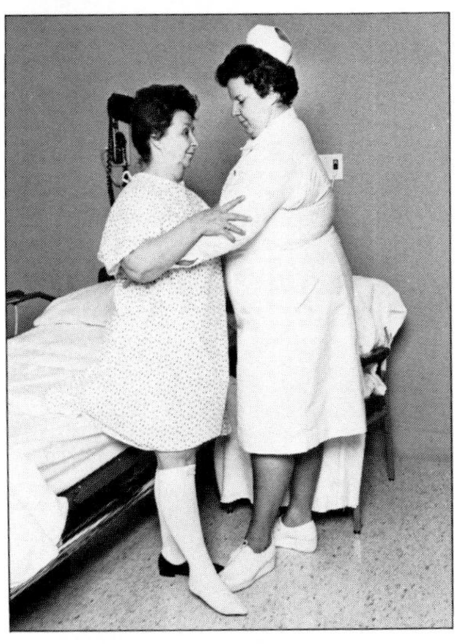

5 Assist her into a standing position, with all her weight resting on her unaffected leg.

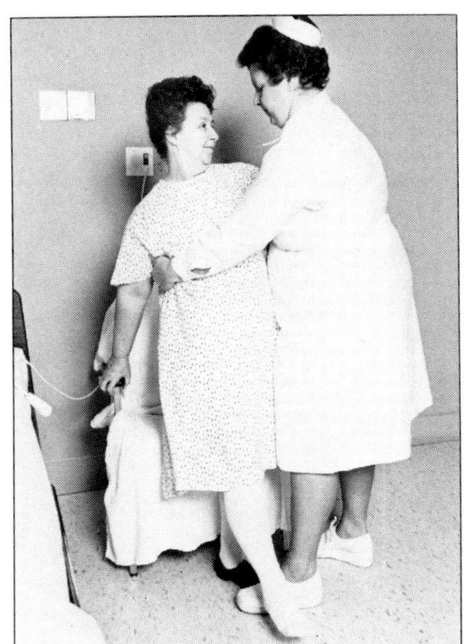

6 Then, help her pivot on that leg. Ask her to reach for the chair's armrests.

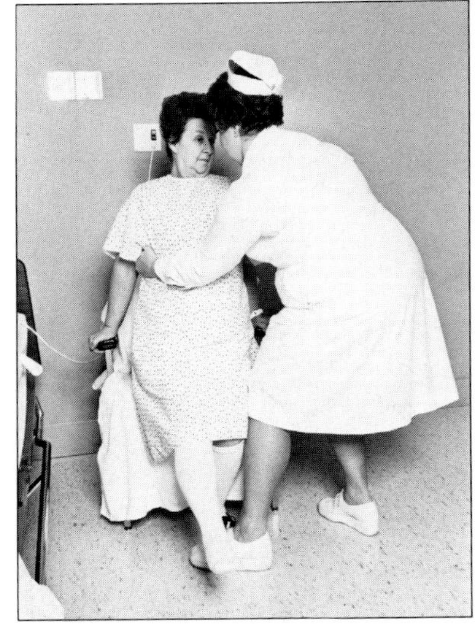

7 Flex your knees and hips, and slowly lower her into the chair. You may elevate her legs on a stool for comfort and to reduce swelling. But, remind her to keep her affected leg straight and her hip slightly flexed.

Nursing tip: If you can't remain with your patient, consider applying a restraint or safety jacket, so she won't fall out of the chair or bend forward too far. Place a call bell within reach. Remember not to leave her sitting too long, or she may become overtired.

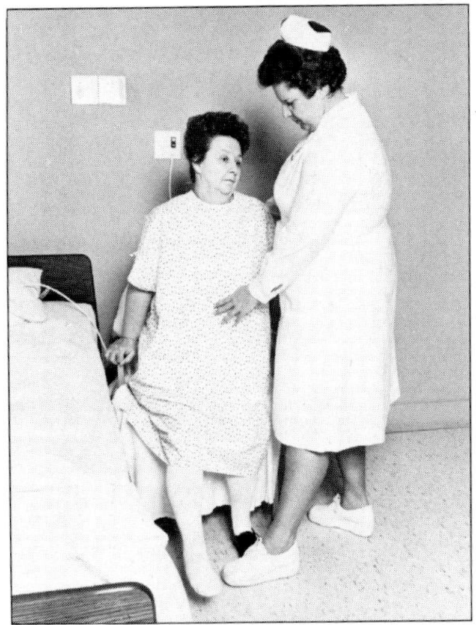

8 When your patient's ready to get back into bed, slide the chair so it's braced against the bed. Have her bend forward from her hips and flex the knee of her unaffected leg at a 90° angle. She should flex her knee as much as possible, while keeping the foot of her unaffected leg flat on the floor.

Now, have her place her hands on the chair's armrests, with her elbows slightly flexed, and come to a standing position, putting all of her weight on her unaffected foot. Be ready to support your patient, if necessary.

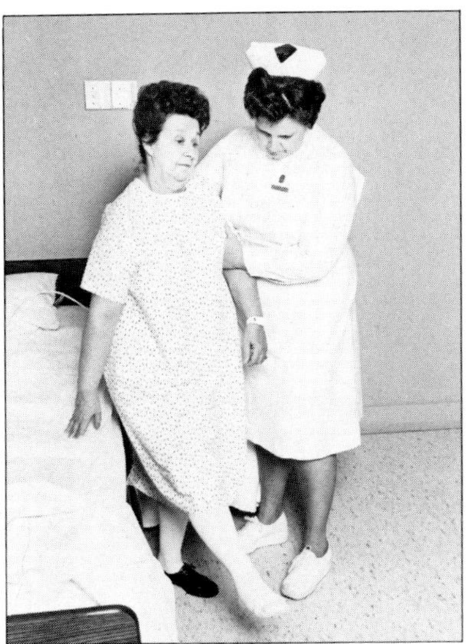

9 Help her pivot back into a sitting position on the side of the bed. Then, reposition her comfortably.

Remember to document the entire procedure and how well the patient tolerated it.

The doctor will determine when the bone's healed enough for it to bear the stress of body weight. When your patient's ready to walk, she'll probably begin by using parallel bars and a walker, before using a quad cane. (For more details on ambulation, see the section on ambulation aids.)

Internal fixation

Learning about electrical bone stimulation

As you know, bone nonunion may occur with internal fixation. If your patient's fracture doesn't heal, the doctor may remove the internal fixation device and perform a bone graft. Or, he may stimulate the bone fragments with electrical current. (In this case, the internal fixation device may not need to be removed.)

Electrical bone stimulation substitutes for normal piezoelectric effect, in which mechanical stress on a solid object induces electrical activity. In healthy bones, exercise produces electrical stimulation, making the bones grow. However, when bone is stimulated by direct current, electronegativity appears to have the same osteoblast-stimulating effect.

The electricity's applied either through magnetic coils placed on the skin at the fracture site, or through implanted electrodes powered by a battery (which may or may not also be implanted). The electrodes may be implanted either by open incision, or percutaneously, using a hand drill.

Percutaneous insertion avoids the problems often associated with extensive surgery. Infection rarely occurs with this implantation method. Also, an internal fixation device may remain in place, as long as the bone stimulator's electrode wires don't come into contact with it. Contact with the metal would disrupt the electrical circuit, hindering osteogenesis.

Cathode wire insertion

During insertion, the doctor implants the four cathode wires of the Zimmer® Direct Current Bone Growth Stimulator (see opposite page) directly into bone tissue (see illustration above).

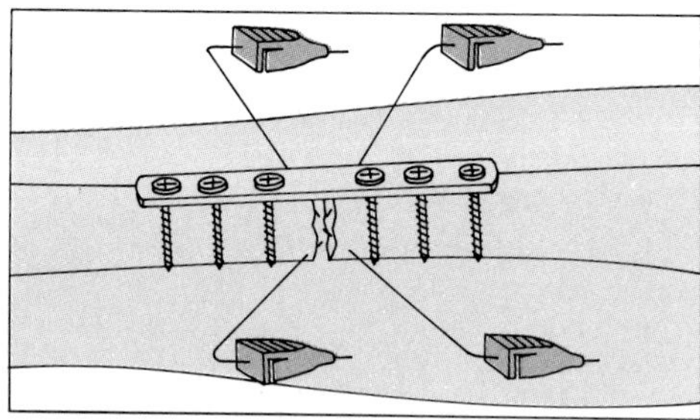

The wires protrude through the patient's skin. The doctor wraps the affected limb with Webril® tape, taking care to leave the wire ends free. Then, he attaches the wire ends to the battery's negative terminals. He places the positive terminal on the skin above the tape. The illustration below shows how the apparatus looks on the leg. The battery transmits a weak current (20 microamperes from each cathode) to the bone. This current is so weak that the patient can't feel it. *Note:* A higher current level would cause tissue necrosis. A lower level could fail to stimulate osteogenesis. After insertion, the affected limb is again wrapped in Webril, which also covers the power pack. The doctor leaves the shorting bar outside the wrap for easy attachment to a power meter. This way, current levels can be monitored. The doctor applies a non-weight-bearing plaster cast around the Webril, again leaving the shorting bar free. The apparatus will remain in place for about 12 weeks.

Patient care

How can you help promote successful healing? Usually, your patient will remain in the hospital for only a day or so after surgery. Make sure he understands that, throughout the 12 weeks of treatment, he must place *no* weight on his affected limb. Otherwise, the cathodes may break. Also, teach him how to apply the anode pad. He must apply a new pad at a new site every other day. Doing so will prevent skin irritation and promote conductivity. Tell your patient to choose a site that won't stress the anode lead wire, and to pull on the *button* when changing the pad, not on the wire itself.

At 4 and 8 week intervals after surgery, the patient will return to the doctor for a power-supply check. His skin around the cast will be inspected and the cast repaired.

The patient should report any signs and symptoms such as pain, burning, throbbing, and hot spots in the cast area (which may indicate thrombophlebitis) as well as an abrupt temperature elevation, chills, or purulent drainage (which may indicate osteomyelitis). The doctor will terminate treatment immediately if the patient has either of these conditions.

After 12 weeks, the doctor will remove the cast and the cathode wires and take X-rays. If the nonunion shows progress toward healing, he'll probably apply a weight-bearing cast around the fractured body part. If nonunion persists, he may have the patient ambulate using a cast or brace for a period of time. Then, if the bone still hasn't healed, he may reinsert cathode wires for another 12-week treatment.

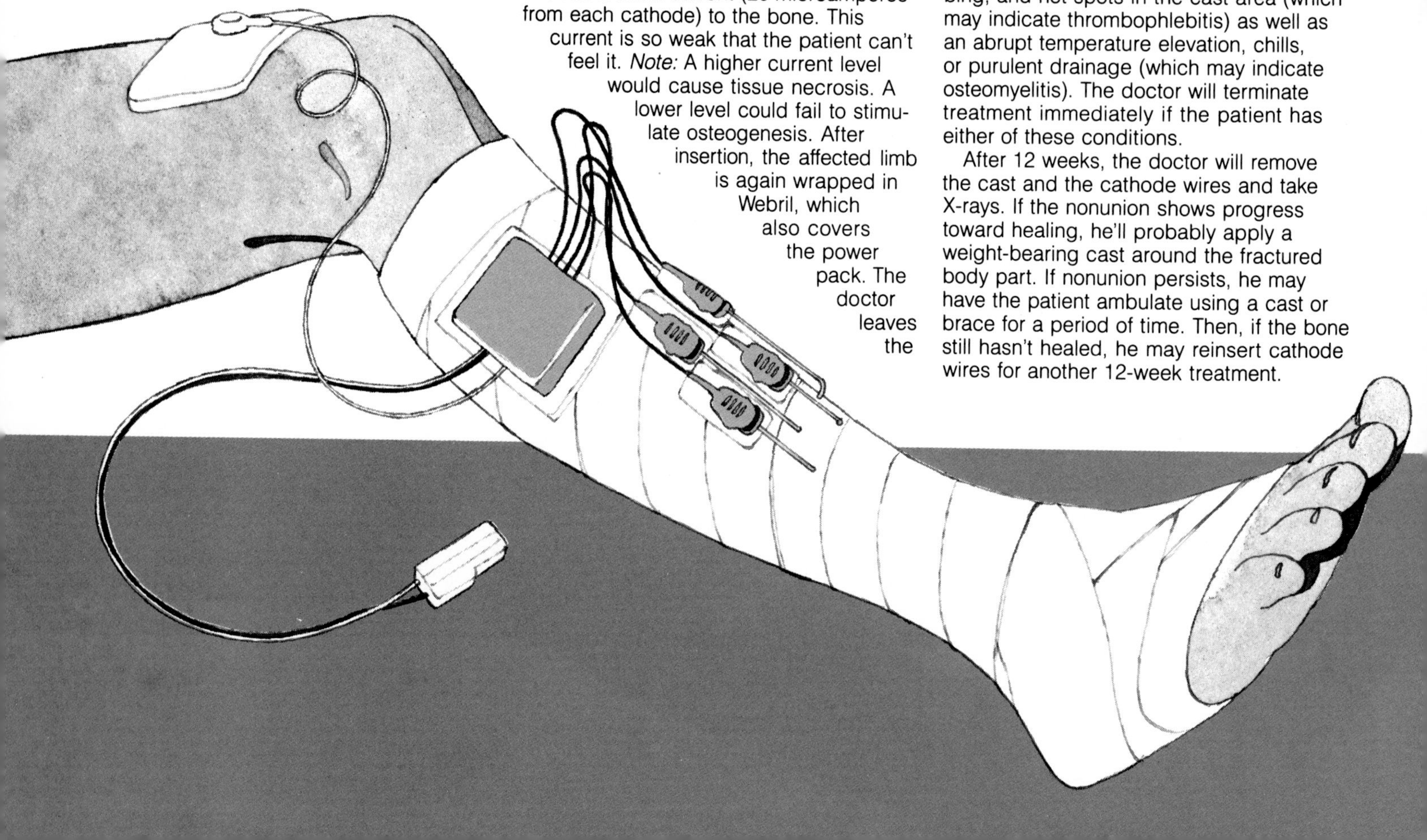

Zimmer® Direct Current Bone Growth Stimulator

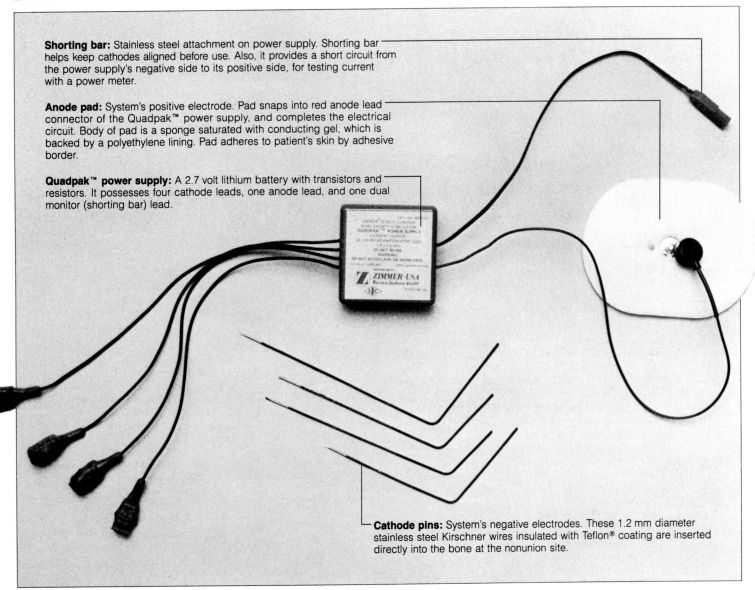

Shorting bar: Stainless steel attachment on power supply. Shorting bar helps keep cathodes aligned before use. Also, it provides a short circuit from the power supply's negative side to its positive side, for testing current with a power meter.

Anode pad: System's positive electrode. Pad snaps into red anode lead connector of the Quadpak™ power supply, and completes the electrical circuit. Body of pad is a sponge saturated with conducting gel, which is backed by a polyethylene lining. Pad adheres to patient's skin by adhesive border.

Quadpak™ power supply: A 2.7 volt lithium battery with transistors and resistors. It possesses four cathode leads, one anode lead, and one dual monitor (shorting bar) lead.

Cathode pins: System's negative electrodes. These 1.2 mm diameter stainless steel Kirschner wires insulated with Teflon® coating are inserted directly into the bone at the nonunion site.

INDICATIONS/CONTRAINDICATIONS

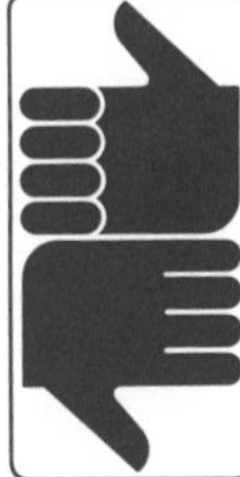

Should your patient undergo bone stimulation?

Electrical bone stimulation is indicated to treat fracture nonunions. However, bone stimulation is contraindicated when the patient has:

- a pathologic fracture, from a benign or malignant tumor.
- a congenital or developmental condition, such as osteogenesis imperfecta.
- an active systemic infection.
- an infection at a nonunion site or at adjacent bone and soft tissue sites.
- thrombophlebitis at adjacent soft tissue sites.
- an active bone-forming disease; for example, Paget's disease.
- sensitivity to nickel or chromium.
- pseudarthrosis.

External fixation

Suppose the doctor decides to apply an external fixation device to your patient's limb. What's your reaction? Are you apprehensive about caring for such a complicated piece of equipment? If so, we can help make it easier for you. Study the fixator illustration and read the care guidelines on the following pages. Then, you'll care for your patient with confidence.

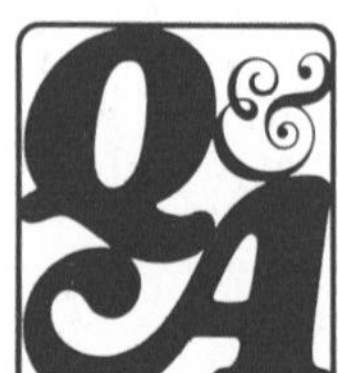

Understanding external fixation

To perform external fixation, the doctor surgically inserts pins through a fractured bone (usually passing the pins all the way through the patient's limb). He'll insert the pins both proximal and distal to the fracture site. He connects the pins to an external framework, which he tightens to align and immobilize the fracture. Within several weeks after surgery, the patient may be walking, with the help of ambulation aids. Following are some questions you may have about external fixation:

Question: When does the doctor apply an external fixation device?
Answer: He uses it to stabilize fractures that are difficult or impossible to immobilize with casts, traction, pins, or plates. For example, he'll use it for a patient who has:

- a massive open fracture, with extensive soft tissue damage.
- a comminuted fracture.
- multiple trauma, with a number of fractures in different body parts.
- an acutely infected open fracture.
- arthrodesis (surgical joint fusion).
- infected nonunion of a fracture.
- a bone graft.

With modification, some form of external fixation can be used on all extremities, the shoulder, and the pelvis.

Question: Why does the doctor use external fixation for the conditions listed above?
Answer: Consider the alternatives:

- Casting probably won't provide adequate visualization of an open wound or access for treatment of an open fracture. Any cast window would have to be so large that it would threaten fracture immobilization. Also, severe open fractures probably couldn't be casted.
- Traction would reduce and immobilize the area securely, but would place the patient at great risk of immobility complications. Also, traction might prolong the exudative stage of wound healing. And, with severe tissue damage, traction is contraindicated.
- Internal fixation might increase soft tissue damage because of the surgical procedure involved. Also, bone fragments in comminuted fractures won't provide adequate anchoring for a pin or plate.
- External fixation, by contrast, provides good wound visualization, access to the wound site, and reduced immobility complications.

Question: What kinds of external fixation devices may the doctor use?
Answer: Several standard models exist: These include the Hoffman, Anderson, Stader, and Haynes devices. In spite of variations, all of these function similarly and require similar nursing care. See the opposite page for details on the Zimmer® Hoffman-type external fixator.

Question: How does the doctor apply the external fixator?
Answer: With the patient under a general anesthetic in the operating room, the doctor makes an incision at each pin site. He positions the pins above and below the fracture. The number, position, and angle of pin insertion depend on the nature of the fracture. The number may range from four to twelve.

The doctor inserts each pin with a hand brace, because use of a power tool could cause bone damage and necrosis. After pin placement, he connects groups of pins to form units by attaching clamps and connecting rods to pin ends. He manipulates these units to align and reduce the fracture. Then, he connects the pin groups with adjustable rods. When these rods are shortened, they pull the pin groups toward each other and hold the pieces of bone in place by exerting pressure on them.

Question: How long does the device remain in place?
Answer: Of course, this varies from patient to patient. Usually, it's in place for a minimum of 4 weeks. For 1 to several weeks, the patient's limb must be suspended, to reduce swelling. After callus formation has begun and soft tissue injuries have healed, the doctor may remove the fixator and apply a brace or a cast. Or, he may leave the pins in place and apply a cast around them. The patient should avoid bearing weight on an injured limb until soft tissue wounds have completely healed and fracture healing is well under way. Even when the fracture is well stabilized, weight bearing may cause movement of the soft tissue against the pin. The doctor will decide whether the patient can bear weight on his limb or must use crutches for ambulation.

Learning about the Zimmer® Hoffman-type external fixator

Are you familiar with the separate components of an external fixator? Do you know what it looks like when it's assembled? If not, study these illustrations.

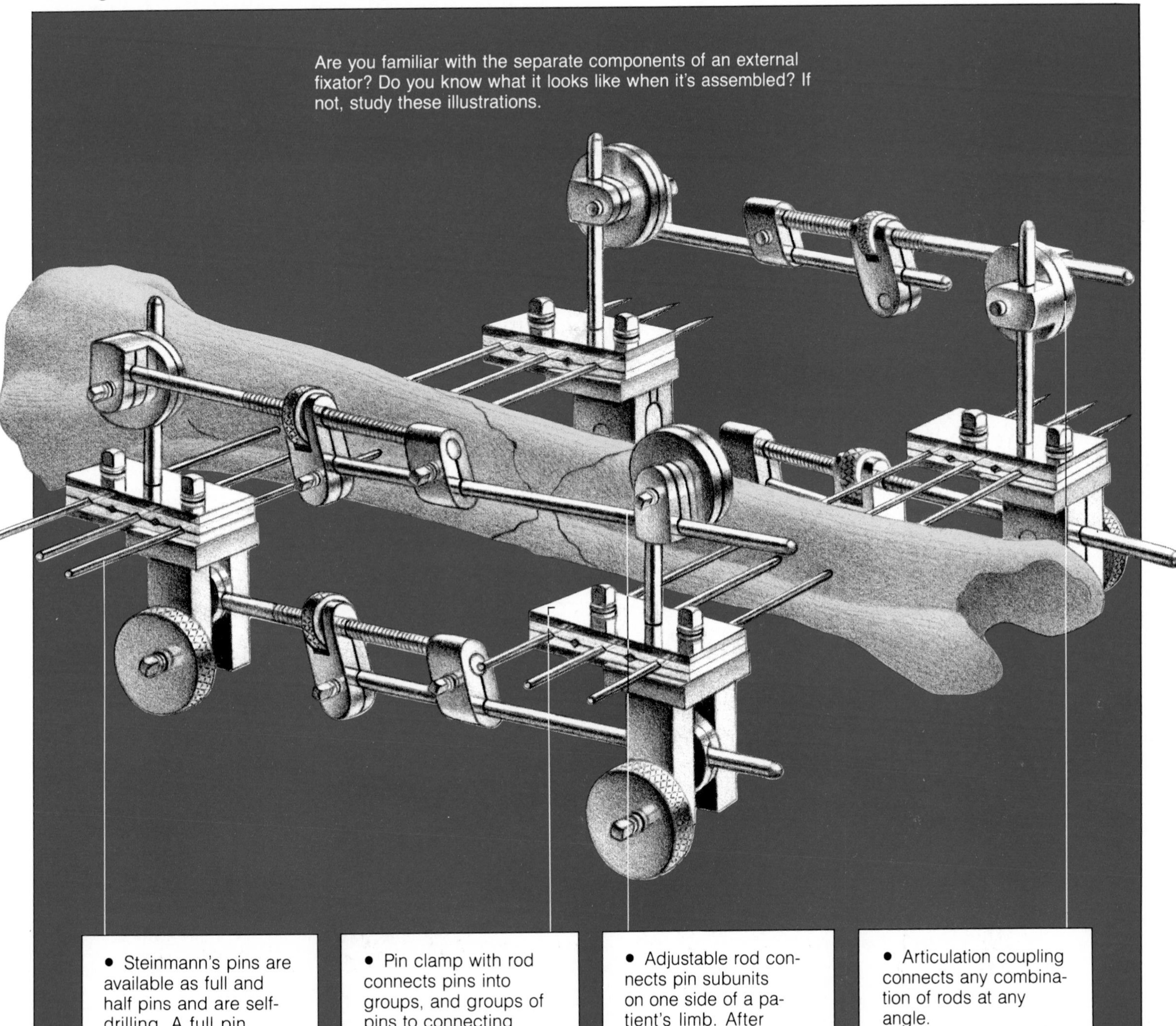

- Steinmann's pins are available as full and half pins and are self-drilling. A full pin (shown here) passes completely through the limb. A half pin passes through the bone, but through soft tissue on only one side of the affected limb.

- Pin clamp with rod connects pins into groups, and groups of pins to connecting rods.

- Adjustable rod connects pin subunits on one side of a patient's limb. After reduction, the rod's adjusted to provide compression and stabilize the fracture site.

- Articulation coupling connects any combination of rods at any angle.

External fixation

Providing postoperative care

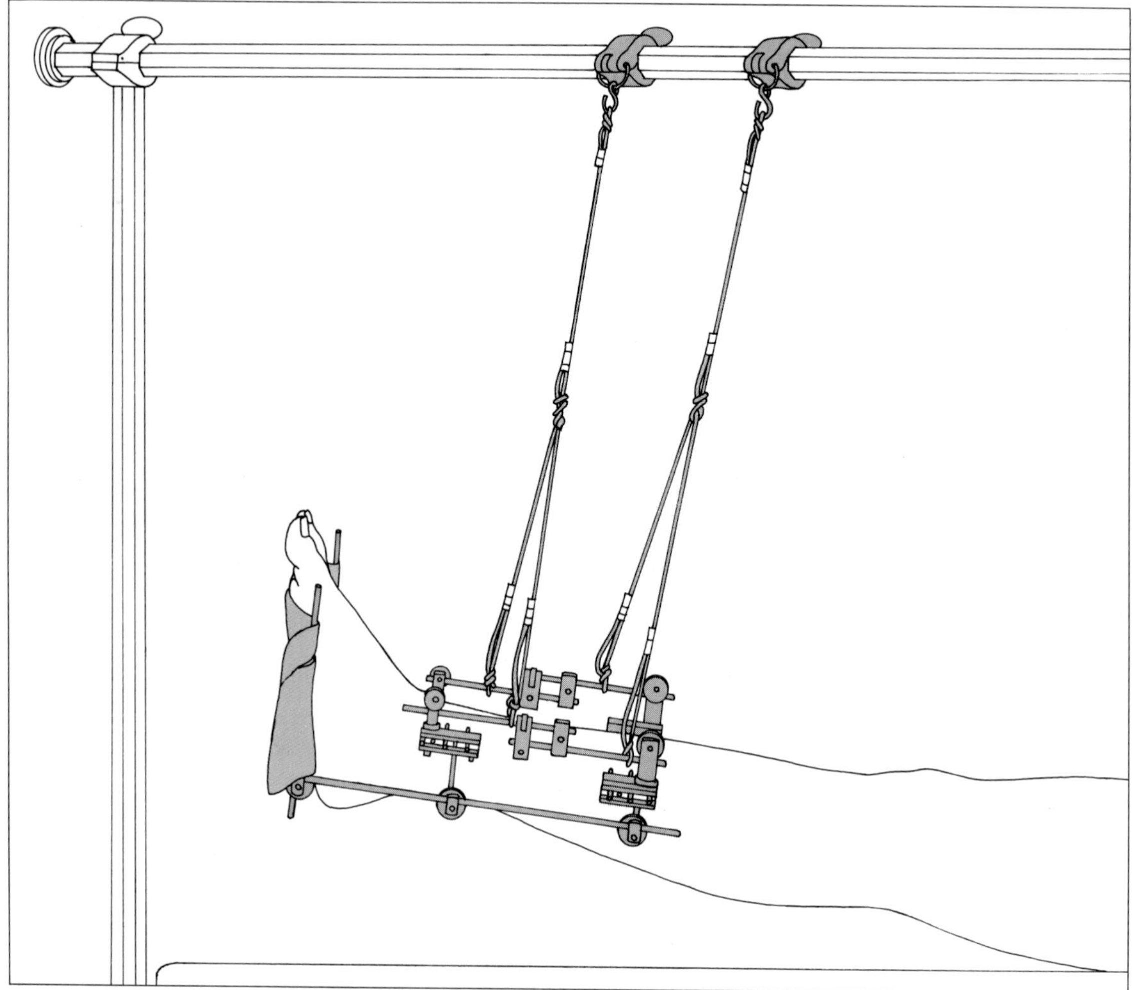

After your patient's had an external fixator applied, be sure to give him the following care:

- To reduce edema, elevate his limb above heart level. Elevation through suspension securely supports the leg, distributes limb weight evenly, and prevents pressure areas. Suspension also permits movement of joints adjacent to the injury.

To suspend his limb, attach traction rope around the device's external frame. Tie the rope to an overhead bed frame. Or, use S hooks to attach the rope, as shown here. You may place supportive pads and protective dressings around the patient's limb.

To prevent footdrop, support the patient's foot securely. The doctor may permit release of the limb from suspension for brief periods of mobility.

- If your patient has an open wound, provide wound care using strict aseptic technique. Avoid touching pins and rods while performing care. If you do, change gloves immediately before continuing.

Change the hard-to-reach dressings under the rods after you've changed other dressings. Use a sterile tongue depressor to manipulate dressings, as necessary. Once you've positioned a dressing around a pin, don't move it around, or you may contaminate the wound.

- Perform pin care, as ordered, at least twice a day in the early postoperative period. Later, it may be performed only once each day. Follow the procedure described on page 84, keeping in mind the information given at right. As soon as possible, transfer pin care responsibility to your patient.
- Provide analgesic medication, as ordered. Because the fixator stabilizes the fracture securely, the patient usually requires only oral analgesics.
- As soon as your patient is oriented and appears receptive, begin the patient teaching outlined on the next page.
- When the swelling has begun to decrease (within a few days to a few weeks after the fracture), you may remove the dressings, as ordered. Begin prescribed active or passive range-of-motion exercises of adjacent joints.

Important: Don't remove the foot support until the patient demonstrates strong dorsiflexion.

Within 4 weeks, elevating the limb on pillows rather than by suspension may be sufficient.

Performing pin care

While performing pin care, examine the skin around the pins for skin tautness (tension), pain, tenderness, and redness from inflammation and infection. Skin tension, in addition to being painful, hinders thorough cleansing and predisposes the skin to necrosis and infection. If tension is severe, the doctor may incise the skin. If that doesn't help, more frequent pin care or extensive debridement may be necessary.

While you're examining your patient's skin, note any crusted serous drainage around the pin site. Gently remove this crust during pin care, to prevent it from obstructing wound drainage. Note any signs of pin looseness, such as increased or purulent drainage, or the pin turning in the skin.

When you provide pin care, avoid prodding the patient's skin. Doing so may cause additional pain, and skin abrasion leading to infection. Cleanse the pins on one side of the patient's leg, working proximally to distally. Then, cleanse the pins on the other side of the patient's leg.

After performing pin care, you may wipe the external frame with a sterile cloth moistened with sterile water. Then, cover the pin ends with pin caps, corks, or rubber plugs from Vacutainer® blood sampling vials.

PATIENT TEACHING

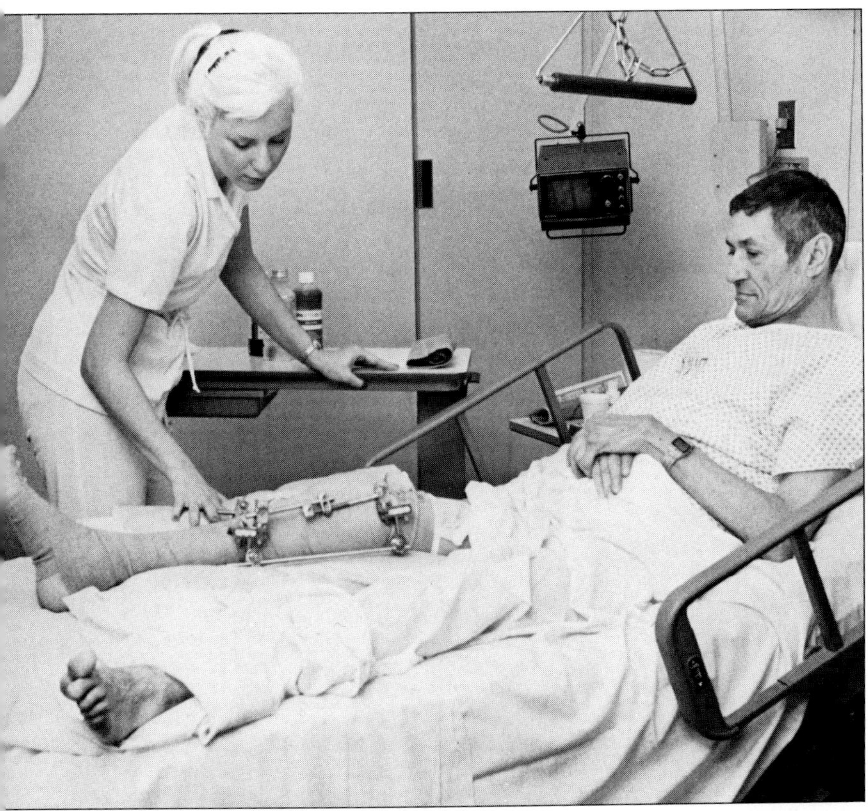

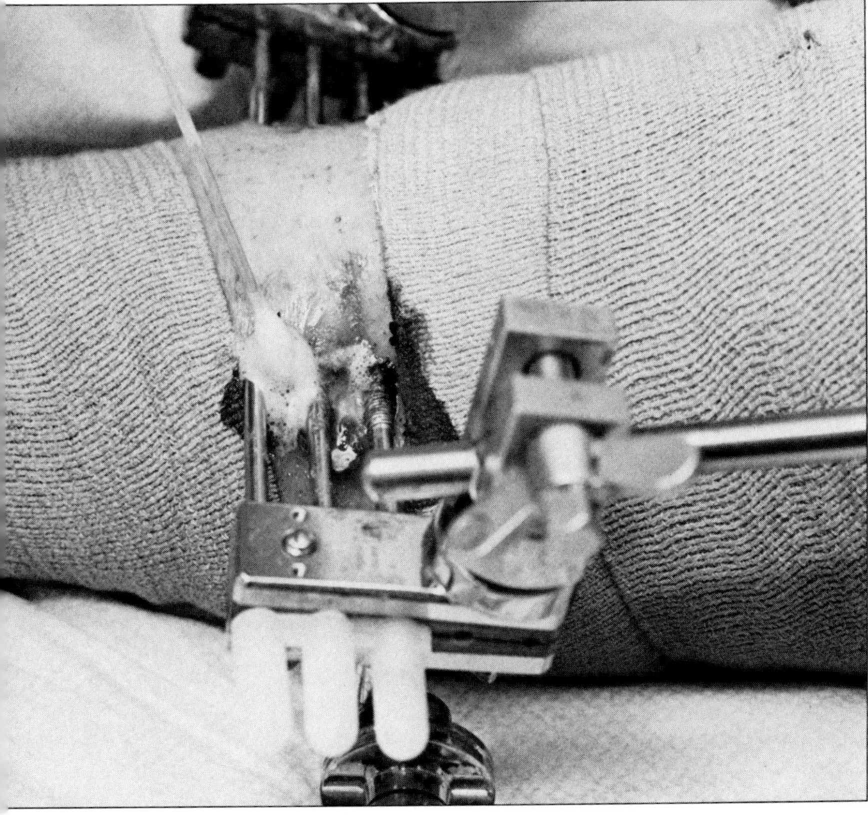

Teaching your patient about external fixation

Because external fixation is usually carried out on an emergency basis following a traumatic accident, patient preparation can't be extensive. Of course, you'll obtain a patient history, and perform a thorough assessment, paying particular attention to your patient's neurovascular status.

After surgery, find an early opportunity (when your patient's fully conscious and relatively pain-free) to instruct him in these important points:

- Your patient may be upset by the appearance of his limb with the equipment in place. Allow him to express his feelings, and provide reassurance that he'll be wearing the device temporarily (even though he may wear it for as long as a year).
- Explain the purpose of external fixation. It stabilizes the fracture securely so the patient has less discomfort and can ambulate early in his recovery period.
- Tell your patient that his nerves and blood vessels have been damaged during his injury. Describe a routine neurovascular check. Warn your patient to notify you of any numbness, tingling, skin color change, or loss of motion in his toes or fingers. Instruct him in the importance of good body alignment to prevent further circulatory impairment.
- Explain how venous blood pooling can impair healing and lead to complications. Tell him that's why you're keeping his leg elevated.
- Emphasize the importance of early mobility. Show him how he can lift his affected limb by grasping the external frame. Depending on his injury, the external fixator may enable him to walk within a few weeks, with the help of an ambulation aid. Teach him muscle-strengthening and range-of-motion exercises for joints adjacent to the injury, and for his unaffected extremity.
- Teach your patient the importance of regularly scheduled aseptic dressing changes.
- Explain that the contact of his soft tissue with the pins produces serous drainage. This drainage is clear, colorless, and odorless, and will dry and crust around the pin sites. Drainage may increase with increasing mobility.

Tell your patient how routine skin care (two to three times each day) around the pins helps prevent infection at pin sites. Show him how to perform pin care. As soon as possible, have him or a family member take over pin care.

- Describe to the patient the early signs of infection: redness, warmth, swelling, tenderness, and drainage. Infection may cause pins to become loose and need replacement.
- Explain that loose pins impair bone alignment and immobilization. Tell him to check the device often for signs of pin loosening, such as increased or purulent drainage, or the pin turning in his skin.
- Warn your patient against tampering with the clamps or nuts. Only the doctor can adjust the fixator.
- Your patient may require further surgery for skin debridement or grafting. If so, prepare him for these procedures as necessary.

Arthroscopy

Why is the knee such a difficult joint to assess properly? Well, for starters, its complex construction contains more ligaments and cartilage than any other joint. Moreover, each ligament or segment of cartilage is vulnerable to damage from disease or injury. To understand more about the knee's anatomy, study the illustration at right.

In addition to understanding knee anatomy, you should be acquainted with diagnostic procedures. One of the most commonly used is arthroscopy. Read on to find out specifics about the arthroscopy procedure, as well as surgical repair that can be performed using this technique.

Commonly injured knee tissues

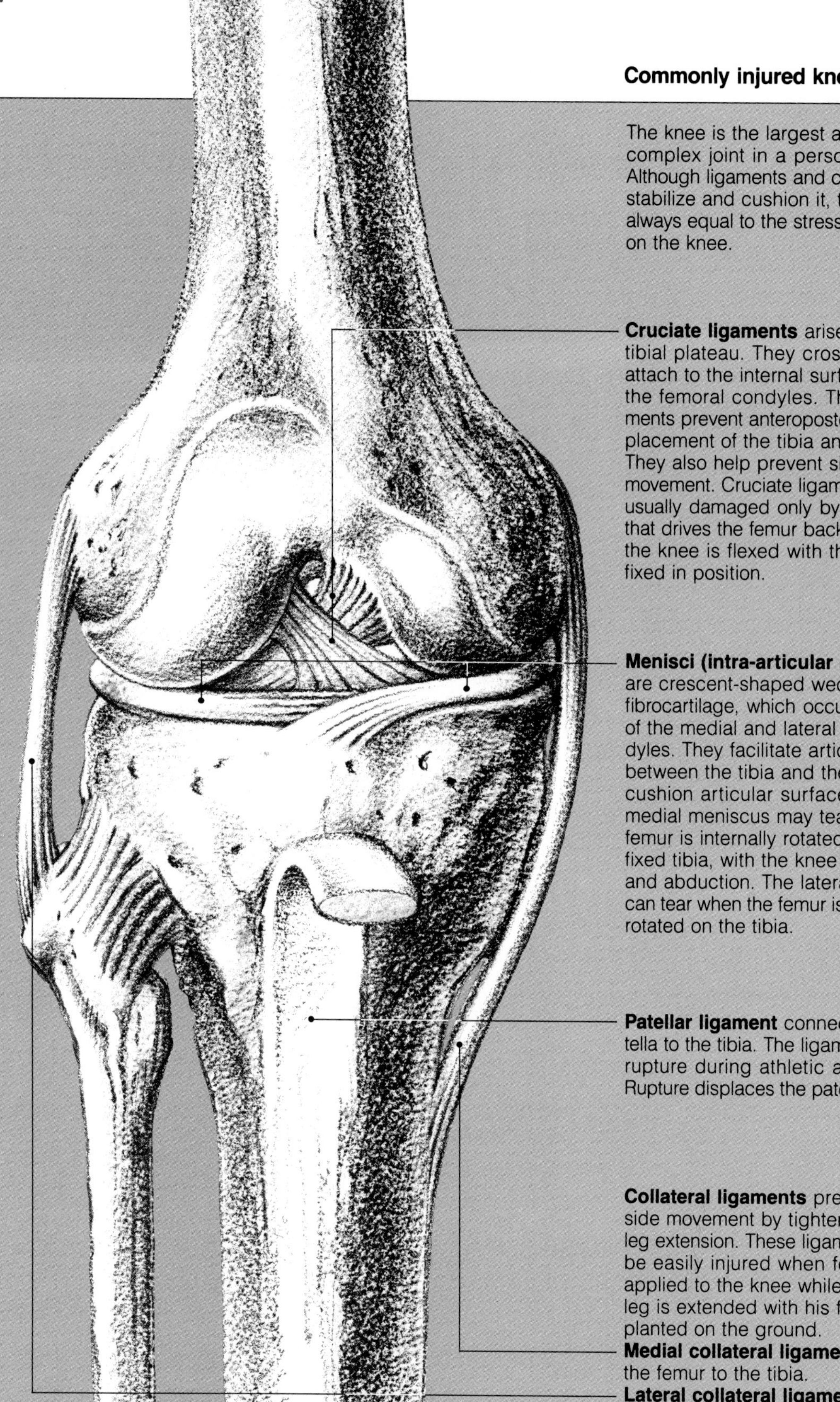

The knee is the largest and most complex joint in a person's body. Although ligaments and cartilage stabilize and cushion it, these aren't always equal to the stresses placed on the knee.

Cruciate ligaments arise from the tibial plateau. They cross and then attach to the internal surfaces of the femoral condyles. These ligaments prevent anteroposterior displacement of the tibia and the femur. They also help prevent side-to-side movement. Cruciate ligaments are usually damaged only by violent force that drives the femur backward while the knee is flexed with the tibia fixed in position.

Menisci (intra-articular cartilage) are crescent-shaped wedges of fibrocartilage, which occur in margins of the medial and lateral tibial condyles. They facilitate articulation between the tibia and the femur, and cushion articular surfaces. The medial meniscus may tear when the femur is internally rotated on the fixed tibia, with the knee in flexion and abduction. The lateral meniscus can tear when the femur is externally rotated on the tibia.

Patellar ligament connects the patella to the tibia. The ligament may rupture during athletic activity. Rupture displaces the patella upward.

Collateral ligaments prevent side-to-side movement by tightening during leg extension. These ligaments may be easily injured when force is applied to the knee while a person's leg is extended with his foot firmly planted on the ground.
Medial collateral ligament connects the femur to the tibia.
Lateral collateral ligament connects the femur and the fibula.

Learning about arthroscopy

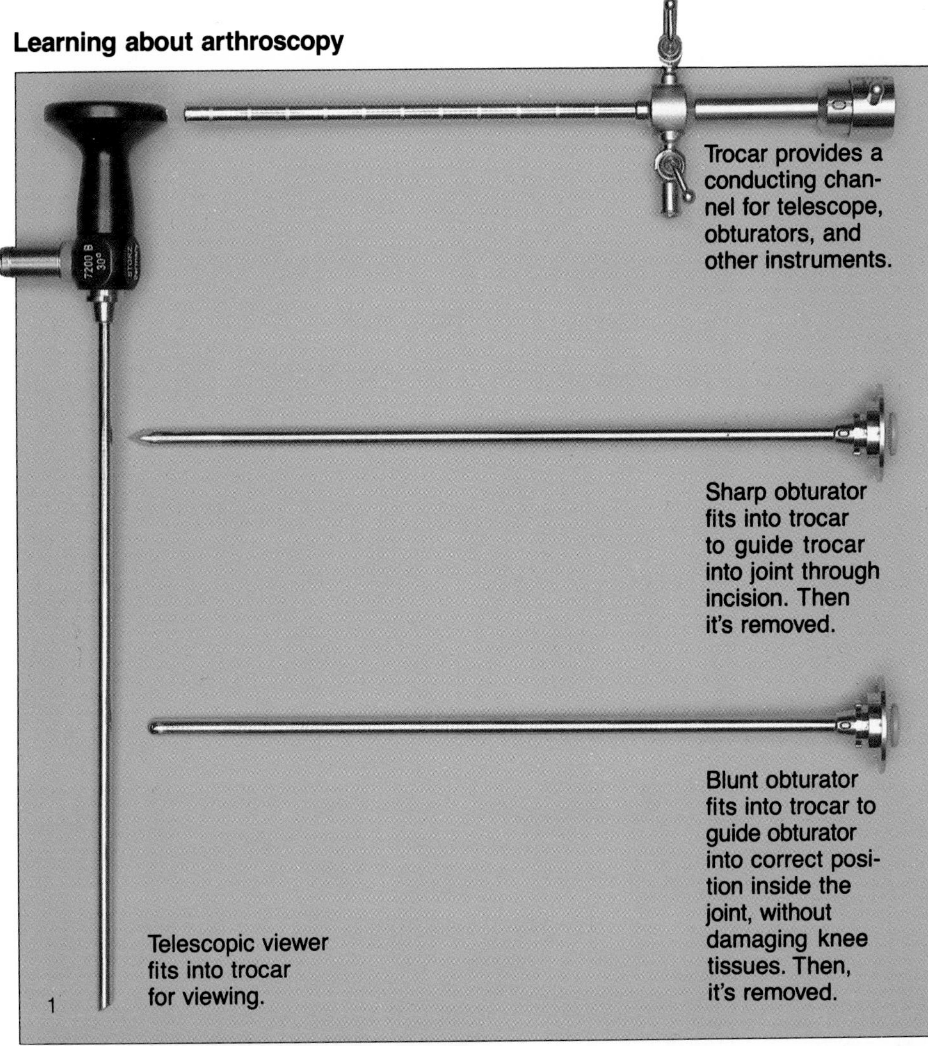
Trocar provides a conducting channel for telescope, obturators, and other instruments.
Sharp obturator fits into trocar to guide trocar into joint through incision. Then it's removed.
Blunt obturator fits into trocar to guide obturator into correct position inside the joint, without damaging knee tissues. Then, it's removed.
Telescopic viewer fits into trocar for viewing.
1

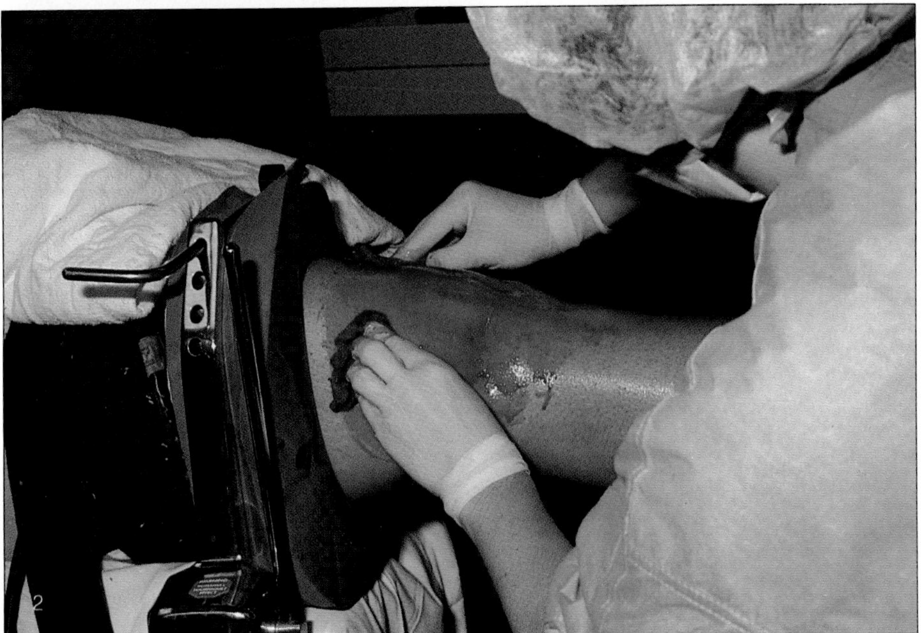
2

When a patient has an acute or chronic knee problem, the doctor has several diagnostic tools at his disposal. First, of course, he'll take a careful history. Then, he'll assess knee range of motion, performing the special maneuvers shown on pages 36 and 37, as well as any other indicated maneuvers. He'll probably obtain X-rays from anterior, posterior, and lateral views. Also, he might remove synovial fluid by needle aspiration, for testing.

However, if these procedures don't provide an accurate diagnosis, the doctor may order either arthrography or arthroscopy.

Arthrography is the X-ray examination of a joint following injection of radiopaque dye. During the test, the doctor instills air, along with the dye, into the patient's joint. Both the air and dye will be resorbed in time; but until they are, the patient may hear unusual noises in her knee. The only contraindication for this procedure is allergy to an iodine-based dye. Consider arthrography strictly a diagnostic procedure, most useful in diagnosing conditions of the posterior and middle third of the medial meniscus.

Arthroscopy is the visual examination of the joint interior, using a fiberoptic lens instrument (see photo 1) attached to a light source. Although arthroscopy originated as a diagnostic procedure, doctors now use it for treatment as well. Because arthroscopy combines both functions, and involves very little knee trauma, its use is increasing. However, it's contraindicated for a patient with a bleeding disorder.

Diagnostic uses

Arthroscopy's particularly useful in diagnosing the following conditions: meniscal disorders, cruciate ligament injuries, collateral ligament rupture, developmental joint changes, degenerative joint conditions, intra-articular tumors, acute sepsis, acute knee conditions, rheumatoid or tubercular synovitis, and problems associated with synovial effusion.

Surgical repair

The doctor can perform any of the following surgeries using the arthroscope and supplementary instruments:

- excising meniscal tears or a meniscus
- removing loose foreign bodies and adhesions
- biopsy of synovial disorders
- partial synovectomy
- draining of a septic joint
- smoothing knee cartilage irregularities from chondromalacia patellae or arthritis.

In the operating room

The doctor may perform arthroscopy with the patient under general, spinal, or local anesthesia. To control bleeding, the doctor will apply a tourniquet to the patient's leg above her knee. Then, he'll position the knee so it's flexed at a 90° angle. He'll prepare the skin with an antimicrobial solution, such as povidone-iodine solution [2]. Just before inserting the arthro-

Arthroscopy

Learning about arthroscopy continued

scope, he'll insert a needle above the kneecap to fill the knee with normal saline solution [3]. Saline solution distends the knee, for better visualization. Next, he'll make a small incision, 5 to 6 millimeters long, for arthroscope insertion. A common arthroscope insertion point is the anterior joint line, below the patella's apex, either medial or lateral to the patellar tendon [4]. After insertion, he may advance the arthroscope up under the patella. When the arthroscope's inserted and positioned, the doctor will connect it to a light system for viewing [5]. He'll also set up an irrigating system, for flushing the knee.

If, after examining the knee joint's interior, the doctor decides to repair some part of the joint, he can replace part of the diagnostic arthroscope instrument with an operating

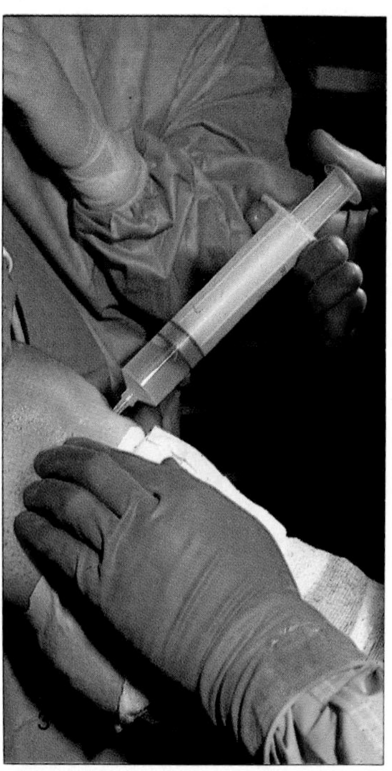
3

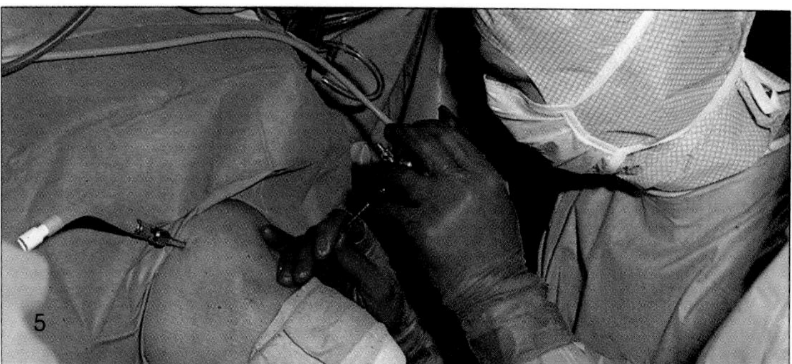
5

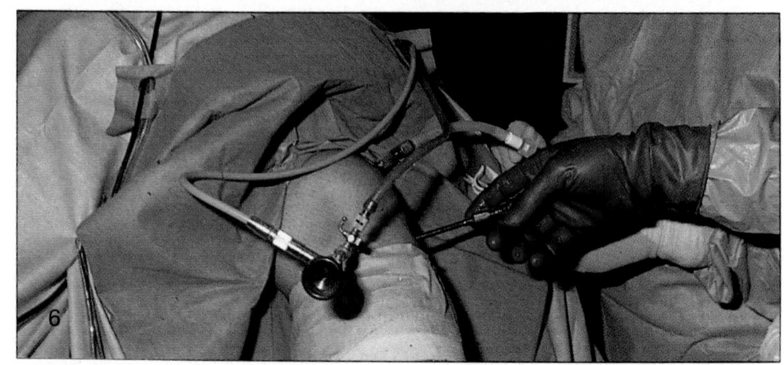
6

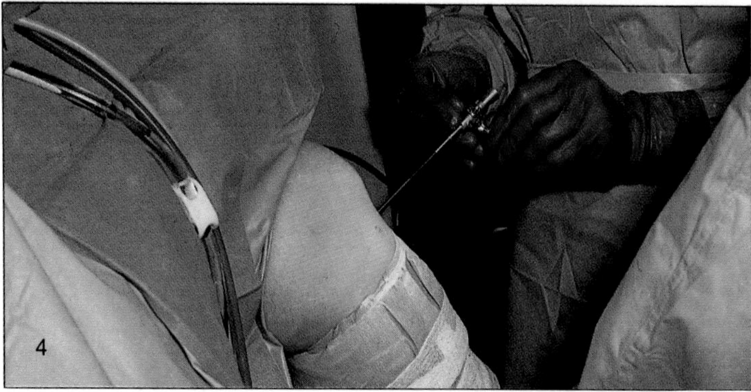
4

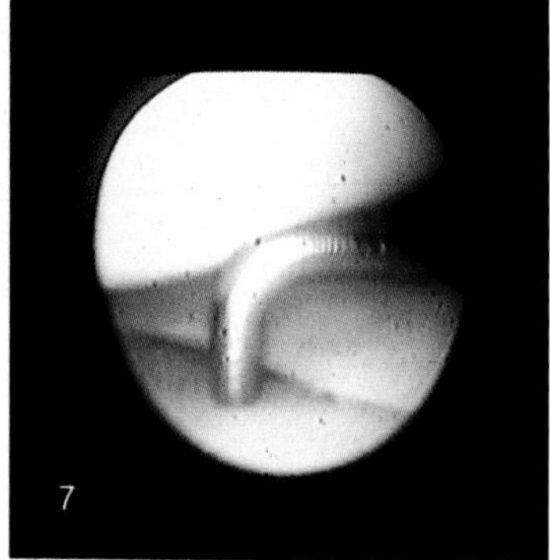
7

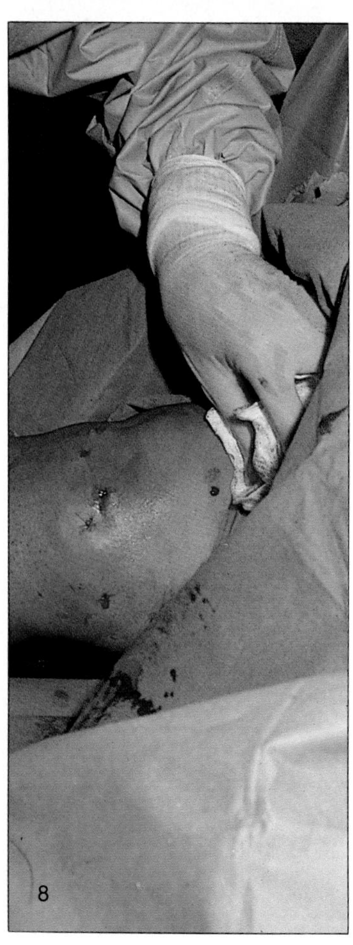
8

attachment. If necessary, he can insert additional instruments, such as hooked scissors or a probe, through a second incision site [6]. The arthroscopic view of the knee joint's interior [7: medial meniscus held by probe] can be projected on a screen.

After surgery

After surgery, the doctor may flush the cavity with saline solution. Then, he'll withdraw the instrument. He also may suture the incision sites, which usually require no more than an adhesive bandage strip to cover them [8]. He may order the knee wrapped with an elastic roller bandage.

After recovering from the general or spinal anesthetic (if used), the patient may return home to recuperate. Walking and ordinary physical activities are allowed immediately and sports activities are allowed within 3 days. Most patients return to normal life within a few days, and require no special physical therapy. Some experience slight joint stiffness for 2 to 3 weeks. Athletes usually resume full athletic activity within 3 weeks.

Complications

Arthroscopy entails few complications. Most are anesthesia-related. But, infection may occur, and occasionally, hemarthrosis. Temporary saphenous nerve damage (though rare) may also be a problem. Instrument breakage, also rare, causes the most serious complication. If a piece of instrument breaks off and remains inside the knee, the doctor must perform immediate arthrotomy (surgical opening of the knee) to remove it.

Suppose arthroscopy leads to no definitive diagnosis. The doctor may then resort to arthrotomy. Because arthrotomy's an involved surgical procedure, requiring a general anesthetic and lengthy convalescence, arthroscopy almost always precedes arthrotomy.

Reconstructive surgery

Does your orthopedic patient have a chronic degenerative joint disease, such as arthritis? Then, you'll want to be familiar with the surgical interventions that can help to relieve your patient's pain and restore joint motion.

Familiarize yourself with the charts on the following pages to learn about common forms of conservative knee and hip surgery. Then, read the detailed information on *total* knee and hip replacement, which may be required when conservative measures fail. This way, you'll be better prepared to give the necessary pre- and postop care.

Common knee-repair surgery

Debridement and synovectomy
Two procedures performed together to relieve pain by excising the synovial membrane and removing diseased cartilage, soft tissue, and bony enlargement from joints. The illustration below shows debridement.

Indication
Persistent synovitis

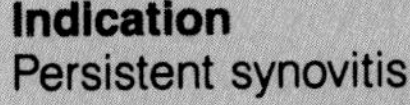

Postoperative considerations
- Patient may have a compression bandage in place or wear an immobilizer.
- Position knee in extension when it's not being exercised.
- Exercises include quadriceps-setting, beginning 1 or 2 days postop, and flexion, beginning 1 week postop.

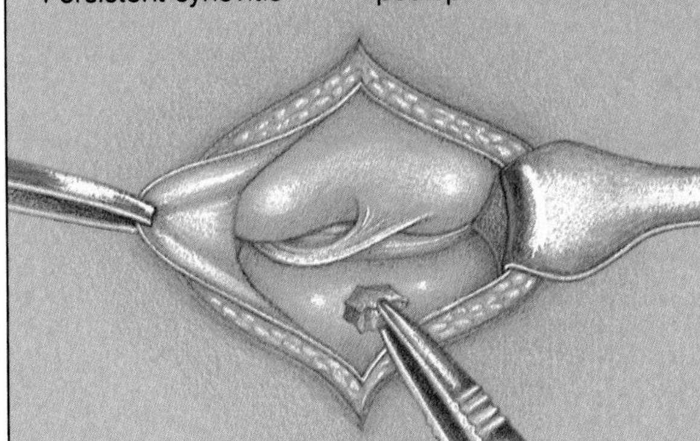

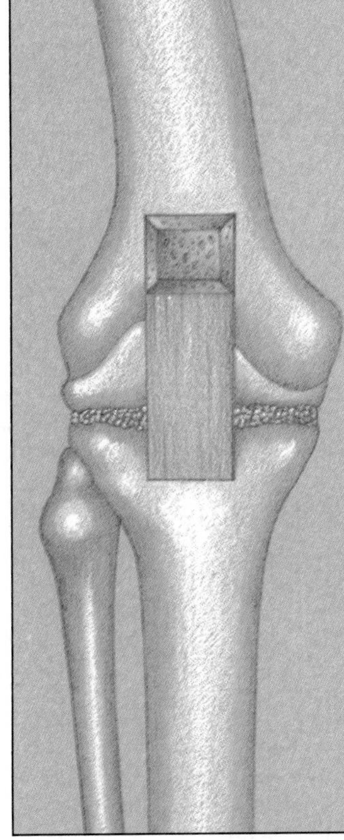

Arthrodesis
Surgical fusion of knee joint to eliminate motion and thereby relieve pain. Involves bone graft, as shown.

Indication
Complete failure of knee prosthesis

Postoperative considerations
- Patient usually returns from surgery wearing a long leg cast.
- Four weeks postop, the patient may begin weight-bearing ambulation, using a cast with a walker-heel attached.

Osteotomy
Surgical removal of a piece of bone to realign bone and shift weight-bearing stress away from a worn area

Indication
Degenerative joint disease, when patient is young and has one healthy articular surface

Postoperative considerations
- Patient usually returns from surgery in a long leg cast.
- Bloody drainage may stain the cast for the first 48 hours.
- Crutch-walking may begin on the third or fourth day postop.

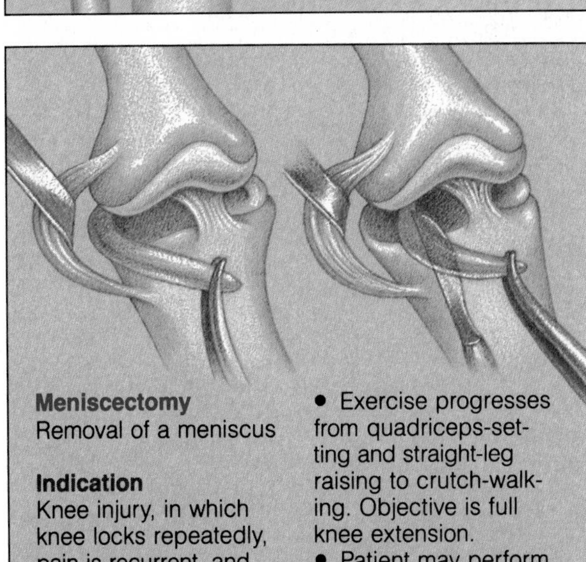

Meniscectomy
Removal of a meniscus

Indication
Knee injury, in which knee locks repeatedly, pain is recurrent, and joint motion is limited

Postoperative considerations
- Dressings range from incision coverings to full leg compression dressings with posterior plaster splints.
- Exercise progresses from quadriceps-setting and straight-leg raising to crutch-walking. Objective is full knee extension.
- Patient may perform non-weight-bearing ambulation on crutches 3 days after surgery.
- Patient may walk without crutches 10 days after surgery, although some doctors prefer use of crutches for 6 weeks.

Reconstructive surgery

Types of total knee prostheses

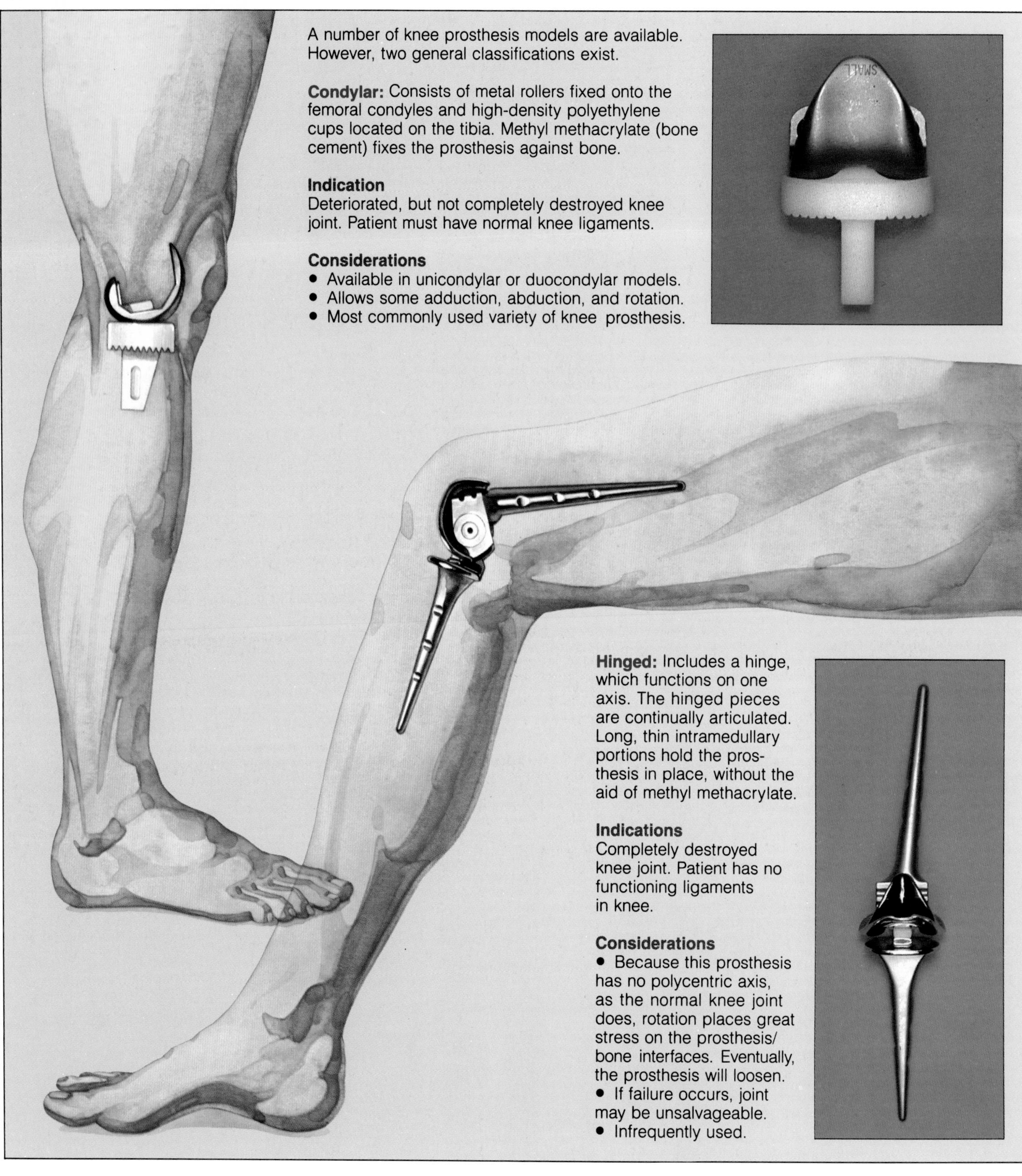

A number of knee prosthesis models are available. However, two general classifications exist.

Condylar: Consists of metal rollers fixed onto the femoral condyles and high-density polyethylene cups located on the tibia. Methyl methacrylate (bone cement) fixes the prosthesis against bone.

Indication

Deteriorated, but not completely destroyed knee joint. Patient must have normal knee ligaments.

Considerations

- Available in unicondylar or duocondylar models.
- Allows some adduction, abduction, and rotation.
- Most commonly used variety of knee prosthesis.

Hinged: Includes a hinge, which functions on one axis. The hinged pieces are continually articulated. Long, thin intramedullary portions hold the prosthesis in place, without the aid of methyl methacrylate.

Indications

Completely destroyed knee joint. Patient has no functioning ligaments in knee.

Considerations

- Because this prosthesis has no polycentric axis, as the normal knee joint does, rotation places great stress on the prosthesis/bone interfaces. Eventually, the prosthesis will loosen.
- If failure occurs, joint may be unsalvageable.
- Infrequently used.

INDICATIONS/CONTRAINDICATIONS

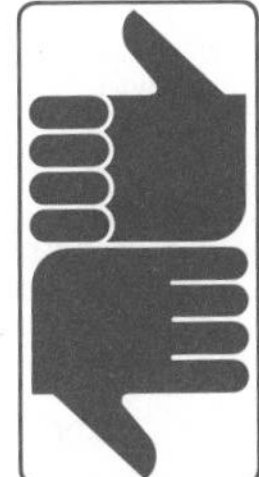

When does your patient need total knee replacement?

Total knee replacement is performed to relieve severe pain, joint contracture, and swelling in a patient who would be ambulatory if it weren't for his knee disorder. Usually it's performed after more conservative measures have failed.

In most cases, total knee replacement works best for older patients. Prosthesis life hasn't yet been accurately determined. But, since they've been in use for 15 years (so it's known they'll last at least that long), 10 to 15 years is the usual estimate. As you can see, a younger patient might require several prosthesis replacements, especially since the more active the person is, the faster the prosthesis will probably wear out.

Total knee replacement may be used for a patient with:

- a disease such as osteoarthritis or rheumatoid arthritis.
- a tumor.
- a condition such as varus/valgus deformity, flexion/extension contracture, or a stiff or fused joint.
- a serious injury such as a severe intra-articular fracture.

Total knee replacement *won't* be used for a patient with:

- a current infection or history of infection in the affected leg.
- a knee with *major* bone loss.
- a knee with poor muscle function.
- a knee with flexion contracture greater than 60°.
- a knee with varus/valgus deformity greater than 40°.
- a history of phlebitis in the affected leg.

Preparing your patient for total knee replacement

Preop preparation involves a thorough nursing history and assessment, standard lab studies, and blood typing and crossmatching. Because a knee-replacement patient may take a lot of aspirin, he'll require lab studies to determine blood coagulability.

Does your patient take other medication regularly? If he's taking antihypertensive drugs or corticosteroids, dosages should be adjusted during the immediate preop, surgical, and postop periods. Administer oral antibiotics as ordered pre- and postoperatively, but administer antibiotics *I.V.* immediately before, during, and after surgery.

Also, you must scrub and shave your patient's affected leg as ordered (see the photostory on the following page). For complete details on preoperative nursing care, see the NURSING PHOTOBOOK CARING FOR SURGICAL PATIENTS.

Patient teaching

In addition to physical preparation, your patient needs to understand the facts about knee replacement. First, explain its purpose. Although knee replacement should diminish his pain greatly, it probably won't eliminate it. However, the prosthesis should increase joint stability, improve limb alignment, and allow greater knee motion and better ambulation.

Don't forget to mention prosthesis limitations. Your patient needs to understand them thoroughly, so he'll make an effort to minimize wear on his prosthesis. Help your patient realize that, although he'll regain at least 90% knee function, his knee won't be a normal healthy one. He should never attempt to use it in activities that place great stress on the joint; for example, football. Excessive wear on his prosthesis may result in surgical replacement, or arthrodesis.

Providing proper nutrition

If your orthopedic patient will be undergoing surgery (or if he has a fracture or a dislocation), make sure he's receiving the nutrition he needs. To ensure proper bone healing, he needs a well-balanced diet containing the full adult requirements of protein, calcium, and vitamins C and D.

What types of foods should you include in your patient's diet? That depends on your patient's general condition, as well as his food preferences, eating habits, and any allergies he may have.

Make sure that at least one third of your patient's protein requirement comes from complete proteins found in meat, milk, cheese, and eggs. Milkshakes, pudding, and nuts provide high-caloric, high-protein between-meal supplements. Also, see that your patient receives adequate amounts of calcium—at least three servings a day of milk, cheese, and eggs. Keep in mind that calcium helps form strong, hard bones.

In addition to protein and calcium, your patient needs adequate vitamin C, from foods such as citrus fruits and juices, potatoes, and cabbage. This vitamin's essential to wound and bone healing because it helps form collagen. As you'll remember, collagen aids in blood vessel and tissue repair. Provide your patient with at least one serving of food rich in vitamin C daily.

Vitamin D is particularly important for orthopedic patients. Why? Because this vitamin helps transfer calcium from ingested food to the bloodstream. It also aids in bone calcification. As you probably know, sunlight is the best source of vitamin D. But if you can't get your patient out on a sunny balcony or terrace, include adequate amounts of eggs, fish oil, and vitamin D-enriched milk and margarine in his diet.

When planning and implementing your patient's diet, remember these important points:

- Consider any chewing problems your patient has; for example, from poor teeth or gums, halo traction confinement, or a jaw immobilizer. Perhaps he's not coordinated enough to feed himself, so you'll have to feed him.
- Closely monitor your patient's fluid intake and output. If the patient perspires heavily, has excess drainage, or his respiratory rate increases, increase his fluid intake accordingly.
- Continually assess and reassess your patient's nutritional status. Make minor adjustments in his diet, as needed, to prevent constipation. For example, use bulk foods such as whole wheat bread, apples, and celery. Give prune juice for its natural laxative effect. Also, make sure your patient drinks six to eight glasses of water daily. Suggest to the doctor a change to pain medications that don't promote constipation. Obtain an order for stool softeners, as necessary.
- Have your patient drink cranberry juice to acidify his urine and prevent calculi.
- Offer your patient a choice of five small meals daily instead of three larger ones.
- Document all your care in your nurses' notes.

Finally, be sure to consult your hospital's dietary department for assistance in planning and implementing your patient's diet, as necessary. Arrange for a visit from a staff dietition. And, before your patient's discharged, arrange for the dietary consultant to talk to your patient and his family about a diet plan for use at home.

Reconstructive surgery

Performing a sterile orthopedic prep and wrap

1 *If your patient's scheduled for knee surgery, the doctor may order sterile orthopedic preps and wraps performed twice before surgery. If the doctor's ordered you to shave the surgical area, you may do so just before the second prep. Follow the procedure given in the* NURSING PHOTOBOOK CARING FOR SURGICAL PATIENTS.

Perform the sterile orthopedic prep and wrap as shown here:

Obtain the following sterile equipment: two metal basins, gauze sponges, 3" roller gauze bandage, towels or drapes, and gloves. Also, obtain antimicrobial solution, nonallergenic tape, sterile water, and a plastic trash bag. Open the plastic trash bag. Place it near your working area for disposing of used sponges. Explain the procedure to the patient. Tell her that the surgical area will remain wrapped until surgery, to keep it as clean as possible.

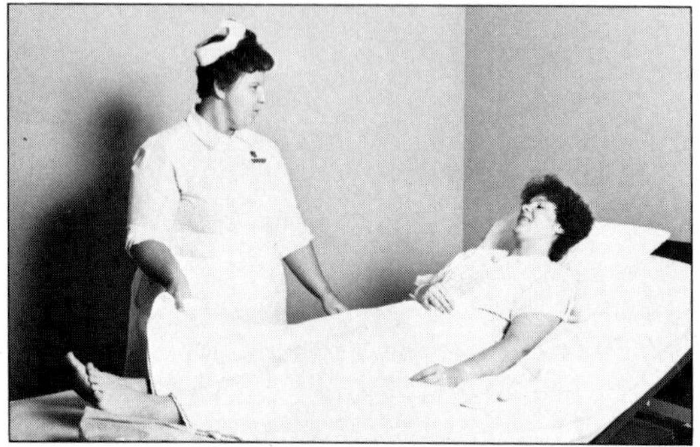

2 Next, wash your hands thoroughly. Using strict aseptic technique, place a sterile towel or drape on a clean, dry surface. Unwrap all sterile equipment and drop it onto this sterile field.

Pour the antimicrobial solution into one basin, and sterile water into the other. Take care not to contaminate the sterile field by splashing liquid.

Grasp a sterile drape by its edges and ask your patient to raise the leg you'll be prepping. Then, place the sterile drape under it, as shown below left. Ask the patient to lower her leg on the drape.

Put on sterile gloves. Then, drape the patient to expose her leg, as shown below right. Keep the rest of her body covered.

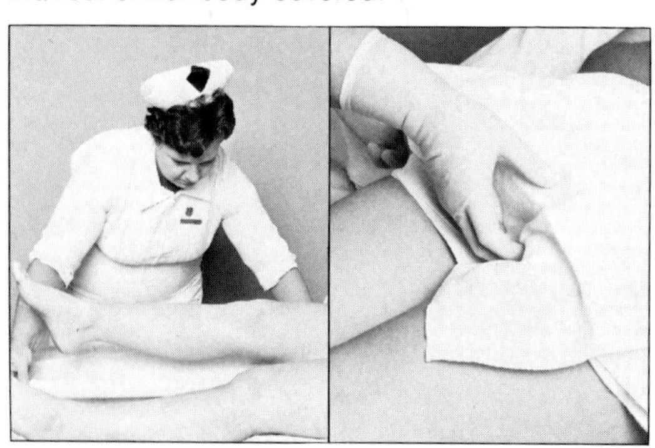

3 Dip a sterile sponge in the antimicrobial solution. Using a circular motion, begin to scrub the patient's knee, as shown below. Start at the proposed incision site and work outward. Remember to create friction as you work, for more thorough cleansing. After 3 minutes, discard the sponge and continue scrubbing with a clean one. Repeat this procedure (using a clean sponge every 3 minutes) until you've scrubbed the surgical area for a total of 10 minutes.

If you're using a potentially irritating antimicrobial scrub (instead of an antimicrobial solution), or if the orthopedic wrap will be in place overnight, reduce the risk of skin irritation by rinsing the patient's leg with sterile water. To do so, dip a gauze sponge in the sterile water, and gently wash the skin you've just cleansed. Then, to prevent chapping, dry the skin with another sterile sponge.

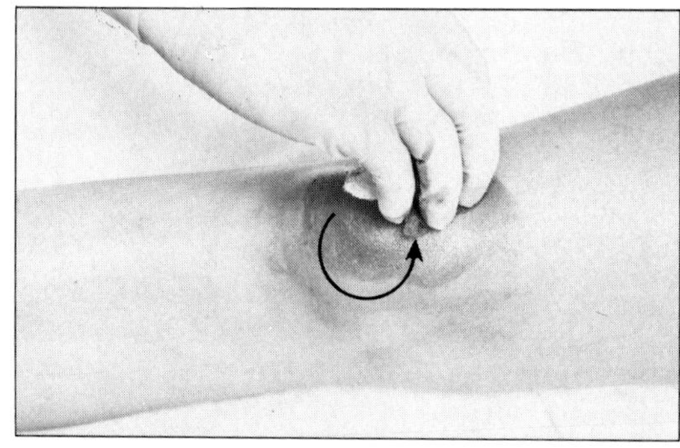

4 To keep the skin as clean as possible, apply a sterile wrap, as the nurse is doing below. Use a sterile drape or towel to cover the surgical area. Fasten the wrap securely with 3" roller gauze. Or, use nonallergenic tape instead.

Remove your gloves. Dispose of the gloves and all other disposable equipment according to your hospital's infection control standards. Thoroughly wash and dry your hands.

Instruct the patient not to touch the prepped skin or move the towel. But, ask her to tell you if her prepped skin begins to feel itchy or irritated. If it does, remove the sterile wrap at once. Quickly assess the patient's skin, and notify the doctor.

Finally, document the entire procedure in your nurses' notes.

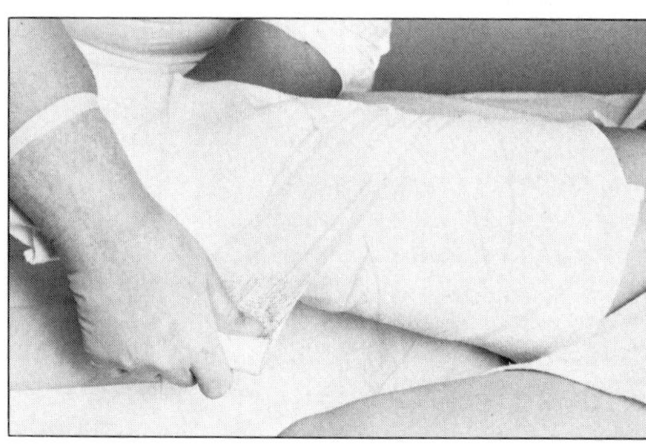

Caring for your patient postop

Your patient will return from surgery with a knee immobilizer, cylinder cast, or posterior splint in place. His knee will be immobilized in extension and remain so for about 48 hours. Whichever device he's wearing, it'll probably be covering a bulky dressing. The dressing may remain in place from 2 to 7 days.

Also, your patient may have a surgical wound evacuator (such as a Hemovac) in place. Perform routine wound evacuator care, using aseptic technique. (For details, see the NURSING PHOTOBOOK CONTROLLING INFECTION.)

Remember to position your patient properly. Elevate his affected leg above his heart level to reduce swelling, by raising the foot of the bed. If your patient's wearing an immobilizer or a posterior splint, place a folded bath blanket under his calf area to keep his heel off the bed, or you may use a heel protector.

Is your patient's leg in a cast? Then, elevate the cast on pillows as it dries. Also, put antiembolism stockings on your patient's unaffected leg to prevent thrombophlebitis.

Throughout the postoperative period, but especially in the first 24 hours, you must monitor your patient's affected leg for excess swelling around his knee or foot; excess bleeding; or any indications of peroneal palsy, such as foot adduction, numbness, tingling, or burning. Because the dressing may prevent you from observing your patient's knee directly (especially for swelling), pay close attention to any complaints of tightness. Make sure no pressure's placed on the popliteal space. Also, perform frequent neurovascular checks.

Exercise and ambulation

Flexion and extension exercises may begin from 1 to 7 days after surgery. Usually, by the time your patient's ready to exercise his leg, the surgical evacuator's been removed, as well as the bulky dressing, splint, or cast. The patient will wear a small dressing over the incision site and his leg may be wrapped in an elastic bandage. From now on, he'll wear the immobilizer at night only. The doctor will order a specific exercise program for your patient which will probably require that he perform the exercises shown below five times, three times a day. You'll supervise these sessions, to make sure he performs his exercises correctly and according to schedule. The doctor may ask you to gently guide the patient's knee into fuller flexion. In doing so, respect your patient's limitations. Never *force* his knee into position or push it beyond normal range of motion.

Note: During exercise, his knee may become swollen or warm. To make sure no infection exists, double-check his incision site for signs and symptoms of infection.

As soon as the doctor orders, usually within the first few postop days, teach the patient how to transfer into a chair, as described on pages 96 to 97.

A few days to a week postop, your patient may begin ambulation, depending on the strength of his quadriceps muscle. He'll usually begin with parallel bars, progress to a walker, then to two canes, and finally to a quad cane. In about 12 days, your patient should have 90 degrees of knee flexion restored and be ready for discharge.

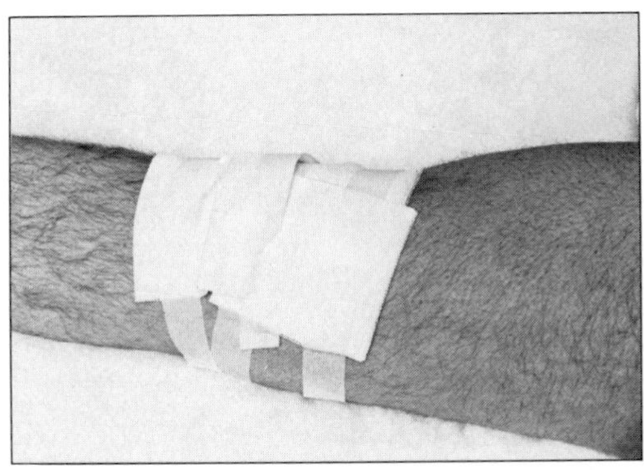

Quadriceps-setting: Position your patient so he's lying on his back in bed. The head of the bed may be flat or elevated. Instruct him to push the back of his affected knee into the bed to fully contract his quadriceps muscles. He should hold this position for a count of five and then relax his leg muscles.

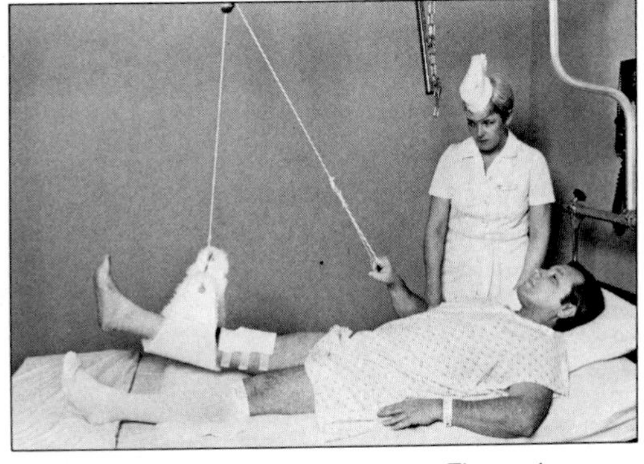

Sling-assisted straight-leg raise: First, place a sling and spreader bar under the mid- to proximal calf on your patient's affected leg. Run the rope through a pulley hanging from an overhead frame. Instruct your patient to extend his leg as he lifts it and tighten his quadriceps muscles.

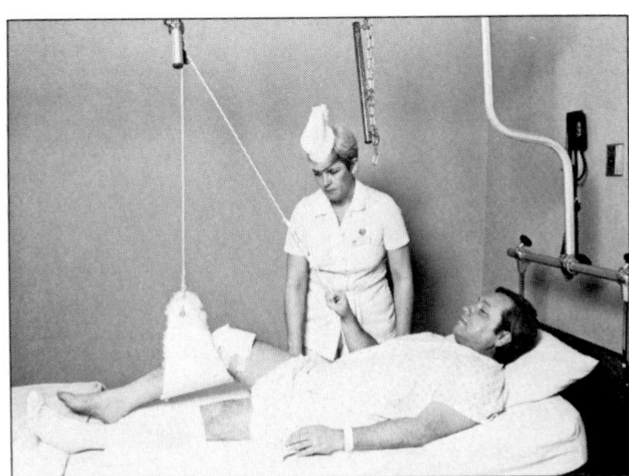

Sling-assisted knee flexion: Suspend your patient's affected leg as described above. Then, have him bend his knee as much as possible, by bringing his heel toward his buttock. Next, have him slowly straighten his leg and lower it in extension.

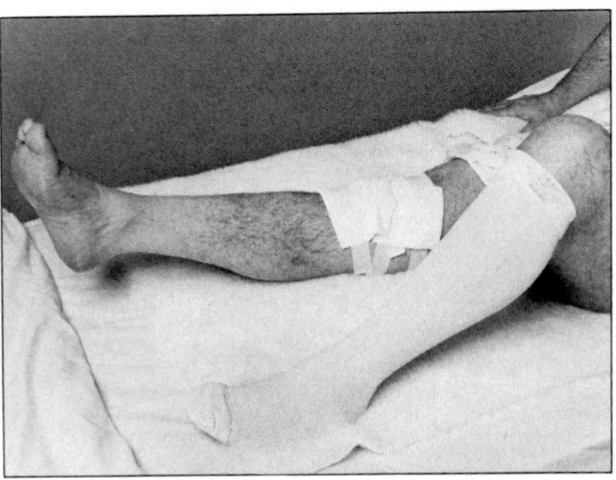

Independent straight-leg raise: Without using a sling, have your patient bend his nonaffected leg so that his foot rests flat on the bed. Now, have him lift his affected leg with his knee in extension, and then lower it again. His toes should point upward.

Complications of total knee replacement

Monitor your patient closely for the following possible complications:

- **Infection:** Because infection may result in prosthesis removal, your patient should receive antibiotics (orally or parenterally, as ordered) before, during, and after surgery. Causes of early infection include contamination during surgery, a break in aseptic technique during wound care, or microorganisms introduced by invasive procedures, such as indwelling (Foley) catheterization. If your patient's temperature increases within the first 72 hours, report it. Check the incision site for any signs of infection: redness, swelling, pain, or purulent drainage. If you suspect a urinary tract infection, question your patient about increased pain or burning on urination.
- **Thrombophlebitis:** Prevent this by keeping your patient's legs elevated to promote venous blood return. Also, have him wear antiembolism stockings and perform leg exercises. Ambulate him as early as possible. Administer heparin sodium (Lipo-Hepin) or aspirin (A.S.A.) if ordered.
- **Prosthesis loosening:** This occurs when the cement/bone interface becomes worn. Loosening causes pain and bone collapse, and necessitates prosthesis revision. Warn your patient not to overuse his joint or force the joint beyond normal range of motion.
- **Mechanical wear of prosthesis:** This may occur over an extended period. A definitive prosthesis life span hasn't yet been determined, though it's expected to last at least 10 to 15 years. Again, warn your patient not to overuse his joint. Keep in mind that treatment alternatives for a worn prosthesis include a new total knee prosthesis or arthrodesis.

Reconstructive surgery

Common hip-repair surgery

Study the following chart. It outlines the procedures used to relieve pain and improve joint motion in a stiffened joint, and to restore stability in an unstable joint.

As you probably know, causes of pain, stiffness, and instability include:

- arthritic or injury-induced inflammation
- acetabulum or femoral head abnormalities after fracture healing
- physiologic changes from aging
- miscellaneous factors contributing to articular cartilage degeneration, such as obesity, hormonal dysfunction, or menopause.

Surgical procedure
Femoral prosthesis: Replacement of degenerated femoral head with an intramedullary or femoral prosthesis. The most commonly used prosthesis is the Austin-Moore prosthesis shown at right.
Indication
Pain from degenerative joint disease of the femoral head. Patient must have a healthy acetabulum and relatively normal muscle function.

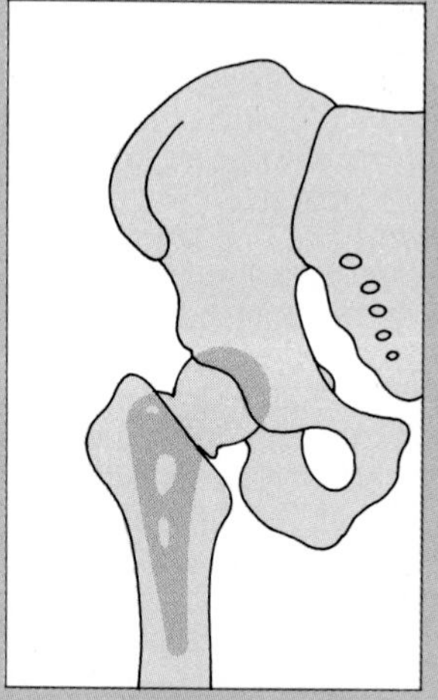

Surgical procedure
Displacement osteotomy: Removal of a bone wedge to shift weight-bearing stresses away from degenerated cartilage onto healthy cartilage. To allow early ambulation, the doctor may insert a blade plate for secure fixation.
Indication
Pain in early stages of degenerative joint disease before motion has been lost

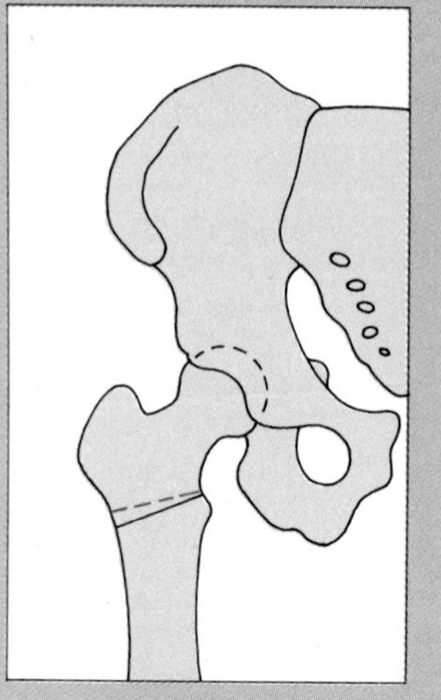

Surgical Procedure
Double-cup arthroplasty: Resurfacing of the femoral head with a metal cup and replacement of the acetabular surface with a plastic cup. The doctor uses methyl methacrylate to cement prosthesis components to bone. Used for younger patient in preference to total hip replacement because revision is simpler, since the doctor removes less bone. Arthroplasty may be revised to total hip replacement, if necessary.
Indication
Pain from degenerated articular surfaces, in a young patient

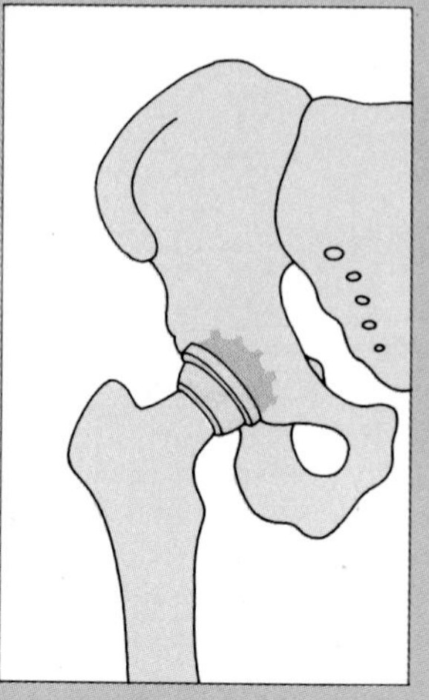

Surgical procedure
Muscle release: Severing of hip muscles and tendons around joint to decrease pressure and pain within joint. Return to full weight-bearing status is a lengthy process, and the success rate is low.
Indication
Severe hip pain from degenerative joint disease in elderly patients who are poor surgical risks and have little prospect of walking again

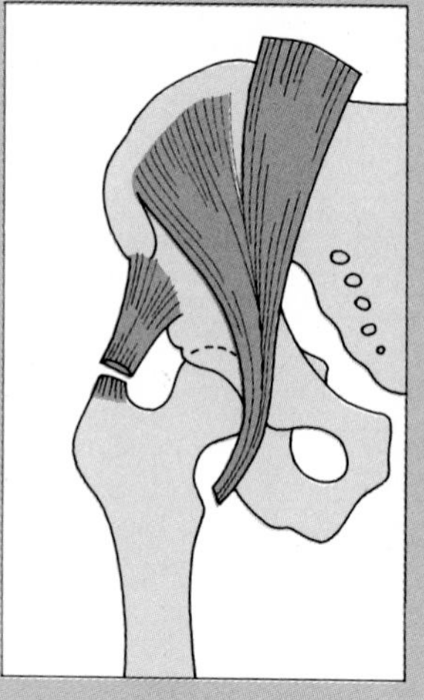

Surgical procedure
Arthrodesis (joint fusion): Surgical fusion of the femoral head to the acetabulum. Surgery relieves pain by eliminating motion. Because surgery results in a stiff hip, more stress falls on patient's back. The doctor may use internal fixation to secure the hip and allow early weight bearing during healing. Resulting joint stability allows the patient to do heavy work (after recovery) that a prosthesis wouldn't allow.
Indication
Pain from degenerative joint disease in a young, potentially active patient with one normal hip and a normal lumbar spine

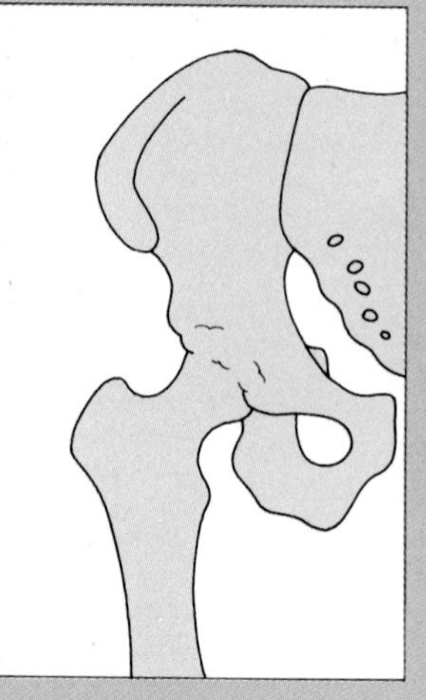

Learning about total hip replacement

When other forms of reconstructive hip surgery have failed, and the patient still suffers incapacitating pain, the doctor may perform total hip replacement. This procedure usually restores joint movement and stability, allowing the patient to ambulate without severe pain.

In choosing candidates for hip replacement, roughly the same age criteria apply as for knee replacement. Usually, a young patient won't receive total hip replacement, because the prosthesis' life span is uncertain. Total hip replacement's contraindicated if your patient has a history of bone infection, or if other problems make him a poor surgical risk.

The prosthesis is considered *total*, in contrast to the procedures listed on the opposite page, because the doctor replaces both joint components. A plastic or metal cup replaces the acetabulum, and a metal femoral head with an intermedullary stem replaces the joint's femoral portion (see the photo and X-ray at right). The doctor cements the prosthesis components in place, using methyl methacrylate. After total hip replacement, a patient eventually regains almost all joint motion. No activities except extreme hip flexion and lifting weights over 50 pounds are prohibited. However, excessive athletic use of the prosthesis is strongly discouraged.

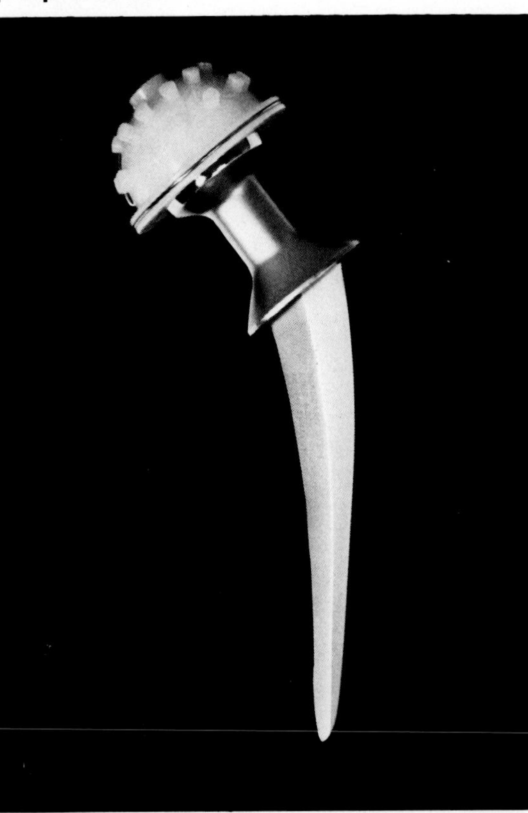

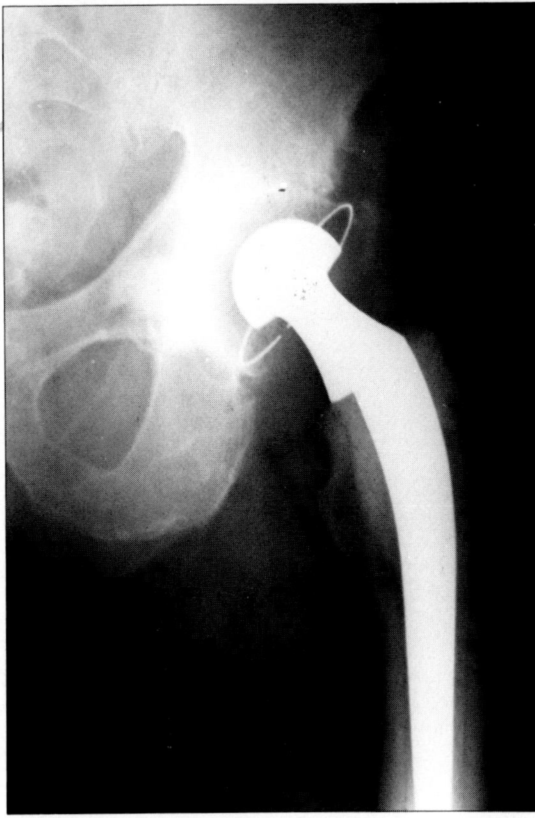

PATIENT PREPARATION

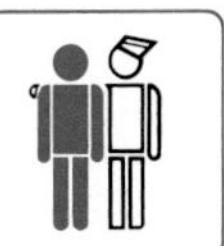

Preparing your patient for surgery

Whenever you care for a patient scheduled for total hip replacement surgery, you'll be responsible for preparing him properly. Explain the surgery, its purpose, and any special equipment your patient may have in place afterwards, such as an I.V. line or indwelling (Foley) catheter.

Instruct your patient in prosthesis function and limitations, as well as proper postop positioning—and activities he'll have to avoid. Teach your patient toe-wiggling, ankle-rotating, quadriceps-setting, and knee-flexion exercises. Arrange a meeting for your patient with the physical therapist who'll be implementing the patient's postop exercise and ambulation program.

Also, follow these preop guidelines as ordered by the doctor:

- Obtain a complete medical history.
- Perform a complete physical assessment on your patient.
- Draw blood for type, crossmatch, complete blood cell count (CBC), and electrolyte determination.
- Prepare your patient for an electrocardiogram (EKG).
- Obtain a urine sample for lab analysis.
- Administer aspirin (A.S.A.), heparin sodium (Lipo-Hepin), or warfarin sodium (Coumadin*) to help prevent deep-vein thrombosis.
- To eliminate any possible infection sources, assess your patient for signs of respiratory infection such as runny nose, coughing, or slightly elevated temperature. Also, closely examine your patient's skin. *Note:* Before admission to the hospital for surgery, the doctor will have ordered a complete dental exam to detect any preexisting infection. If your patient's a woman, she'll probably also have had a gynecologic exam.

About 24 hours before surgery, follow these steps:

- Administer fluids and antibioitics, I.V., as ordered by the doctor.
- Prepare your patient's skin, as described on page 110.
- Take your patient's vital signs, as ordered.
- Check to be sure type-and-crossmatched blood is on hand.

While your patient is undergoing surgery, prepare his bed with a firm mattress and hang a trapeze on an overhead frame. Finally, remember to document all preop preparation, including any patient teaching, in your nurses' notes.

*Available in both the United States and in Canada

Reconstructive surgery

Providing patient care after total hip replacement

Your patient will probably return from surgery with a compression dressing and a surgical evacuator (Hemovac™) or other drainage device in place. To reduce postop swelling, he may have several icebags placed above and below his incision site.

General postop care is similar to that for a hip internal fixation patient (see pages 94 to 97). In addition, follow these specific guidelines:

• If your patient's elderly, be prepared for pallor, chills, low blood pressure, and a rapid pulse in the immediate postop period. Monitor his vital signs every 30 minutes. Once his signs are stabilized, check them every 4 hours for 24 hours. *Note:* Icebags above and below your patient's incision site may contribute to his chilliness. If so, cover him with extra blankets.

• Keep accurate intake and output records. Diuresis, from increased fluids administered during surgery, may occur during the first 24 to 48 hours postop. Diuresis may cause sodium depletion leading to disorientation. Report any signs of disorientation immediately to the doctor.

• Routinely inspect the patient's dressings for signs of purulent drainage. When you empty the surgical evacuator or change dressings, use strict aseptic technique. After the dressing's been removed, inspect the incision daily for signs of infection, including redness, swelling, warmth, tenderness, odor, or purulent drainage. *Remember:* Infection may necessitate prosthesis removal.

For complete details on wound care, see the NURSING PHOTOBOOK CARING FOR SURGICAL PATIENTS.

• Encourage frequent coughing and deep breathing, as well as use of an incentive spirometer.

• Administer medication, as ordered (see pages 135 and 136). If narcotic injections are ordered for pain, give them in the patient's unaffected hip and thigh, to help prevent contamination of the incision site. After a few days, the doctor may order oral nonnarcotic analgesics.

Muscle spasm may cause pain, especially if the patient's leg has been lengthened. If so, the doctor may order Buck's extension or Russell traction, as well as muscle relaxant medication to relieve muscle spasm. *Note:* If your patient has rheumatoid arthritis, other joints may also be causing pain. Anti-inflammatory medication, such as aspirin (A.S.A.), may provide relief.

Continue to administer anticoagulants and antibiotics, as ordered.

• Position your patient correctly. During bed rest, which may last 3 to 7 days, positioning is critical to prevent prosthesis dislocation. Your patient must spend most of his time lying on his back with his affected leg abducted. As ordered, use an abductor pillow or splint, balanced suspension in abduction, Buck's extension, or a double sling. For the first 24 hours postop, keep the foot of your patient's bed raised 15°. The head may temporarily be elevated 30° to 45° for meals. Never raise it any higher. Also, never raise it for an extended period of time. During the first few days postop, keep your patient's hip and knee flexion on his affected side to a minimum.

Note: For an elderly patient, consider using a special bed, such as a Roto Rest® bed.

• Turn your patient so he lies on his affected side for 2 hours out of every 8 hours. This position helps keep the prosthesis securely within the acetabulum. If you turned him to his unaffected side, his affected leg might slip off a pillow, causing adduction and dislocating his prosthesis.

Note: To minimize pain, some doctors prefer to turn the patient about 20° to his unaffected side (with his affected leg maintained in abduction).

• Gradually increase your patient's activity level, as ordered by the doctor.

• During bed rest, encourage your patient to perform toe-wriggling and ankle-rotation exercises on both legs. He may perform quadriceps-setting and knee flexion on his unaffected leg every 1 to 2 hours during the day. Encourage range-of-motion exercises in his unaffected joints.

The patient's ambulation and exercise program will progress through several stages, much of which the physical therapist will oversee. However, you'll be called upon to assist your patient with early ambulation (as in the following photostory) and to supervise some of his exercise sessions. (See the exercise instructions on the following pages.)

Helping your patient stand

1 *The doctor will determine when your patient can enter the first stage of his exercise and ambulation program. The patient's first task, which may be ordered several days after surgery, is to stand by the bed with the support of a walker. The physical therapist may help the patient do this, using a tilting table. Or, you may be responsible for helping him, with the assistance of a co-worker.*

Remember: Schedule the activity for 20 to 30 minutes after you've given pain medication. Also, keep in mind that your patient's affected leg must remain abducted without hip flexion or external rotation.

To help your patient stand, do the following: First, place antiembolism stockings on both his affected and unaffected legs. Then, put supportive shoes with nonskid soles on both feet. Position a walker near his bedside, on the side of his unaffected leg.

Next, place the trapeze at the proper height for the patient. Have your co-worker stand at the same side of the bed as your patient's affected leg. *Remember:* You'll be turning the patient toward his *un*affected leg.

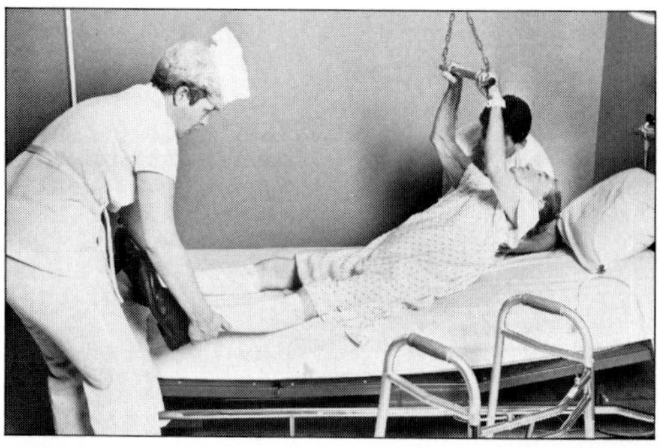

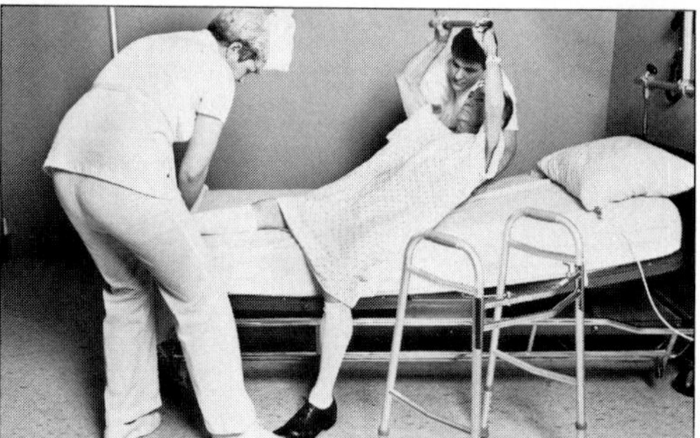

2 Next, ask your co-worker to help the patient slowly move his upper body toward the side of the bed. The patient will remain partially reclining with his hips in extension.

Ease the patient's lower body to the side of the bed, until his foot (on the unaffected leg) can reach the floor. Remind him not to flex his affected hip. *Important:* Never pull on your patient's affected leg while you're easing him to the bedside.

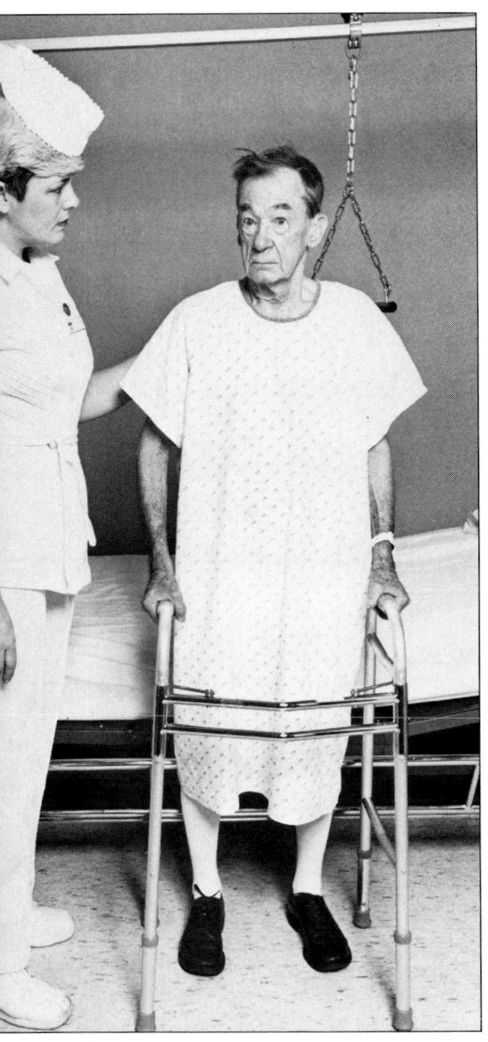

3 Now that your patient has his foot on the floor, assist him to a standing position. Place the walker directly in front of him, so he can grasp it as soon as he's upright.

Note: Your patient may feel dizzy or faint. If so, slowly lower him back to bed. Encourage him to take deep breaths. After about 15 minutes, have him try standing again. Encourage him to stand up straight, take deep breaths, and look straight ahead.

Providing no osteotomy was performed during prosthesis insertion, the patient may bear full weight on his affected leg.

After about 5 minutes of standing, help your patient back into bed by reversing the steps given above. Reposition him comfortably. Document the procedure and your patient's response to it.

Helping your patient exercise

The physical therapist will teach and supervise most of your patient's exercise program. But you'll supervise your patient's activities in between physical therapy sessions. On the second or third postop day, the patient may begin walking with a walker, two quad canes, or between parallel bars. Encourage him to approximate a normal gait when he walks, flexing both hip and knee on his affected side during the swing phase of his gait. On the third day he may be taught transfer from a walker or quad cane to a wheelchair or armchair. Next, he'll be taught transfer to a toilet adapted with a high seat and grab bars, or to a portable elevated commode. *Note:* Some doctors don't permit the patient to sit until 1 or 2 weeks after total hip replacement surgery.

Remember: When you assist your patient in and out of bed for transfer or ambulation, always have him lead with his unaffected leg. Doing so allows the patient to help himself as much as possible.

On about the fourth postop day, your patient will enter a new phase of activity: performing active independent exercises with his affected leg. He'll probably perform these three times a day, twice in the physical therapy department and once in his bed in the evening, under your supervision. Depending on your patient's condition, the physical therapist may teach him some or all of the exercises shown here. When you supervise your patient, have him repeat each exercise five times.

Pendulum flexion: Suspend your patient's leg in a sling attached to a rope. Run the rope through a pulley. Tell him to flex his

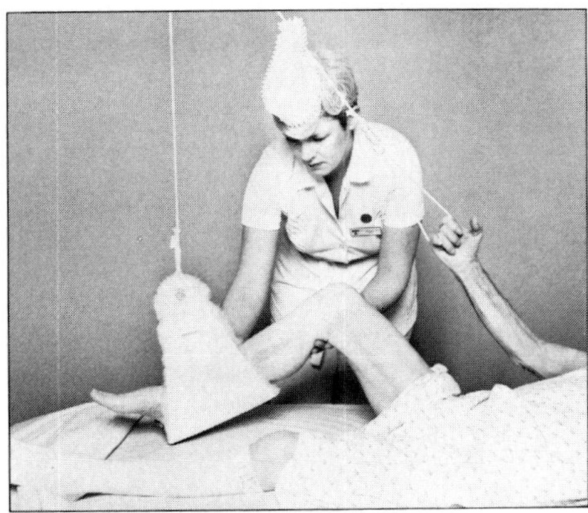

knee, pulling his heel to his buttock. Then have him straighten his leg slowly and steadily.

Pendulum abduction: Suspend your patient's leg as described above. Ask him to slowly push his leg outward, heel first. He should hold this position for a few seconds, and then pull back slowly and steadily.

Stomach lying: Turn the patient prone, with his legs in abduction. Position his legs so his toes hang over the end of the mattress

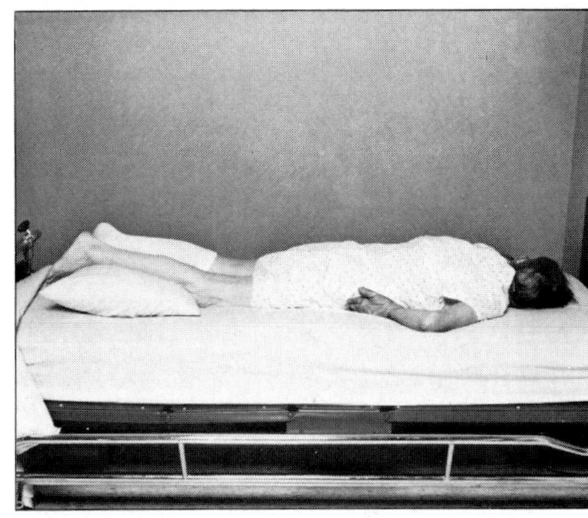

or a pillow. Have him turn his head toward his unaffected side, and maintain this position for about 30 minutes. For momentary relief from this position, he may turn his head toward his affected side and lift his hip off the bed for a few minutes. Then, he should resume the ordered position.

The next activity level includes the following exercises:

Powdered sheet or powderboard flexion: If you don't have a powderboard, lightly powder the patient's sheet to reduce friction.

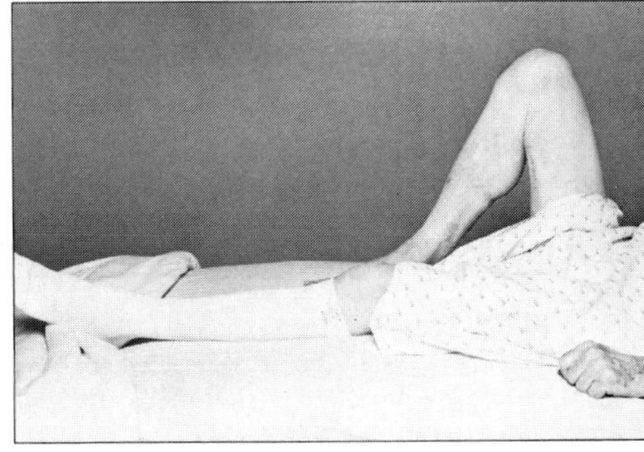

Instruct the patient to lie supine, with both legs resting on the powdered sheet. Have him first slide his heel toward his buttocks and then push his leg flat again, slowly and steadily. His unaffected leg may bend somewhat as he does so.

Powdered sheet or powderboard abduction: Tell the patient to rest his legs on the powdered sheet. Then, instruct him to first push his heel outward and then pull it back in, slowly and steadily.

Reconstructive surgery

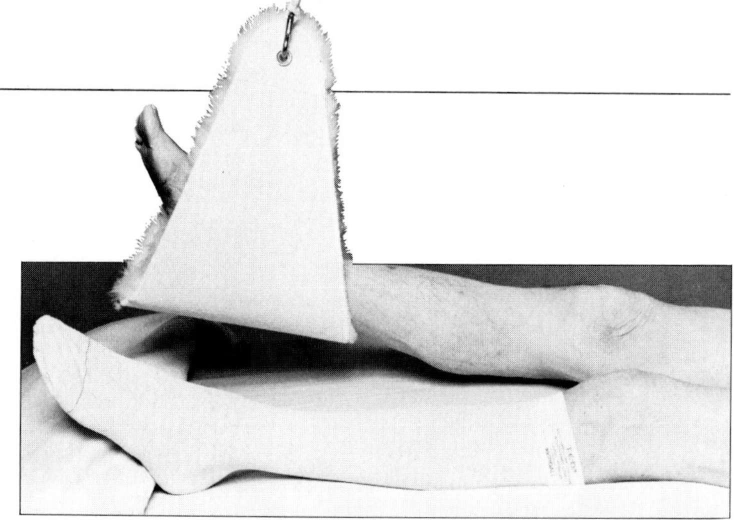

Helping your patient exercise continued

The next activity level includes:

Spring extension: Suspend your patient's leg in a sling as shown at right. Attach the sling to a spring and a pulley. Tell him to pull his foot down to the powdered sheet with his leg extended. Then, have him lift his leg back up slowly and steadily. Don't allow his leg to bounce up and down.

Bedpan exercise: Instruct your patient to lie supine on the bed. Tell him to raise his hips (as if he's getting on a bedpan), and hold the position for a few seconds. Then, encourage him to slowly lower his hips back to the bed.

PATIENT PREPARATION

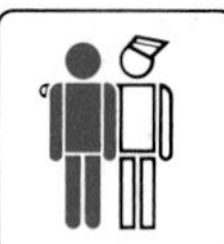

Preparing your patient for discharge

With the physical therapist's guidance (according to doctor's orders), your patient's activity level will gradually increase in preparation for discharge. He'll be ready for discharge when he's progressed to using crutches or a quad cane, when he has sufficient muscle control to position his hip properly during all activities, and when he can function independently enough to perform most necessary maintenance activities at home. *Note:* If necessary, make arrangements to refer your patient to outside agencies for assistance.

Before he goes home, make sure your patient thoroughly understands the hip movement and positioning precautions listed in the home care aid below. Photocopy the aid, and give him a copy to take with him.

Using terms he'll understand, tell him he can resume sexual activity, as long as he avoids positions that cause his hip to rotate internally, adduct past neutral, or flex past 90 degrees.

Also, make sure your patient receives a pamphlet outlining his specific exercise program. Make the necessary arrangements for regular visits to the physical therapy department. The physical therapist will continue evaluating the patient's home exercise program after his discharge, and will modify it as the patient's strength increases. After 6 to 8 weeks, the patient may begin a resistive exercise program. He'll continue to use an ambulation aid for some time after discharge, to eliminate limping, which places stress on his hip. Eventually, he should be able to walk without the use of an aid.

In preparing your patient for discharge, be sure to teach him the following signs and symptoms of prosthesis dislocation:

- sudden, sharp pain, accompanied by clicking or popping sound at joint
- edematous hip
- shortened leg, with foot in external rotation
- loss of control over leg motion, or complete loss of leg motion.

Instruct your patient to contact the doctor immediately or go to the hospital emergency department if he suspects hip dislocation. The sooner the dislocation's treated, the easier it will be to reduce. Also, the reduction procedure will involve less risk to the patient. Reduction may require a sedative only. Or, surgical reduction under general anesthesia may be necessary.

Inform your patient about his visit schedule. Most patients return for an outpatient checkup in 1 week, followed by checkups at 3-month, 6-month, and yearly intervals.

Home care

How to position your leg after total hip surgery

Dear Patient:

Because you've had hip surgery, you'll need to be particularly careful about leg movements. For the next 3 months, observe the following *dos* and *don'ts.*

- Don't cross your legs, whether you're lying, sitting or standing.
- Do place a pillow between your legs when you lie on your unaffected side, with your affected leg uppermost.
- Don't sit on low stools, low chairs, or low toilets. You may need to use cushions or pillows to raise chair seats. Also, you may consider renting or buying a raised toilet seat or special commode.
- Do sit only in chairs with arms. You'll need chair arms to help you stand up.
- Do move to the edge of your chair before getting up. Place your affected leg in front of your other leg, which should be well under the chair. Keep your affected leg in front while getting up.
- Don't reach down to the end of your bed to pull up your covers. This flexes your hip too much.
- Don't bend down to pick up things from the floor, or to reach into lower cupboards or drawers.
- Do keep your affected leg facing front at all times, whether you're sitting, lying, or walking. Never turn your hip or knee inward or outward.

Laminectomy

Let's say you're caring for a patient with a suspected herniated disc. The doctor decides to perform a laminectomy. Do you know why this surgical procedure's performed? What diagnostic tests may be ordered? Why the doctor may simultaneously perform a spinal fusion?

Do you really know all you should about a laminectomy? For example, do you know how to assess drainage on your patient's dressing after surgery? Why an overbed trapeze may be dangerous for a postop laminectomy patient? How to teach your patient to sit up properly after his laminectomy?

If you're unsure about the answers to these questions, study the next few pages. You'll find detailed information, photos, and illustrations that'll help you gain a better understanding of laminectomy. In addition, we've included a home care aid to give your patient.

Learning about a herniated disc

If your patient's scheduled for a laminectomy, he probably has a herniated disc (also called a ruptured or slipped disc or a herniated nucleus pulposus). Wondering what causes this disorder? Strain, degenerative joint disease, or trauma may force all or part of the intervertebral disc's soft center (the nucleus pulposus) through the disc's weakened or torn outer ring. As you can see in this illustration, the protruding disc may compress the spinal nerve root or the spinal cord itself. Keep in mind that the most common areas for disc herniation are the L_4 to L_5 and L_5 to S_1 interspaces. Only about 5% of disc herniations occur in the cervical vertebrae.

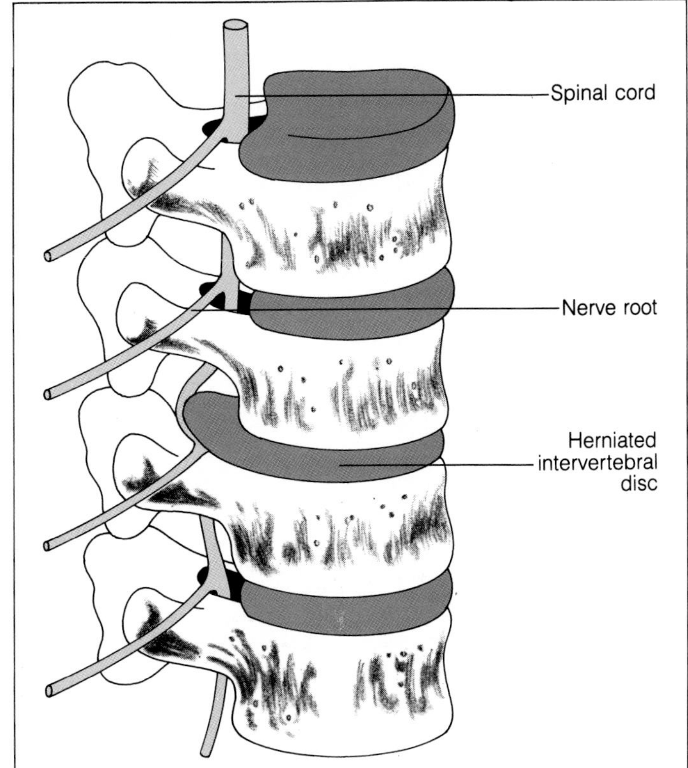

How does a disc herniation affect your patient? Most patients experience low back pain, sometimes accompanied by muscle spasms which may radiate to the buttocks, legs, and feet. A herniated disc may also cause loss of sensory or motor function or muscle power in the area innervated by the compressed nerve root. And, if the herniated disc is located in a cervical vertebra, your patient may complain of neck stiffness and pain radiating down his arm to his fingers. This pain may be further aggravated by coughing, sneezing, or straining.

In most cases, the doctor will initially order conservative medical management for the patient with a disc herniation. For example, he may order several weeks of bed rest (possibly in pelvic or cervical skin traction, if the pain's severe). He may also order moist heat applications, specific exercises, and diet management (especially if your patient's overweight). In addition, he may prescribe analgesics and a muscle relaxant for pain control. He may also prescribe an anti-inflammatory analgesic, such as aspirin, to help control inflammation-associated pain and edema-associated pain at the injury site.

After several weeks of treatment, the doctor will reassess the patient's condition. If the conservative treatment hasn't worked, and if the pain persists, the doctor will probably order diagnostic procedures, such as myelography. Then, he may perform a laminectomy to correct the condition.

What you should know about a laminectomy

As you may know, a laminectomy involves the surgical removal of a portion of the lamina. When that's accomplished, the protruding disc fragments are removed to relieve pressure on the nerve root or spinal cord.

But, suppose your patient requires additional vertebral stability because of his occupation, or the extent of the injury. Then, the doctor may perform a spinal fusion along with the laminectomy.

Note: A patient may have a spinal fusion without having a laminectomy.

During a spinal fusion the doctor will reinforce the patient's spine by fusing bone chips (from the patient's anterior or posterior iliac crests, or tibia), or by inserting a metallic rod, screw, or plate.

Of course, you'll be responsible for preparing your patient for the laminectomy (and/or spinal fusion), and caring for him afterwards.

Review what the doctor has told your patient about the surgery and answer any questions your patient may have. Explain to him what to expect after surgery. Be sure to gather as much information as possible about your patient, including past medical history, present condition, day-to-day activities, and his expectations following surgery.

Also, take this opportunity to teach deep breathing techniques, logrolling, proper posture, how to get out of bed, and strengthening and range-of-motion exercises. Stress that these procedures will help prevent complications and speed recovery.

As part of your daily routine (before and after surgery), assess your patient's pain, muscle power, motor and sensory status, and circulatory status. Administer medications, as ordered. (For more detailed information on caring for your patient before and after surgery, see the following pages.)

Document your care in your nurses' notes.

Laminectomy

Understanding diagnostic tests

Before your patient's laminectomy, the doctor will perform several diagnostic tests to confirm the existence and location of the disc herniation. Exactly which tests the doctor chooses depends on your patient's condition and the hospital's equipment.

Learn how to prepare your patient for these tests by reading this chart carefully.

Note: Because testing procedures vary from hospital to hospital, familiarize yourself with *your* hospital's specific procedures.

Test
Myelography
Purpose
To visualize the spinal column and determine exact location of herniated disc

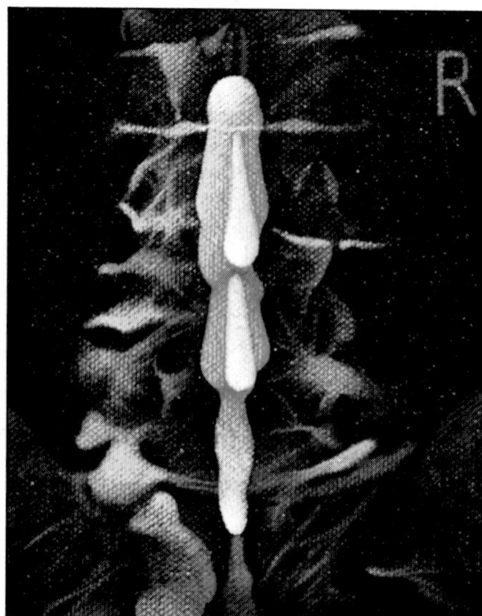

What to tell your patient
"Provided you're not allergic to iodine or seafood, or pregnant, you'll be asked to sign a consent form. Then, the doctor will order clear liquids for your breakfast the day of the test. I'll give you a sedative before the test to help you relax. Then, you'll go to the X-ray room and lie on your abdomen on a special tilt table. The doctor will inject anesthetic into the skin of your lower back to numb it. When the skin is numb, he'll insert a special needle and withdraw a small amount of spinal fluid from your spinal column. If he's able to withdraw fluid, he'll know the needle's positioned properly. Now, he'll inject dye into your spinal column. After the dye's injected, the technician will fasten the tilt table's straps so you're securely held in place. Then, he'll move the tilt table into seven or eight different positions. As the table moves, the technician will take X-rays of the dye passing through your spinal column. The doctor will study these X-rays to observe the spinal column's inner structure and identify any abnormalities that are present.

"After the procedure, you'll return to your room. Depending on which dye the doctor used, your bed will be positioned with the head either flat or elevated. I'll tell you how long you have to stay in bed, and let you know when it's okay to get up. Remember to keep your head against the bed when you're lying down. Also, you'll need to drink plenty of liquids."

Test
Spinal X-ray
Purpose
To identify disc space narrowing
What to tell your patient
"You'll go to the X-ray room and stand close to the X-ray machine, or lie on a table under the X-ray machine. The X-ray beam will be absorbed or deflected by your body's internal structure and then recorded by the machine. Next, the doctor or technician will move the machine slightly and repeat the procedure. Eventually, they'll take enough pictures of your vertebral column to help visualize any bony abnormalities."

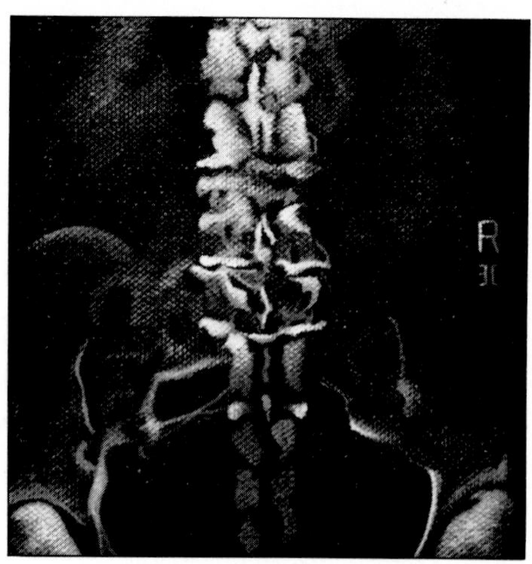

Test
Straight-leg-raising
Purpose
To diagnose a herniated disc
Note: The doctor willl consider this test positive if the patient complains of posterior leg pain, not back pain, as his leg's raised.
What to tell your patient
"You'll lie flat on your back. The doctor will place one hand at the base of your spine and his other hand under your ankle. Then, as you keep your leg straight, he'll slowly raise it. He'll repeat this procedure on your other leg."

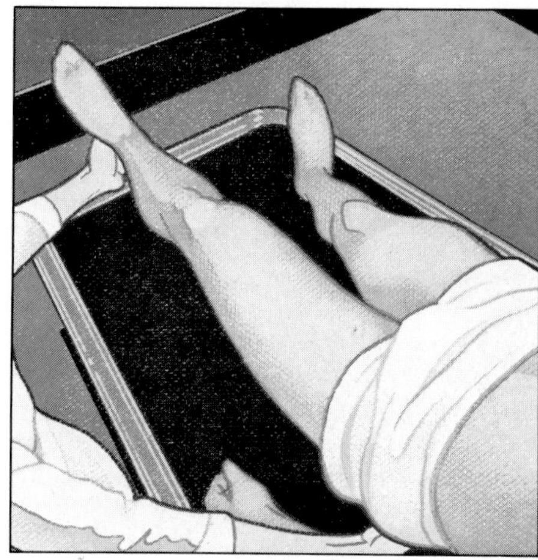

Test
Kernig's sign
Purpose
To diagnose a herniated disc
Note: The doctor will suspect spinal root compression if, after the leg is flexed and then extended, the patient complains of pain and the doctor notes resistance and loss of ankle and knee-jerk reflexes.
What to tell your patient
"You'll lie flat on your back. The doctor will place one hand on your knee and the other hand under your ankle. He'll flex your thigh and knee to a 90° angle and then straighten your leg."

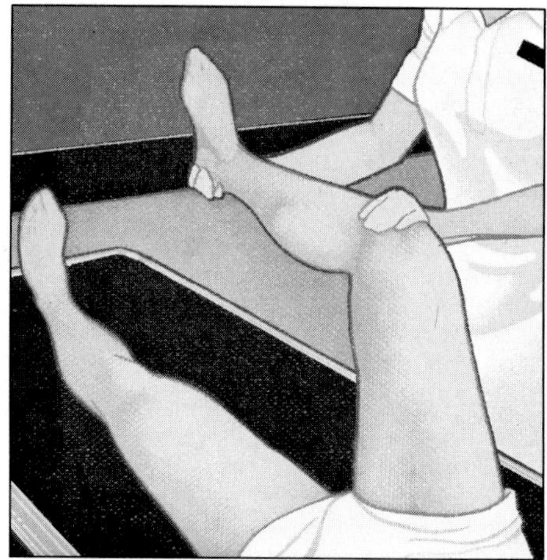

After a laminectomy: Caring for your patient

1 *Thirty-one-year-old Edith Griznik will be returning to your unit from the recovery room. She's just had a laminectomy in the L_4 to L_5 vertebral area. Before she returns, prepare her bed with a firm mattress. Or place bed boards between the mattress and the frame. Place a sheepskin over the bottom linens. Also, be sure to remove the trapeze from her bed frame, so she won't use it to move around. Her back must remain completely straight.*

She'll return from the recovery room with an I.V. in place, a surgical evacuator (such as a Hemovac) and a dressing at her wound site, and antiembolism stockings on her legs. To properly care for her, follow these steps:

Begin by reassuring Ms. Griznik. Explain each procedure as you perform it, even if she seems groggy from the anesthetic.

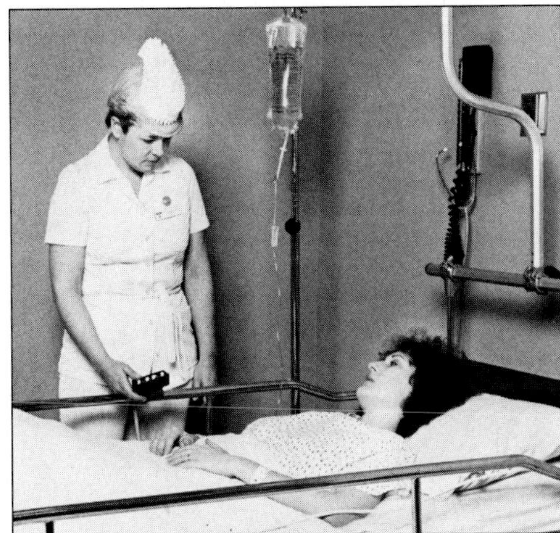

Place Ms. Griznik in a low Fowler's position. Depending on doctor's orders, keep the bed flat or tilt the head at a 20° to 30° angle. Place a pillow under her head and shoulders. Is she having muscle spasms? If so, place pillows laterally under her legs. But take care to avoid extreme knee flexion or pressure behind her knees.

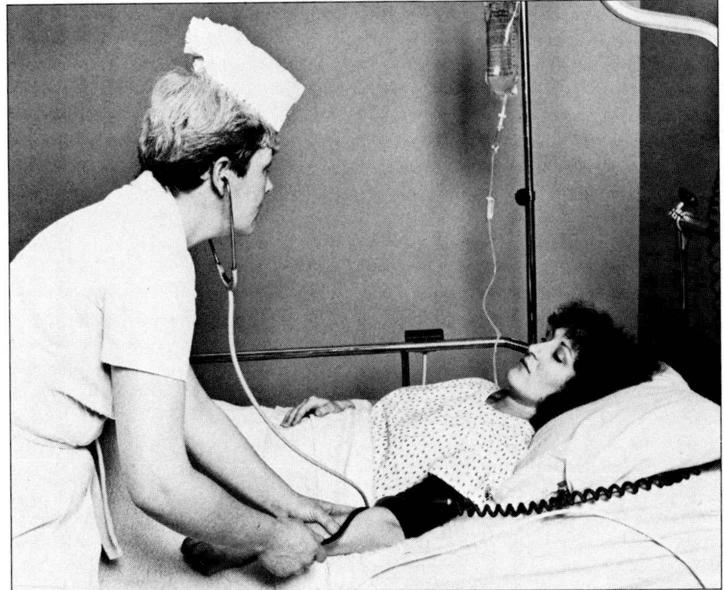

2 Now, take Ms. Griznik's blood pressure, pulse, respiration rate, and temperature. Document your findings. For the first 24 hours after surgery, your patient's temperature may be elevated because of blood in her subarachnoid space or respiratory complications such as atelectasis. Notify the doctor.

Continue to take Ms. Griznik's vital signs frequently, until they stabilize. Then, take them every 2 to 4 hours.

3 After taking vital signs, check her dressing for excess drainage. To do so, insert your hand between her back and the bed. Feel the dressing and bed linens to determine whether they're wet or dry. Notify the doctor if the dressings are wet.

Also, note the amount and color of the drainage in Ms. Griznik's surgical evacuator. Immediately following surgery, expect a small amount of bloody drainage. In addition, check the entire length of the drainage tubing, as the nurse is doing here. If the tubing's twisted, straighten it to prevent blockage.

Note: To ensure even, constant suction, be sure the surgical evacuator bulb's compressed.

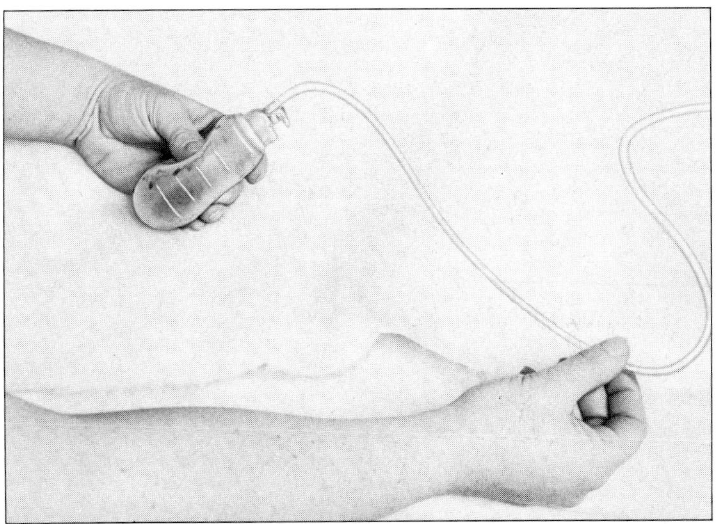

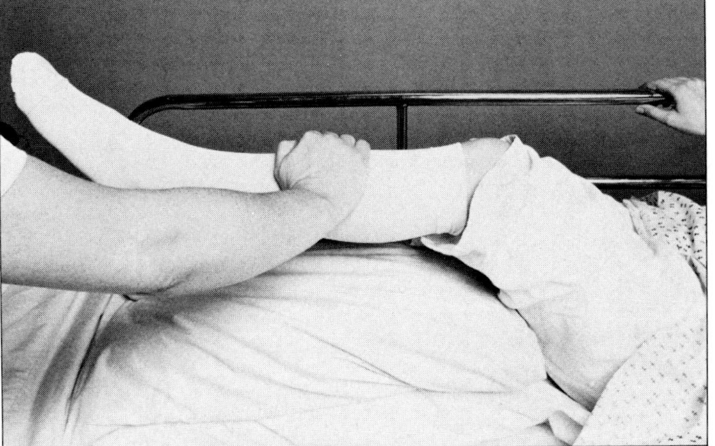

4 Assess muscle power as shown here. (For guidelines, see page 39.) Next, remove your patient's antiembolism stockings. Now, perform a complete neurovascular check (see page 24). As you do, assess Ms. Griznik's legs for pulse, color, warmth, and capillary refill. Replace her antiembolism stockings. Perform another neurovascular and muscle-power assessment in 1 hour. After that, repeat your checks along with the vital sign checks, or as ordered.

Compare all your findings with the preoperative data baseline. But be sure to take into consideration any medication she may be receiving. Report any changes in your patient's condition to the doctor immediately.

Laminectomy

After a laminectomy: Caring for your patient continued

5 When the doctor says it's okay to turn your patient (usually 2 to 8 hours postop), logroll Ms. Griznik onto her side. Now you can closely examine her dressing. Encourage her to take slow, deep breaths as you logroll her. For more information on logrolling, see the NURSING PHOTOBOOK CARING FOR SURGICAL PATIENTS. *Note:* Instruct your patient to make no attempt to logroll by herself (or assist you in logrolling) until her surgical evacuator's removed.

When she's turned on her side, note the amount and color of drainage (if any) on her dressing. Very little drainage should be present. Outline the stain, as shown here. Record the date, time, and your initials within the outline. Continue to check Ms. Griznik's dressing each time you reposition her. Turn and reposition her every 2 hours.

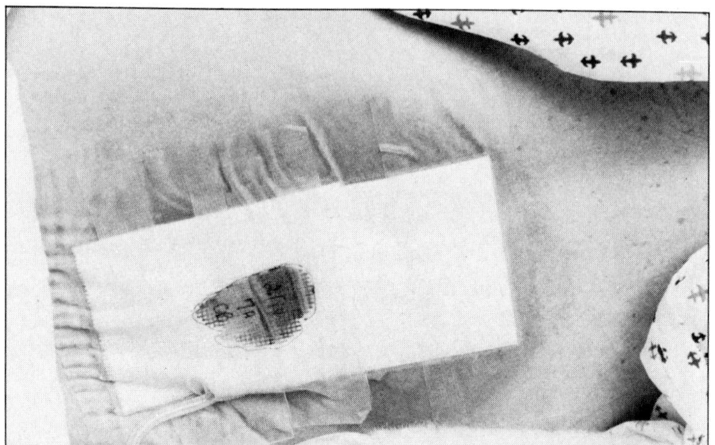

6 If, after 6 to 8 hours postop, she hasn't urinated, assess and palpate her abdomen for distention. Offer her a bedpan. If she can't urinate, let water run from a faucet within her hearing for a few minutes. Or, pour warm water over her perineum. If she still can't urinate, notify the doctor. He may order straight catheterization.

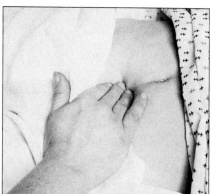

7 Encourage your patient to take deep breaths and use an incentive spirometer. Have her cough only if you have a doctor's order. Coughing may be contraindicated.

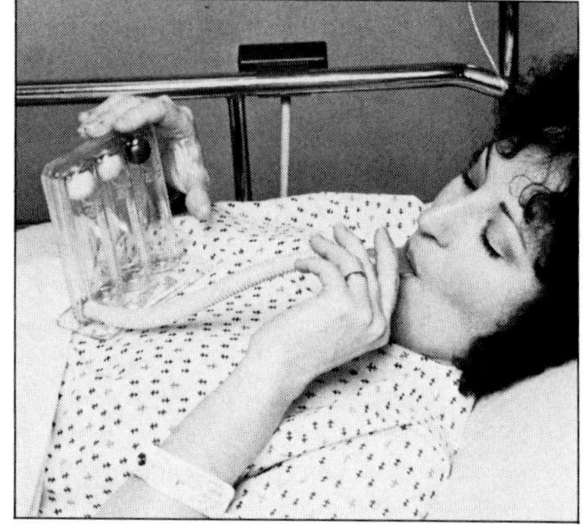

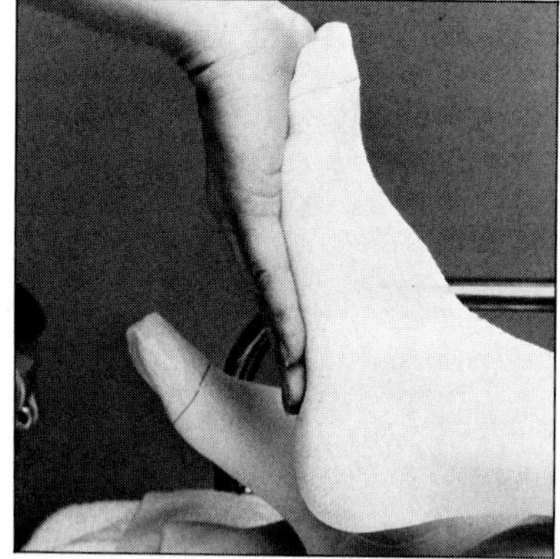

8 To promote venous blood return, have Ms. Griznik perform simple foot exercises, such as foot flexion. You may provide resistance against the sole of her foot, using your hand or a footboard. *Important:* Your patient must avoid extreme knee flexion.

Have her repeat these exercises every 2 hours, or as ordered.

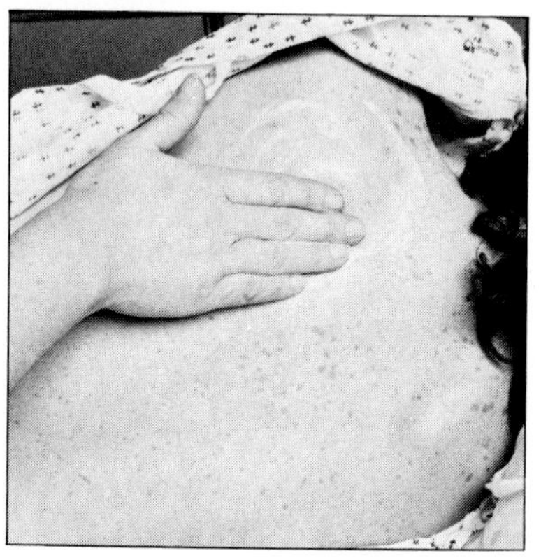

9 When you turn your patient, massage her back and other skin areas. Closely examine her skin, especially at bony prominences, for redness, edema, or other signs of developing pressure areas. Continue to check her skin every time you turn her.

Administer analgesics, as ordered, to help relieve pain in her buttocks, lower back, legs, and wound site.

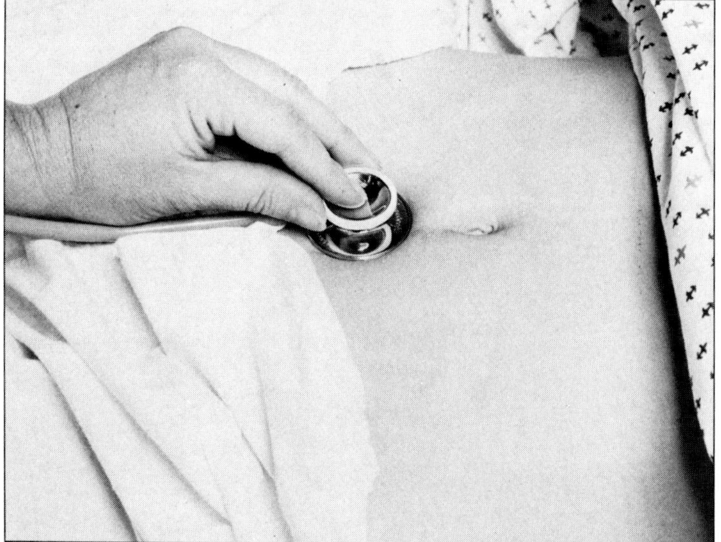

10 Auscultate Ms. Griznik's abdomen every 8 hours for bowel sounds. When the sounds return (about 24 to 48 hours after surgery), notify the doctor. He'll probably instruct you to begin giving fluids and food orally. *Note:* Once she's able to tolerate fluids, obtain an order to discontinue her I.V. Be sure to record the intake amount as well as her fluid tolerance. To help avoid constipation, provide a diet with plenty of fluids and bulk. Request an order for stool softeners, if indicated.

Document all procedures in your nurses' notes.

After a laminectomy: Getting your patient out of bed

1 *Twenty-four hours have passed since Edith Griznik's laminectomy. The doctor's left orders to get Ms. Griznik out of bed today. To assist her, follow these guidelines:*

First, explain the procedure. Then, place a straight-back chair close to her bed. Lower the entire bed as far as possible. Raise the head of the bed to low Fowler's position.

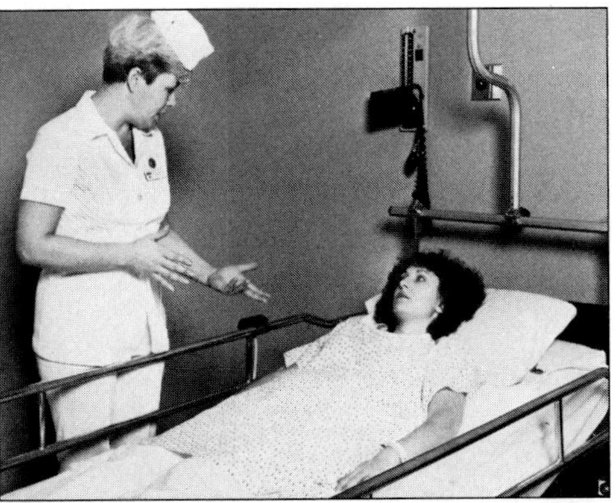

2 Now, prepare to logroll Ms. Griznik toward the edge of the bed, so she's facing away from you. Hold the sheepskin close against her lower back to splint the incision site. Encourage her to help by grasping the side rail and pulling herself onto her side.

For details on logrolling, see the NURSING PHOTOBOOK CARING FOR SURGICAL PATIENTS.

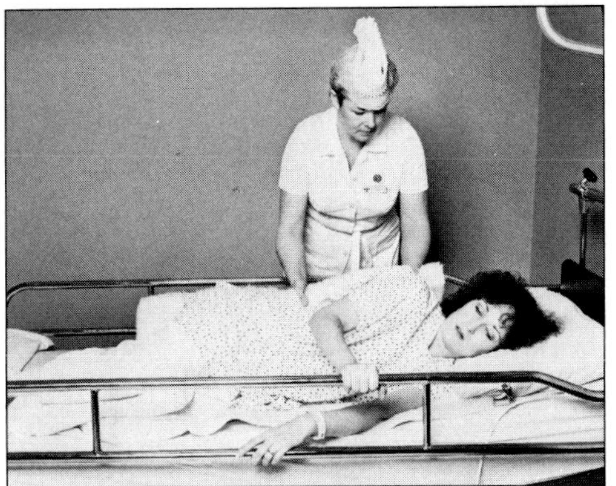

3 When Ms. Griznik's close to the edge of the bed, lower the side rail, positioning yourself to prevent her from falling.

Now, have her raise herself into a sitting position by pushing against the mattress with her upper hand as she swings her legs over the side of the bed. Encourage her to breathe deeply. Be sure to support her incision site, as shown here.

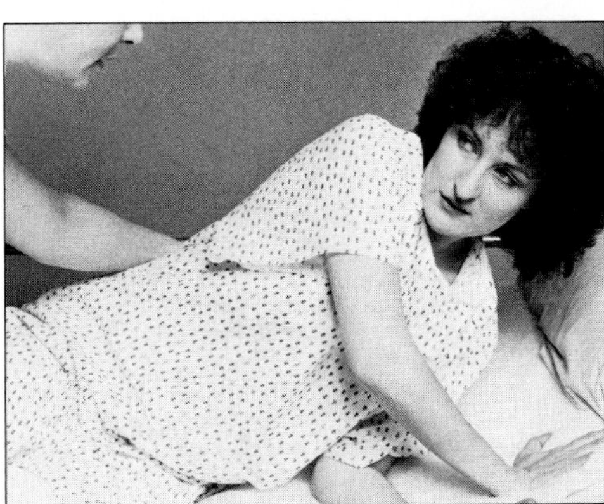

4 Place your patient's slippers or shoes (with nonskid soles) by her feet, and have her slip them on. Assist her, as necessary, and encourage her to relax. Tell her to take several more slow, deep breaths.

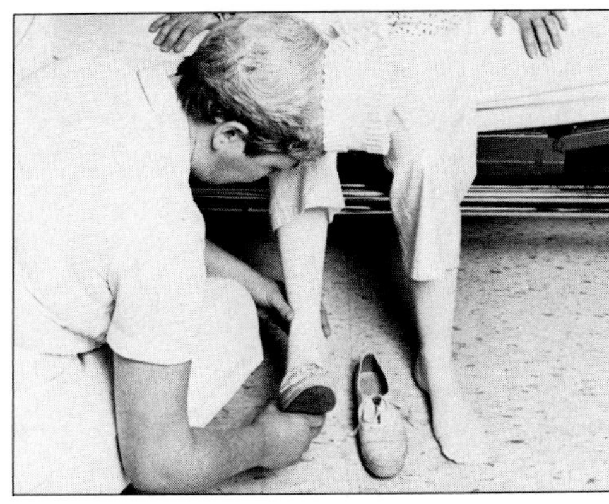

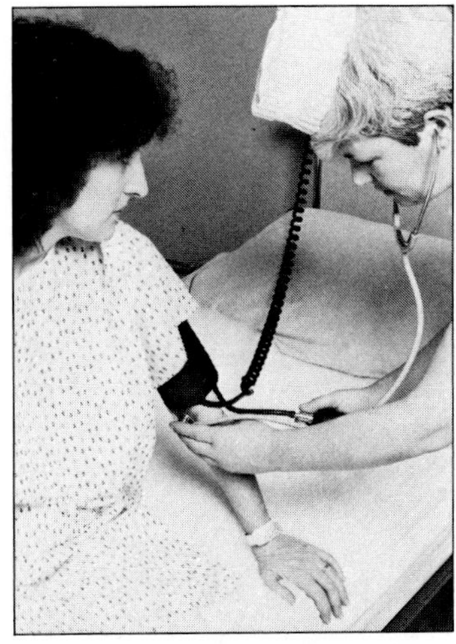

5 Check her blood pressure and pulse. Also, ask your patient how she feels. Note her facial color and expression as she responds.

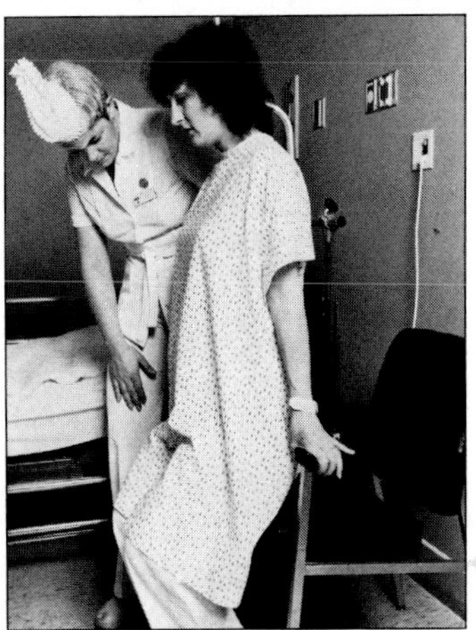

6 If everything's okay, have her raise herself to a standing position by pushing against the bed with her palms. Remind her to keep her back straight and look straight ahead. Splint her incision site.

When she's standing, have her take a few steps. She should feel for the chair with the back of her knees as she reaches back for the chair arm.

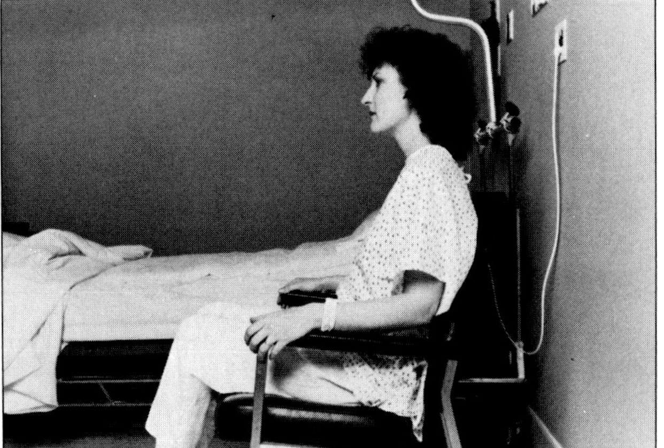

7 Help her slowly lower herself into the chair, keeping her back straight while you support her incision site. Make sure she elevates her knees to hip level or slightly higher to avoid stress on her lumbar spine. Don't leave your patient unattended in the chair.

To assist her back into bed, reverse the above procedure. Encourage progressive ambulation, as ordered.

Document all care in your nurses' notes.

Laminectomy

Home care

After a laminectomy: How to care for yourself

Dear Patient:

Because you've just had back surgery, you must take special precautions to help speed your recovery. Above all, never overexert yourself. In addition, your nurse has filled in the doctor's specific instructions on the following list. Read it carefully. If you have questions, talk to your nurse. Then, when you go home, make a special effort to follow the guidelines listed here:

- Restrict your activities. For example, you may go up and down the stairs __times a day. Ride in a car as little as possible during the first weeks, because the vehicle motion may create back pain. Also, wait at least __weeks before driving a car.
- Do not lift or carry anything that's heavier than 5 pounds (2¼ kg) for __weeks. Don't engage in strenuous physical activity for at least __weeks or you'll experience back pain.
- Avoid sexual activity for __weeks after surgery.
- Take a shower __days after surgery. But before taking a tub bath, get your doctor's okay.

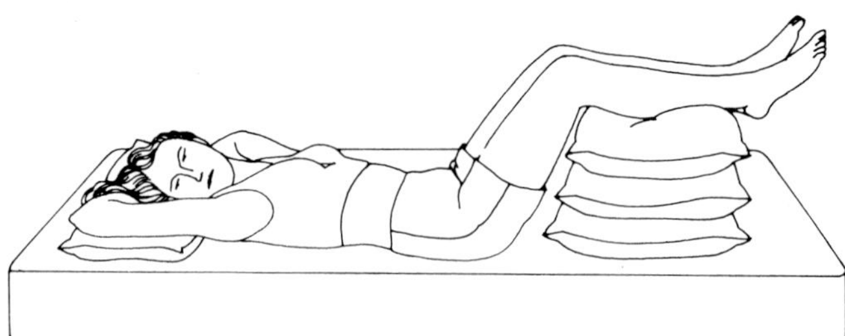

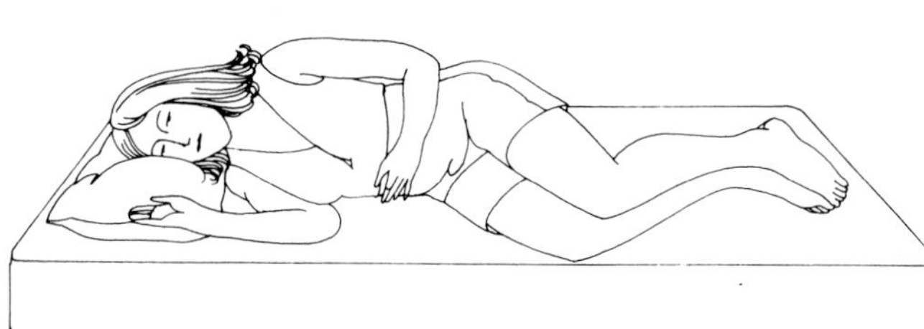

- Spend at least __hours a day in a bed with a firm mattress. When lying on your back, elevate your legs on pillows. If you prefer lying on your side, bend your knees. Position a small pillow under your head and neck to avoid straining your neck, shoulders, and arms. *Never lie on your stomach.*
- Ask a family member to check your incision site once a day. If he notices drainage or redness, or you notice increased incisional pain, call your doctor.
- To strengthen your arm and leg muscles, continue the exercises you learned in the hospital.
- When stooping down, bend your knees, keeping your back straight.

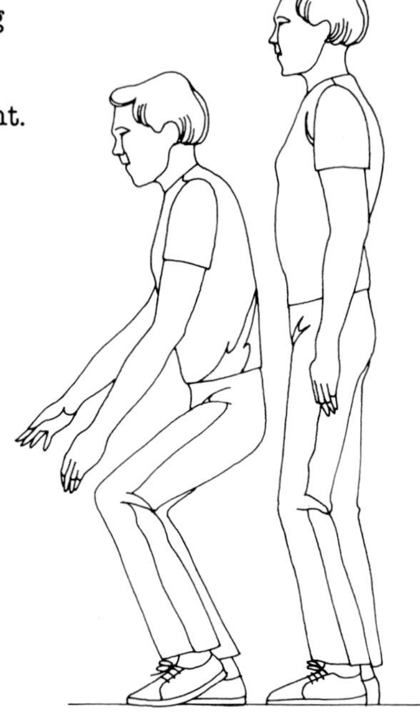

- When sitting, support your feet on a footstool with your knees at hip level or higher.

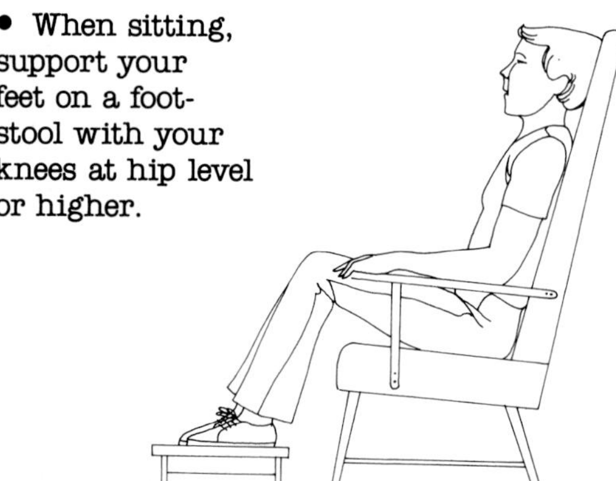

- Remember to return to your doctor on ______ for a checkup.

Amputation

Blake Toben just returned to your unit after having his leg amputated below the knee. The doctor has decided on a delayed prosthesis fitting. In addition to providing for your patient's physical needs, you'll be expected to help him—and his family—cope emotionally. In the pages that follow, we'll detail special guidelines and precautions you'll need to know. We'll tell you:

- what to do if your patient's cast slips off.
- how to bandage a stump, whether it's above or below the knee.
- how to assess stump drainage.
- how to teach stump care to a patient with a leg amputation.
- how to help your patient cope with the loss of a leg or arm.

In addition, we'll explain two amputation methods and review common amputation sites. Study the following pages carefully.

Learning about amputation

The doctor will perform an amputation because of trauma, infection, vascular disease (such as arteriosclerosis), congenital deformity, thermal injury, or severe chronic pain. As you probably know, during the procedure, the doctor'll remove part or all of the patient's bone, as well as the soft tissue at, above, or below a joint at the designated amputation site. Two amputation methods exist (see illustrations at right): *closed or flap* (doctor forms skin flaps to cover the bone stump), and *open or guillotine* (doctor severs tissues and bone at the same level without forming skin flaps). If the reason for your patient's surgery is infection, or your patient has a high risk of infection (for example, he has a partially severed toe from a lawnmower accident), the doctor may perform an open amputation.

In most other situations, however, the doctor will perform a closed amputation, implanting drains at the wound site. The closed amputation usually heals faster, allowing for earlier prosthesis fitting. Keep in mind the doctor may place a plaster cast over a closed amputation. That way your patient can be fitted with a prosthesis immediately.

How will the doctor decide the exact amputation site? That depends on the following: your patient's overall physical condition, age, muscle strength, learning ability, his extremity's remaining ability to be functional, the blood supply to the remaining stump, and the specifications for proper prosthesis fitting. Remember, the doctor's primary consideration is to amputate as little of the arm or leg as possible.

The information that follows will familiarize you with all levels of amputation presently being performed:

- Partial foot: removal of one or more toes and part of the foot.
- Total foot: removal of the foot below the ankle joint.
- Ankle (Syme's): removal of the foot at ankle joint.
- Below the knee (BK): removal of leg 5" to 7" (12.7 to 17.8 cm) below the tibia. Procedure allows patient to use prosthesis without a knee hinge.
- Knee disarticulation: removal of patella with quadriceps brought over femur end; or patella fixed to a cut surface between condyles (called Gritti-Stokes amputation).
- Above the knee (AK): removal of leg from 3" (7.6 cm) above the knee.
- Hip disarticulation: removal of both leg and hip, or leg and pelvis. Procedure's performed only on patient with malignant tumor, extensive injury, or gangrene.
- Hemipelvectomy: removal of leg and half of pelvis. *Note:* Procedure's performed only on patient with malignant tumor, extensive injury, or gangrene.
- Fingers: removal of one or more fingers at hinge or condyloid joints.
- Wrist disarticulation: removal of hand at wrist.
- Below the elbow (BE): removal of lower arm about 7" (17.8 cm) below the elbow at the junction between the middle and lower third of forearm.
- Elbow disarticulation: removal of lower arm at elbow.
- Above the elbow: removal of arm from 3" (7.6 cm) above the elbow.

Closed amputation

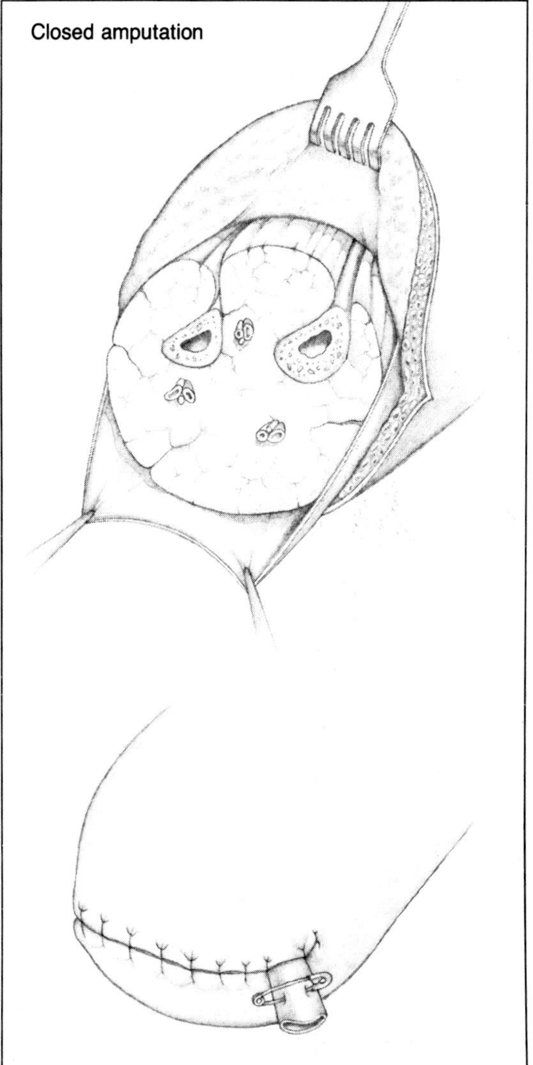

Open amputation

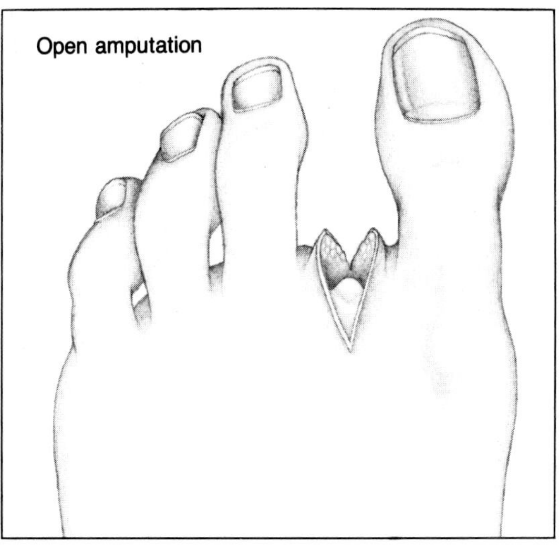

Amputation

After an amputation: Caring for your patient

After an amputation, your nursing care responsibilities for your patient depend on when he'll be fitted for a prosthesis. Expect a patient who has a prosthesis fitted in the operating room immediately after surgery to have a plaster cast, with a metal joint imbedded in the distal end, applied over his stump. The patient's temporary prosthesis fits into this joint. On the other hand, a patient scheduled for a prosthesis fitting after the stump heals will have his stump wrapped in an elastic bandage to mold and shape it.

As you know, the longer a patient's immobilized, the more likely he is to develop complications. Always try to get your patient out of bed and ambulating within 48 hours—regardless of when he's fitted with his prosthesis. If a patient's fitted with a prosthesis immediately after surgery, he may be able to bear weight on his prosthesis, using a walker.

If the patient's scheduled for a delayed prosthesis fitting, he may also be able to use a walker. You may need to use the stand-pivot transfer to assist him to the walker. Be sure to administer pain medication, as needed.

Usually, the sooner a patient can walk—with the aid of crutches or a walker—the quicker he'll adjust successfully to his amputation. In many cases, ambulation may give him the confidence he needs to achieve the goals he sets for himself. Be sure to offer your patient emotional support, and praise him for his efforts. *Note:* When your patient's in bed, instruct him to move around as much as possible. Have him perform the exercises on pages 133 and 134, as ordered.

Depending on your hospital's policy and the doctor's orders, adapt these postop guidelines to your patient's needs:

- Check vital signs and stump drainage every 30 minutes until the patient's condition stabilizes. Using a felt-tipped pen, mark the drainage on your patient's cast or dressing. Be sure to initial it and note the time.
- If the doctor orders, elevate your patient's stump continuously for 24 to 48 hours, to decrease edema. *Important:* If your patient has vascular problems, the doctor may order the end of the bed lowered, to improve circulation to the legs.
- Place an antiembolism stocking on his unaffected leg. After the first 24 to 48 hours, the doctor may order you to position your patient prone to help prevent flexion contractures.
- Perform frequent neurovascular checks.
- Encourage your patient to turn every 2 hours, or as ordered.
- Check your patient's skin for signs of breakdown, such as loss of skin color or swelling, especially around the incision site. If you see any problems, notify the doctor.
- Instruct and encourage your patient to perform range-of-motion and muscle-strengthening exercises several times a day.
- Administer analgesics for pain, as needed.
- Encourage your patient to do as much for himself as possible. Praise him for his efforts.
- Document all care in your nurses' notes.

In addition, *if your patient has a cast on his stump:*

- Be alert for cast slippage as stump swelling decreases. If the cast slips off, wrap an elastic roller bandage around the patient's stump immediately, following the guidelines on pages 125 or 126.
- Be prepared to assist the doctor with cast removal and application, as needed. The doctor will usually change the patient's cast several times during healing to compensate for stump shrinkage.
- Petal cast edges, as needed. For more cast care information, see pages 59 to 68.

If your patient has a dressing on his stump, change the dressing, using strict aseptic technique, as needed or as ordered.

How to help your patient cope with an amputation

"I never know how to start the conversation." Sound familiar? Whenever you're caring for a patient who's had an amputation, those first few words about it can be the hardest to say. But helping your patient and his family cope emotionally, as well as physically, is an important part of your nursing responsibility.

Begin by assessing your own feelings and emotions. Are you able to accept your patient's condition realistically—yet with a positive attitude? If you're having difficulty, consider asking a co-worker to take over for you. Remember, any uneasiness or frustration you feel will be communicated to your patient and his family.

As you perform your patient's daily care, try to evaluate his feelings. If you sense that he wants to talk, sit down and chat for a few minutes. Keep in mind that reaction to an amputation varies from individual to individual. Your patient may feel anger or fear. He may deny or accept his condition. In addition, your patient's family will have to adjust to his condition.

Try to understand the effect your patient's amputation has on his emotions. Encourage family involvement and support as much as possible. And don't hesitate to express your support for your patient and his family. Let them know you care.

Now, here are some specific guidelines to remember when caring for a patient who's had an amputation:

- Try to find out what your patient and his family know about his condition. You'll want to make sure they clearly understand what the doctor's told them.
- Explain the reason for your patient's amputation, and any procedures that may be necessary for his continuing care. Doing so will help both the patient and his family know what to expect.
- Clear up any misconceptions the patient or his family may have. Find out how your patient and his family feel about the amputation. Encourage them to verbalize their feelings of denial, anger, fear, or sorrow.
- Help the patient and his family understand phantom-limb sensations. Tell them the sensations the patient may be experiencing in his missing arm, leg, fingers, or toes, feel real. At times they feel painful. Explain that this condition is normal and may continue for some time.
- Stress to the patient's family the importance of encouraging and supporting the patient as he does things for himself—rather than doing things for him.

Remember: Performing small, easy-to-accomplish tasks will give your patient more confidence and motivate him to be increasingly independent.

And finally, in your nurses' notes, document your observations, all patient teaching, and the reactions of your patient and his family. That way, other nurses who care for your patient can build on your foundation when they provide care.

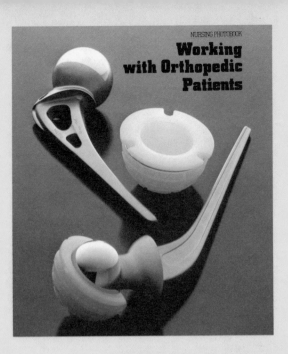

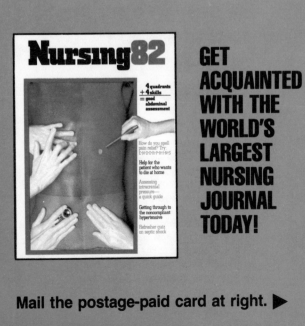

NO POSTAGE
NECESSARY
IF MAILED
IN THE
UNITED STATES

BUSINESS REPLY CARD
FIRST CLASS PERMIT NO. 2080 HICKSVILLE, N.Y.

POSTAGE WILL BE PAID BY ADDRESSEE

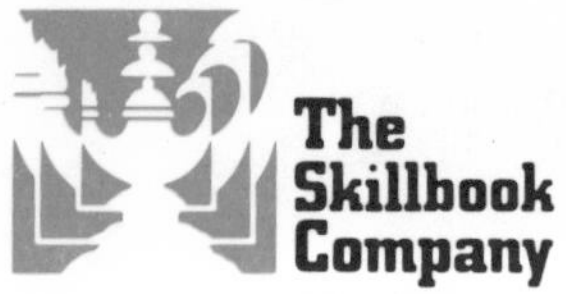

The Skillbook Company
6 Commercial Street
Hicksville, N.Y. 11801

Introduce yourself to the brand-new NURSING PHOTOBOOK™ series

...the remarkable breakthrough in nursing education that can change your career. Each book in this unique series contains detailed *Photostories*... and tables, charts, and graphs to help you learn important new procedures. And each handsome PHOTOBOOK offers you • 160 illustrated, fact-filled pages • brilliant, high-contrast photographs • convenient 9"x10½" size • durable, hardcover binding • carefully chosen bibliography • complete index. Watch the experts at work showing you how to... administer drugs... teach your patient about his illness and its treatment... minimize trauma... understand doctors' diagnoses... increase patient comfort... and much more. Discover how you can become a better nurse by joining this exciting new series. You can examine each PHOTOBOOK at your leisure... for 10 days *absolutely free!*

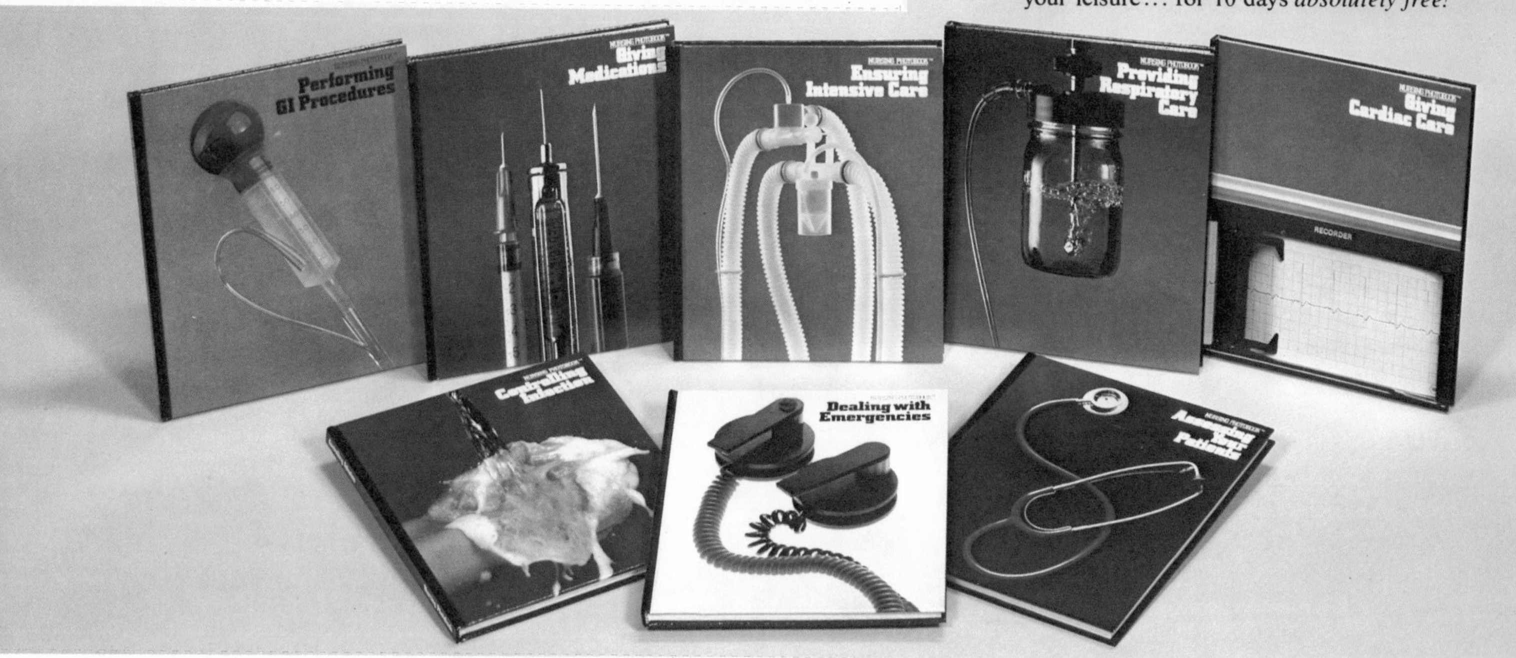

NO POSTAGE
NECESSARY
IF MAILED
IN THE
UNITED STATES

BUSINESS REPLY CARD
FIRST CLASS PERMIT NO. 182 MANASQUAN, N.J.

POSTAGE WILL BE PAID BY ADDRESSEE

Nursing82®
One Health Road
P.O. Box 1008
Manasquan, N.J. 08736

Be sure to mail the postage-paid card at left to reserve *your* first copy of *Nursing82.*

Nursing82 gives you clear, concise instruction in "hands-on" nursing. Every issue brings you in-depth clinical articles about the newest developments in nursing care—what's being discovered, researched, treated, cured. You'll learn about the new procedures, new techniques, new medications, and new equipment that will mean more skills and knowledge for you...better care for your patients!

Order your subscription today!

Stump bandaging after an above-the-knee amputation

1 *Joseph Donaghue, a 62-year-old truck driver, who's an uncontrolled diabetic, has a varicose ulcer that's not responding to treatment. Several days ago, the doctor amputated his left leg above his knee. Now the doctor asks you to bandage his stump. You may use a Jobst® custom-made stump shrinker as a substitute for wrapping. Or, you may follow these steps.*

Begin by explaining to your patient that the bandaging procedure will help reduce swelling and shape his stump for a prosthesis. Also, tell him you'll teach him the procedure as you perform it. Then, place him in a low or semi-Fowler's position, or have him sit on the edge of the bed. Wash your hands. *Note:* For details on applying an elastic roller bandage, see pages 42 and 43.

Now, remove the elastic bandage. Obtain a 4" (10.2 cm) clean elastic bandage. Remove any dressing and discard it. Wash your hands again. Check your patient's leg for signs of circulatory impairment or infection. Notify the doctor if any signs are present. Otherwise, redress the wound.

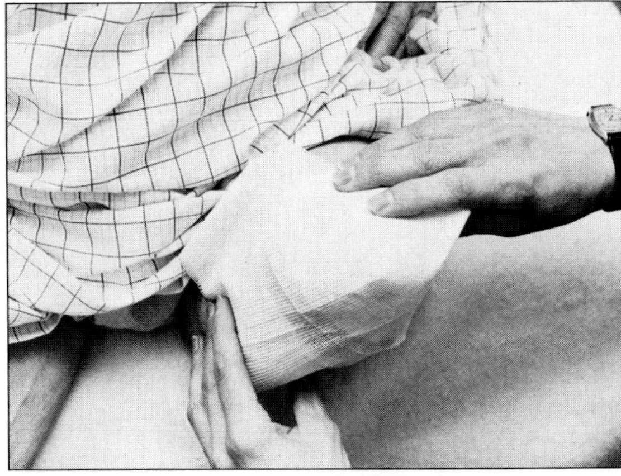

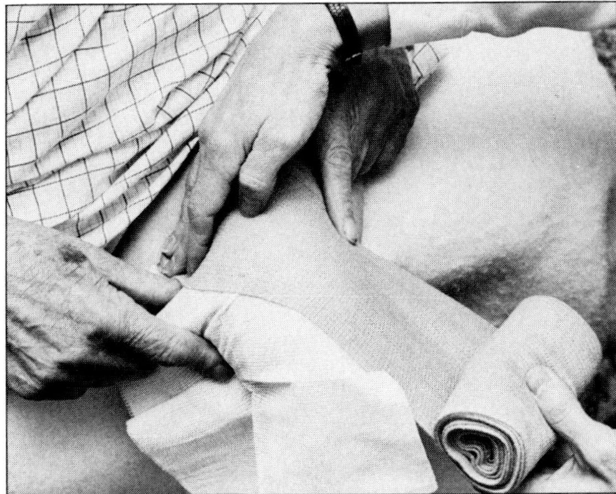

2 Hold the end of the elastic bandage at the top anterior surface of your patient's leg. Or, ask your patient to hold the bandage, if he can. Then, bring the bandage diagonally downward toward the distal end of your patient's stump, as shown here.

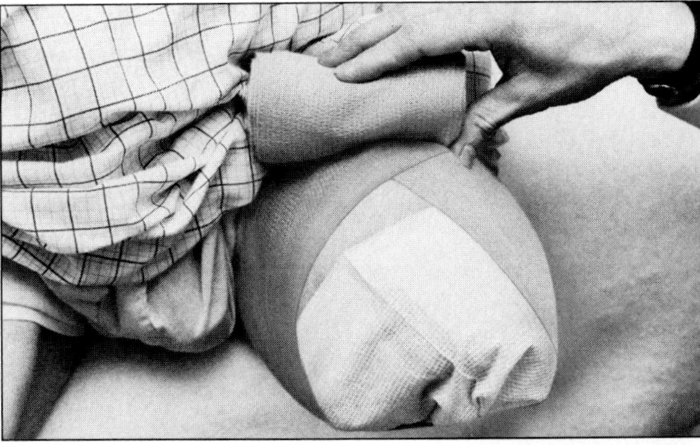

3 Applying even pressure, bring the bandage diagonally upward, close to the groin area.

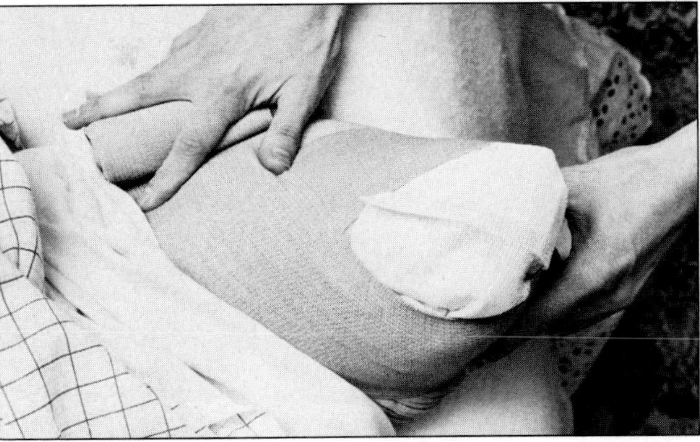

4 Next, secure the bandage end. To do this, make a figure-eight turn with the bandage, wrapping it around the top of your patient's leg, downward under his stump, and back to the groin area, as shown. Then, repeat the figure-eight turn two times.

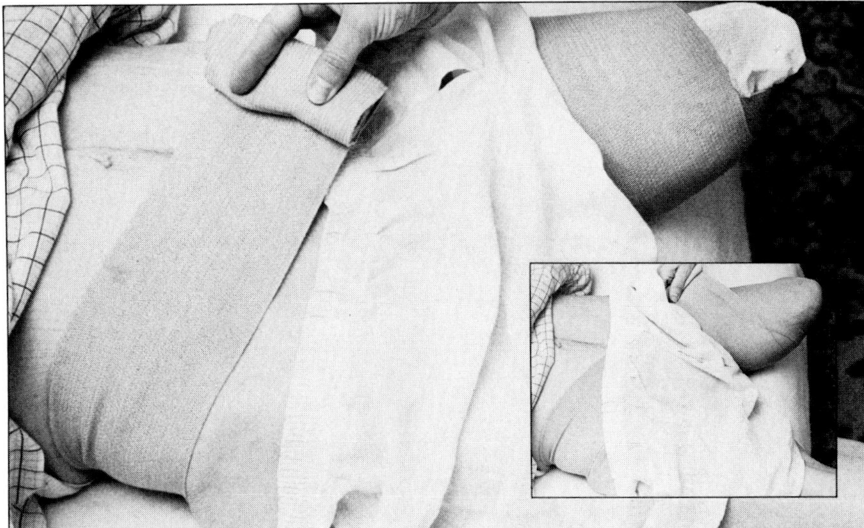

5 Now, bring the bandage diagonally under your patient's buttocks to the opposite iliac crest, and then diagonally back toward his stump, as shown. [Inset] Making figure-eight turns, wrap the bandage around your patient's stump, until it's completely covered, as shown.

Finally, secure the bandage with clips, safety pins, or adhesive tape. If you're using clips or safety pins, make sure they're on the stump's anterior side. Doing so prevents possible pressure areas.

Document the rebandaging procedure in your nurses' notes. *Note:* If you're caring for a patient with an above-the-elbow amputation, adapt this wrapping procedure to meet that patient's particular needs.

Amputation

Stump bandaging after a below-the-knee amputation

1 *Has your patient had a below-the-knee amputation? If so, you'll need to teach him how to properly wrap his stump.* First, place him in low or semi-Fowler's position, or have him sit on the edge of the bed. Then, perform steps 1 and 2 on the previous page. After you've shown him how to wrap the bandage, allow him to practice, as the patient's doing in this photostory.

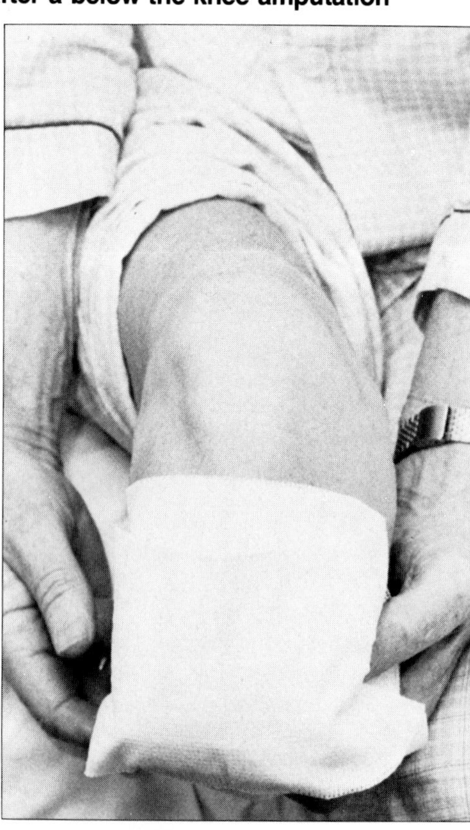

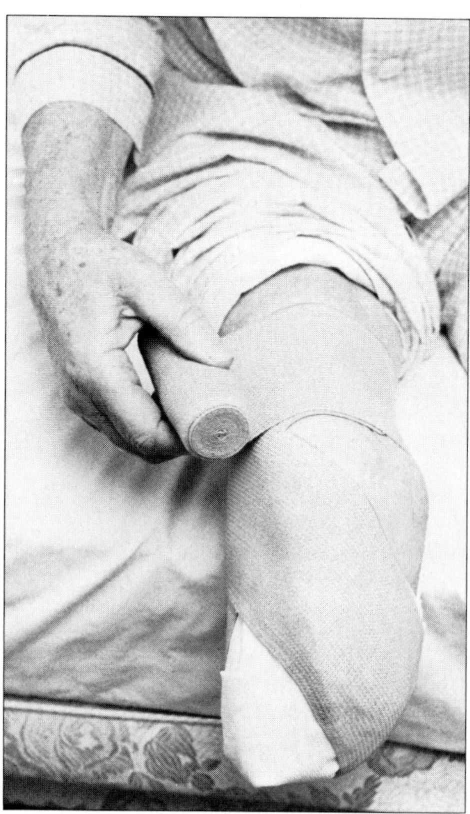

3 Then, your patient should bring the bandage above his knee, to begin making a figure-eight turn. To ensure proper venous blood return, he should apply less tension on the bandage above his knee than on the end of the stump.

[Below] Have him continue the figure-eight turn to cover his stump end and knee.

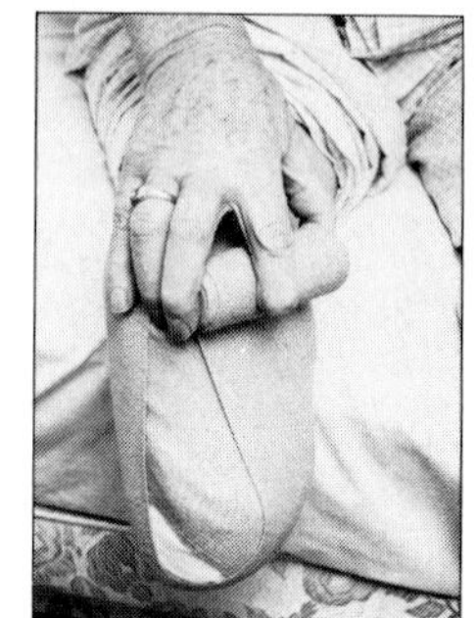

2 First, with one hand, the patient should hold the end of the elastic bandage just above the bend of his knee. With his other hand, he should bring the bandage downward to the distal end of his stump. Tell him to be careful not to fold or crease the elastic bandage.

When he reaches the end of his stump, he should bring the bandage upward in a diagonal direction.

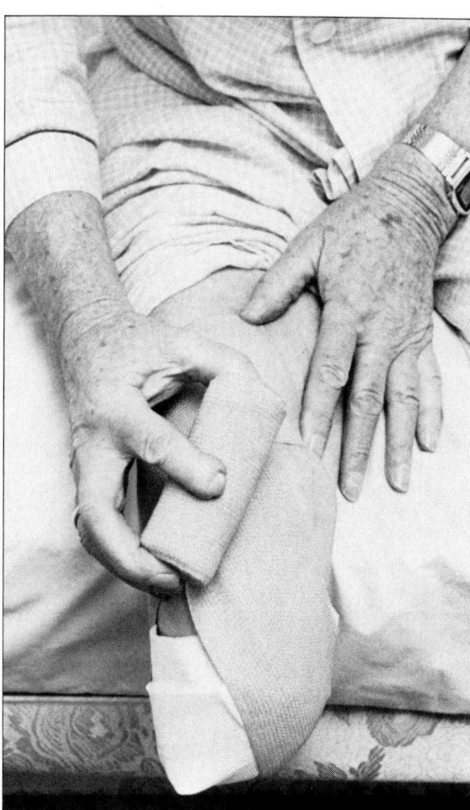

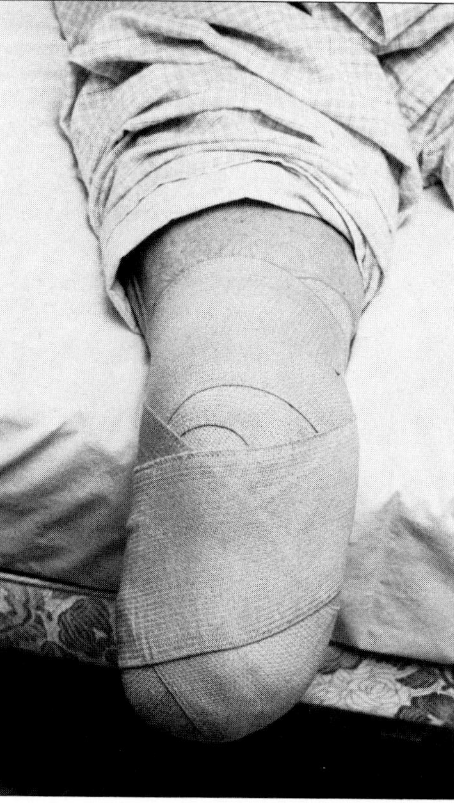

4 Then, he'll repeat the figure-eight pattern two more times until the stump and knee are completely covered. He'll secure the bandage with clips, tape, or safety pins.

Document the entire procedure, including your patient teaching, in your nurses' notes. *Note:* If you're caring for a patient with a below-the-elbow amputation, adapt this wrapping procedure to meet that patient's particular needs.

Home care

Going home after amputation

Dear Patient:
Now that you're ready to go home, be sure to follow these instructions. They'll help speed your recovery and ensure that your new prosthesis fits and functions properly. Here's what to do:

1 Inspect your stump once a day. Use a mirror to help you see all surfaces. Call your doctor if your incision appears to be opening, looks red or swollen, feels warm, is painful to the touch, or you see drainage.

Suppose you see a blister, raw spot, or cut on your stump. Your prosthesis may need an adjustment. Call your prosthetist immediately, and follow his instructions. Don't cover the irritated area with gauze, tape, or a Band-Aid®. And never try to adjust the prosthesis by yourself.

Clean your stump daily, using a washcloth and mild soap, such as Ivory®. Rinse the area with warm water and dry it thoroughly. To ensure proper prosthesis fit, do not apply rubbing alcohol, oil, or body lotion to your stump.

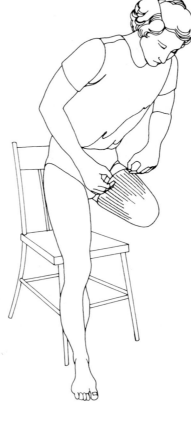

2 Before applying your prosthesis, slip a specially made sock (synthetic or woolen, whichever you prefer) over your stump. Make sure the sock fits properly, and smooth out any wrinkles. To avoid skin irritation, never apply a sock that's been mended, or has tears, holes, or seams. Wash the sock daily and dry it thoroughly. Remember, if your sock's woolen, allow it to air-dry. A woolen sock will shrink in a dryer.

When the doctor says it's okay, you'll begin wearing your prosthesis all day long. Doing so will help mold your stump. However, expect your prosthesis to need adjustments from time to time. Remember, as your stump heals, it should shrink, because the swollen tissue is returning to normal. But, if your prosthesis begins to feel too tight, remove it, and elevate your stump for short periods during the day. If the prosthesis continues to feel too tight and you notice increased swelling, call your doctor. Suppose the prosthesis feels too loose. In that case, make an appointment to see your prosthetist.

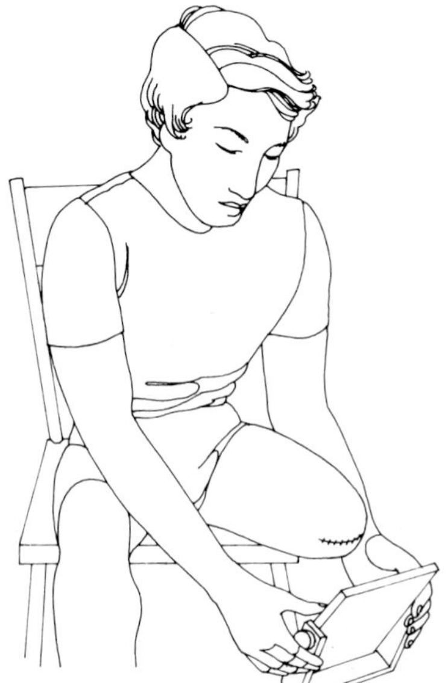

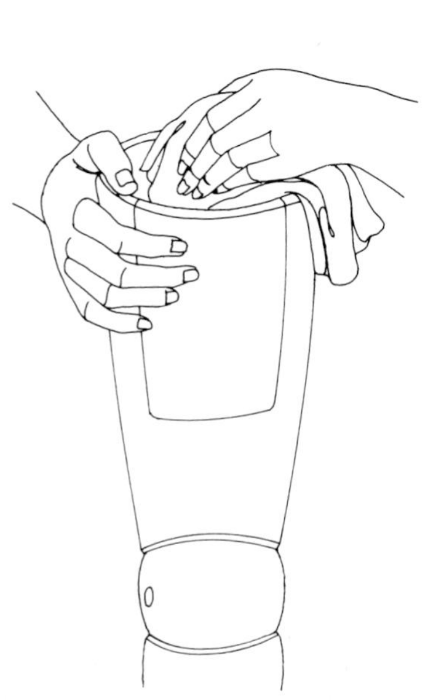

3 When you remove your prosthesis after a day's wear, use a damp cloth to wipe out the inside. Thoroughly dry it with a towel. Never immerse your prosthesis in water. Water will eventually deteriorate the prosthesis' leather and joints.

In addition to the instructions given above, read and follow the manufacturer's instructions that came with your prosthesis. Also, be sure to return to your prosthetist for a yearly check.

Finally, continue to perform the arm or leg exercises the nurse taught you in the hospital.

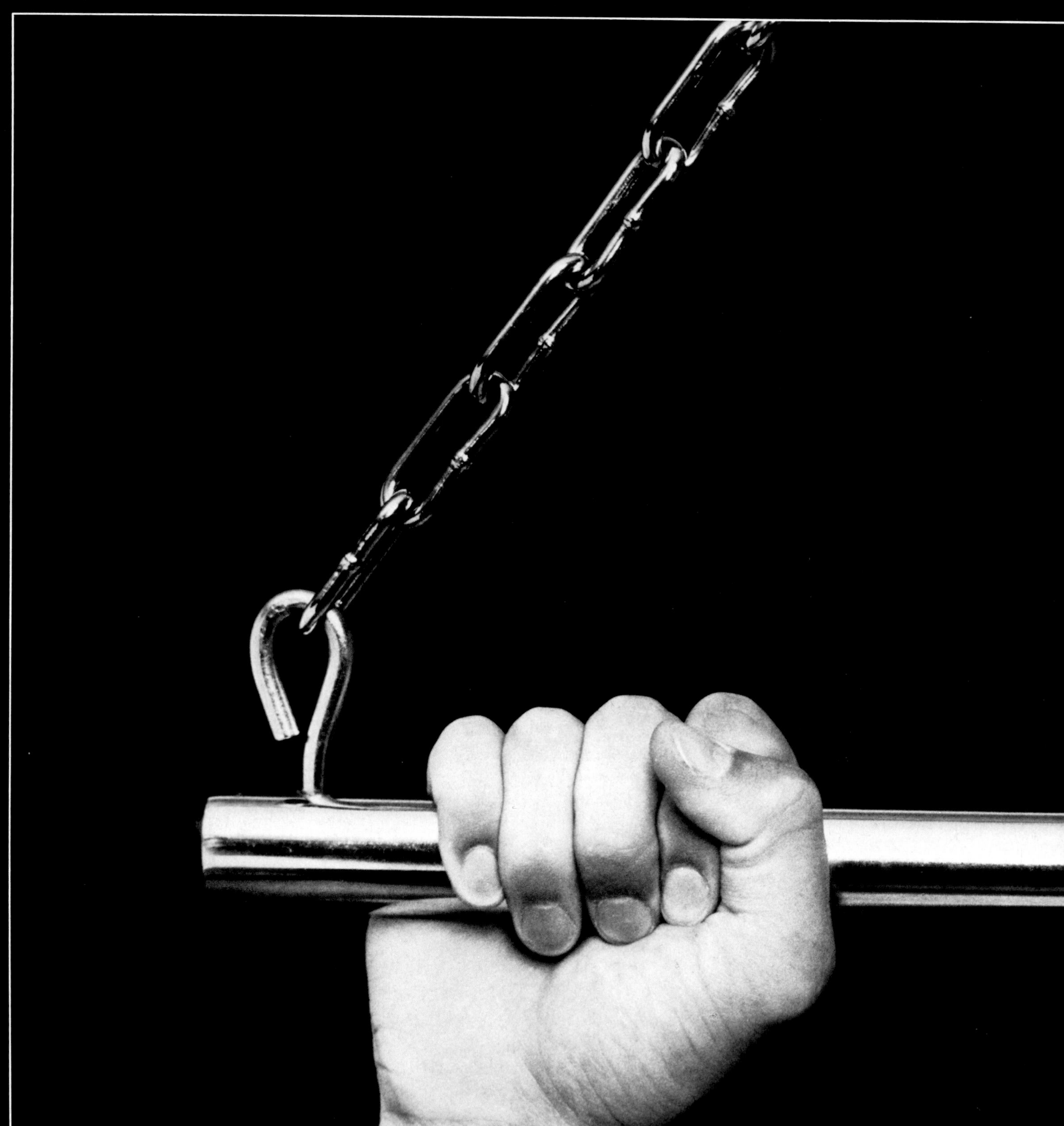

Preventing Complications

Common complications
Pain control
Positioning aids
Ambulation aids

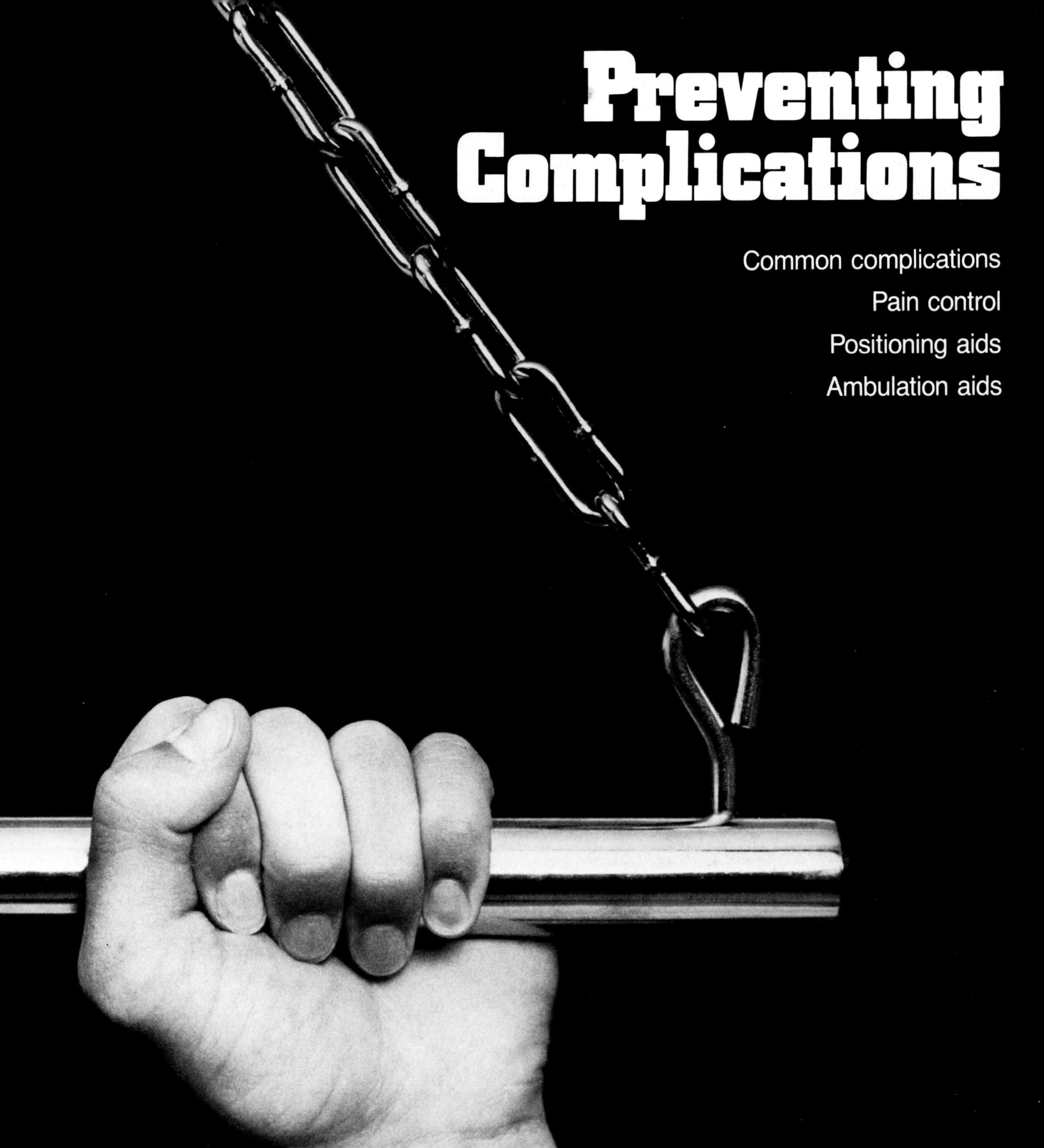

Common complications

How much do you understand about the complications your orthopedic patient's most likely to experience? For example, do you know the causes of malunion in a fractured bone? How to detect the onset of gas gangrene? The signs and symptoms of fat embolism? You'll find answers to these questions, and more, in the text at right.

Then, in the pages that follow, we'll briefly outline immobility complications and show you how to help prevent them through exercise.

Use the information presented here to help promote proper healing and speed

Understanding bone-healing problems

Does your patient have a bone fracture? Then, he's vulnerable to three fracture complications: *delayed union, malunion,* and *nonunion.*

In *delayed union,* callus formation is retarded, so the fracture fails to mend within the normal healing time. Factors contributing to this complication include:

- inadequate fracture immobilization
- repeated fracture manipulation
- infection of the fractured bone
- infection of the surrounding tissues (as in an open fracture)
- defective metabolism, especially protein metabolism
- vitamin C or vitamin D deficiency.

Delayed union is a temporary condition; healing eventually will occur. Treatment involves maintaining proper immobilization during the healing process. Tibia and femur fractures, when complicated by delayed union, may heal faster if weight-bearing's combined with immobilization. External fixation, for example, allows this.

Malunion means a fracture has healed incorrectly, leaving the bone deformed, weak, and possibly causing pain. Malunion may limit range of motion. Contributing factors include:

- inadequate fracture reduction
- an improperly applied cast
- a cast that has softened, permitting bony fragments to move.

If the doctor detects malunion *before* healing's complete, he can realign the bone fragments. If he detects malunion *after* healing's complete, he'll have to surgically correct the malunion to obtain a more

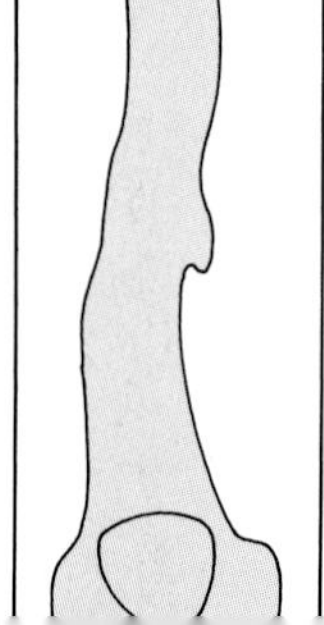

rection procedure could cause delayed union or nonunion.

In *nonunion,* the fracture never mends. Instead, a false joint (pseudarthrosis) may form at the fracture site, causing excessive bone mobility, decreased joint motion *proximal* and *distal* to the fracture site, gradual muscle atrophy, and pain with weight bearing.

What causes nonunion? Any of the following:

- inadequate immobilization
- inadequate fracture reduction
- poor blood circulation to the fracture site
- bone fragmentation, which allows soft tissue to intervene between bone fragments
- loss of bone tissue, especially from necrosis.

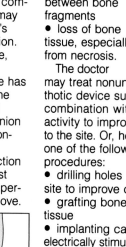

The doctor may treat nonunion with an orthotic device such as a brace, in combination with increased activity to improve blood supply to the site. Or, he may perform one of the following surgical procedures:

- drilling holes near the fracture site to improve circulation
- grafting bone to supply bone tissue
- implanting cathode wires to electrically stimulate bone growth.

What can you do to help prevent these three complications? Whatever the immobilization device your patient's using, monitor him to assess and maintain proper immobilization. Increase activity only as directed by the doctor. Encourage range-of-motion exercises, as ordered. Provide strict aseptic wound care

Identifying infection signs and symptoms

Infection can affect the healing process in any orthopedic injury. When left untreated, infection can spread through soft tissue and destroy bone, causing irreparable damage and in some cases, death.

Recognizing infection's signs and symptoms is important to early detection and treatment. As you care for your patient, observe him for systemic signs and symptoms of infection, such as fatigue, malaise, slightly elevated temperature, and nausea. Also, look for localized signs and symptoms, such as redness, swelling, and pain. Always take particular care when assessing a patient with:

- an open fracture
- a wound under a cast
- an external fixator
- pins for skeletal traction
- a surgical wound.

Here we'll discuss two serious infection problems associated with orthopedic injuries: osteomyelitis and gas gangrene. Read the following information carefully.

Osteomyelitis

This infection may occur when pyogenic bacteria, such as *Staphylococcus aureaus,* invade the patient's injured bone or soft tissue surrounding the bone. Usually, the bacteria reach the bone as a result of erosion from a neighboring infection, by direct contamination, or from a systemic infection.

As the infection progresses, pus accumulating at the infection site may form an intramedullary abscess. In osteomyelitis, the abscess generally forms at the tip of a long bone, where it exerts pressure inside the bone. Pressure spreads the infection, leading to bone destruction

Or, the infection incubates and, in time, gradually works its way out by abscess and sinus tract formation.

Look for the following signs and symptoms that accompany osteomyelitis:

- localized redness, warmth, and edema over the involved bone
- tenderness in soft tissue over the involved area
- severe, continuous pulsating pain in the affected bone or the adjacent joint region from pus under pressure in the bone. This pain is usually aggravated by motion.
- sudden fever
- tachycardia
- nausea
- general malaise
- elevated ESR (erythrocyte sedimentation rate)
- leukocytosis, indicated by white blood cell count (WBC)
- presence of causative organism in wound or blood culture.

Administer broad spectrum antibiotics, as ordered, until blood or wound cultures identify causative organism. Then, administer ordered antibiotic specific for the organism. Surgical incision and drainage will relieve the pressure from a localized abscess within the bone and periosteum. The doctor may also order you to irrigate the wound, using low pressure suction. He'll probably immobilize the affected bone with a cast, traction, or bed rest. Administer analgesics, and oral and I.V. fluids, as ordered. Maintain strict aseptic technique when changing dressings and irrigating wounds. Wash your hands before and after giving patient care. *Remember:* Isolation may be indicated. Follow your hospital's policy.

Gas gangrene

Gas gangrene occurs most often in deep wounds (especially those in which tissue necrosis further reduces oxygen supply) or in wounds grossly contaminated following trauma. Anaerobic wound culture reveals gram-positive *Clostridium* species bacteria.

If your patient has gas gangrene of his wound, you'll probably see, feel, or hear crepitation from carbon dioxide and hydrogen gas bubbles, which are metabolic by-products of necrotic tissue. Other signs and symptoms include:

- severe, localized pain
- edema
- discoloration (often dusky-brown or reddish)
- formation of bullae (large blisters), and necrosis
- frothy, foul-smelling drainage
- eventual rupture of wound, revealing dark red or black necrotic muscle
- extreme apprehension
- moderate fever, usually below 101° F. (38.3° C.)
- hypotension
- tachycardia
- tachypnea.

Provide the following nursing care:

- Observe your patient for signs of ischemia in the affected limb, such as cool skin temperature, pallor or cyanosis, sudden severe pain, edema, and loss of pulses.
- Observe affected area carefully for inflammation of cellular tissue (cellulitis), and muscle tissue (myositis), indicated by redness, warmth, and tenderness. For cellulitis, apply warm compresses, as ordered. If you detect signs of myositis, the doctor must immediately surgically debride all affected tissue and necrotic muscle.
- Administer high-dosage antibiotics I.V., as ordered.
- Wear sterile gloves when changing dressings and maintain strict aseptic technique at all times.
- Dispose of wound drainage matter according to your hospital's infection control policy.
- Provide hyperbaric oxygenation after debridement, as ordered.

Hyperbaric oxygen therapy

If your patient develops gas gangrene, or persistent osteomyelitis, the doctor may order hyperbaric oxygen therapy. This therapy provides an oxygen-rich environment to help destroy the anaerobic organisms that cause gas gangrene. Also, it promotes quicker healing, partly by improving circulation and stimulating capillary development.

To give hyperbaric oxygen therapy, you'll use a specially designed chamber. In the chamber, the patient can receive 100% oxygen concentration at greater than normal atmospheric pressure. By increasing barometric pressure within the chamber, you can give him double or triple this concentration.

Two types of chambers exist: a monoplace and a multiplace. The monoplace chamber holds only one patient. You'll place him on a stretcher that slides into the chamber. Since oxygen's piped directly into the chamber, the patient won't need an oxygen mask.

Monoplace chambers don't allow you to attend the patient directly. However, they do have a communication system that lets you talk to him. And, some chamber models are partially transparent acrylic, allowing you to see the patient during treatment.

The multiplace chamber accommodates several patients and staff members. The staff members breathe piped-in compressed air. Patients receive 100% oxygen through a tight-fitting aviator mask or hood. Or, you may apply it directly to the affected area, using a bag or cup.

Caution: Never use hyperbaric oxygen therapy for patients with untreated pneumothorax; emphysema with carbon dioxide retention; untreated metastatic cancer; epilepsy; history of thoracic or ear surgery, or upper respiratory infection.

When using a hyperbaric chamber, take these precautions:

- Warn your patient that when treatment begins, he may feel pressure in his ears, as though he were in an airplane. Tell your patient to swallow, yawn, or move his jaw from side to side to relieve this discomfort.

  Note: Some patients must undergo a myringotomy to prevent ear damage.
- Warn your patient that he may experience visual changes, such as nearsightedness or double vision. Normal vision will return after each therapy session.
- Because concentrated oxygen's highly flammable, reduce static electricity by warning anyone who enters the chamber to wear all-cotton clothing. In addition, make sure all bed linens and towels

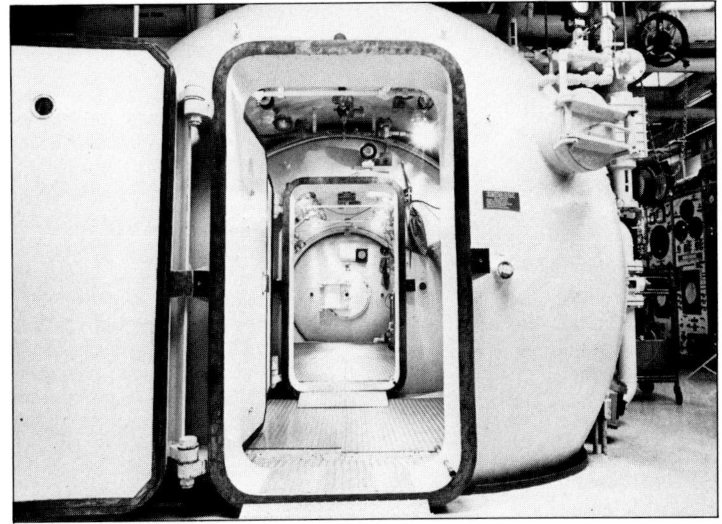

Common complications

Hyperbaric oxygen therapy continued

are 100% cotton and that the pillows are feather-filled.

- Don't allow pens, hearing aids, petroleum-based products, matches, or smoking materials inside the hyperbaric chamber.
- To protect your patient against high noise level in a multiplace chamber, place earmuffs on his ears.
- Keep the patient in the chamber only as long as ordered.
- Don't administer 100% oxygen at pressures higher than three times that of sea level. Doing so can cause central nervous system (CNS) toxicosis, indicated by apprehension, visual changes, muscular twitches, and convulsions. If your patient develops any of these signs or symptoms, notify the doctor. He may order treatment stopped.

Note: Central nervous system toxicosis usually precedes pulmonary toxicosis, which can cause substernal chest pain, patchy atelectasis on chest X-ray, and decreased performance on pulmonary function tests.

- Be aware of the complications that can develop from repeated treatments. These include: spontaneous pneumothorax; air embolism (from your patient holding his breath during the decompression phase); CNS and pulmonary toxicity; labored breathing; and barotrauma (ear and sinus compression).

Learning about fat embolism

Q&A

Perhaps you've heard about fat embolism, a common complication of long-bone fractures or surgery, or multiple fractures. But, you may not know enough about it to detect it in your patient. Following are some questions you might have.

Question: What exactly is fat embolism?
Answer: A fat embolism is an accumulation of fat particles (emboli) which obstruct blood flow and cause inflammatory reactions around affected blood vessels. Some emboli lodge in blood vessels of the patient's lungs, while smaller globules may filter through the lungs and circulate to other body areas, such as the brain.

Question: What causes fat embolism?
Answer: Researchers have formulated several theories about fat embolism development, but none are conclusive. A fat embolism may develop after pressure changes in the fractured bone's interior. The pressure change may force fat molecules out of the bone marrow and into the systemic circulation. A second theory states that the emboli form when fat emulsions in blood plasma combine with platelets.

Question: How can I detect a fat embolism in my patient?
Answer: Signs and symptoms usually occur within 24 to 72 hours following the fracture or surgery. However, they may appear up to 7 to 10 days after it. Fat emboli may circulate to lungs within minutes after release from the marrow, causing dyspnea, air hunger, and tachypnea from hypoxia. Emboli may also affect the central nervous system causing confusion, restlessness, combativeness, and coma. Flat petechiae, which fail to blanch when you apply pressure, develop above the patient's nipple line. Evidence of hemorrhage and exudate may appear in your patient's retinae. Other signs and symptoms may include cyanosis, elevated temperature, and oliguria.

Lab tests may reveal more evidence of fat embolism, such as a sudden drop in hemoglobin; elevated levels of free fatty acids; low arterial oxygen tension; and microscopic fat particles in sputum and urine. The most definitive of the diagnostic tests is a cryostat test, which reveals the fat droplets in frozen sections of blood clots.

Severe cases of fat embolism may rapidly lead to coma and death. However, signs and symptoms may remain subtle and undetected.

Question: How does the doctor treat fat embolism?
Answer: Treatment primarily addresses the signs and symptoms; for example, you'll probably administer oxygen. Occasionally, the patient may require endotracheal intubation and mechanical ventilation if signs and symptoms worsen. Also, the doctor may order administration of anti-inflammatory medications, diuretics for pulmonary congestion, or parenteral infusions of low-molecular dextran.

Question: What is my role in caring for a patient who's predisposed to fat embolism?
Answer: Because the causes of fat embolism haven't been clearly defined, neither have preventive measures. One measure that may help prevent it is to splint the fracture immediately after injury. Perform frequent, thorough assessments of a patient at risk for fat embolism. Immediately report any signs and symptoms to the doctor.

Note: A patient with long-bone fractures or long-bone surgery who goes into shock, is more vulnerable to developing fat emboli. Provide rapid treatment for shock.

Reviewing common immobility complications

As you know, patients with orthopedic injuries usually require limb immobilization. Sometimes, they need extended bed rest. But, although limiting movement may help a fracture or other injury to heal, immobilization can also negatively affect many of your patient's body systems.

Here's a list of body systems, and the complications that can affect each one:

- *Integumentary (skin)*—pressure areas, decubitus ulcers, and infection
- *Skeletal*—disuse osteoporosis
- *Muscular*—contractures, decreased muscle tone, backaches, muscle atrophy
- *Cardiovascular*—decreased myocardial tone, venous blood stasis, thrombus formation, orthostatic hypotension, and pulmonary edema
- *Respiratory*—atelectasis and hypostatic pneumonia
- *Gastrointestinal*—anorexia, ileal stasis, paralytic ileus, distention, stress ulcers, constipation, and diarrhea
- *Genitourinary*—urinary retention, renal calculi, and urinary tract infection
- *Psychological*—regression, dependency, withdrawal, loneliness, and sexual frustration that may lead to emotional outbursts or abnormal behavior.

Remember, your primary goal is to prevent these complications through conscientious nursing care. But, if you do detect complications, adjust your nursing care to meet patient needs.

To review both prevention and treatment measures, refer to the NURSING PHOTOBOOKS ENSURING INTENSIVE CARE, PROVIDING EARLY MOBILITY, and COPING WITH NEUROLOGIC DISORDERS. Also, to help prevent complications, teach your patient the general strengthening exercises given on the following pages.

Reviewing commonly prescribed exercises

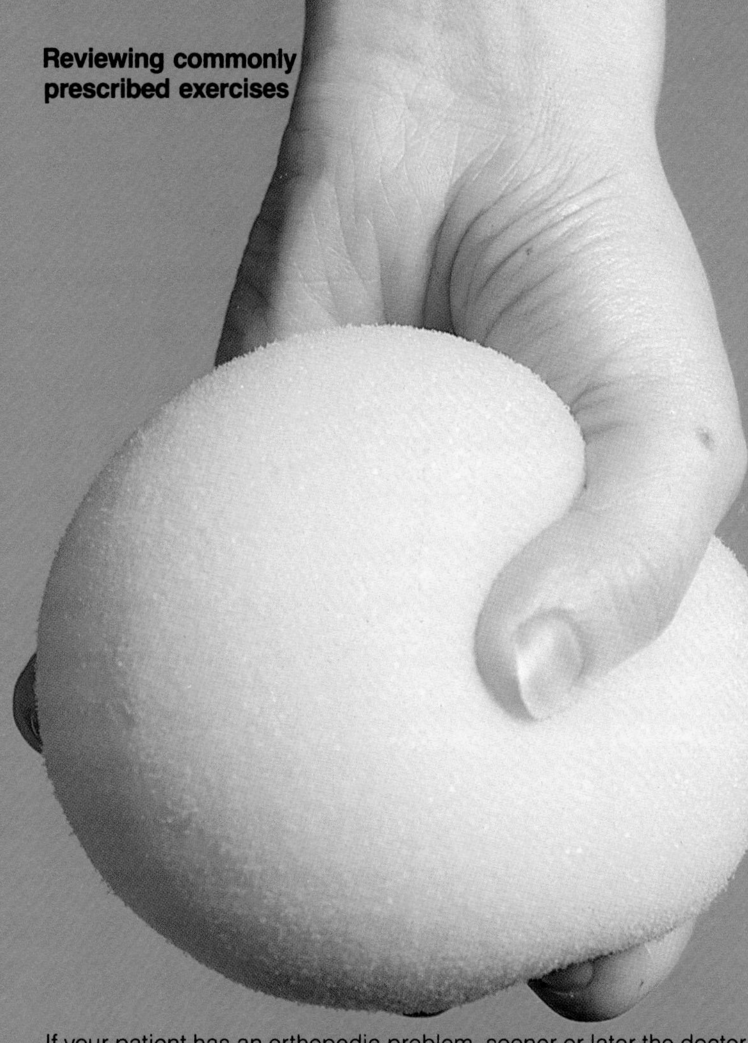

If your patient has an orthopedic problem, sooner or later the doctor will order an exercise program. These exercises will help maintain muscle tone and build muscle strength, preventing muscle atrophy and contractures.

When designing an exercise program for your patient, expect the doctor to consider your patient's personal preferences, age, physical condition, and strength.

In carrying out the program, you and the physical therapist will follow the doctor's orders closely. Be sure to assess the patient's needs and the equipment available in the hospital as well as at home.

Remember to document all patient teaching and your patient's reaction to it, in your notes.

We've detailed eight commonly prescribed exercises here. By familiarizing yourself with these exercises, you'll be better prepared to help your patient, if necessary. But, always keep in mind these important points:

- Stress to your patient the importance of doing the *exercises* and *repetitions* exactly as ordered by the doctor.
- Instruct your patient to stop immediately and tell you, the doctor, or the physical therapist if she feels pain or meets resistance while doing any of her exercises.
- Never encourage her to perform any exercises not ordered by the doctor.

Has the doctor ordered hand exercises for your patient? He may want her to squeeze a rubber or sponge ball, as shown above.

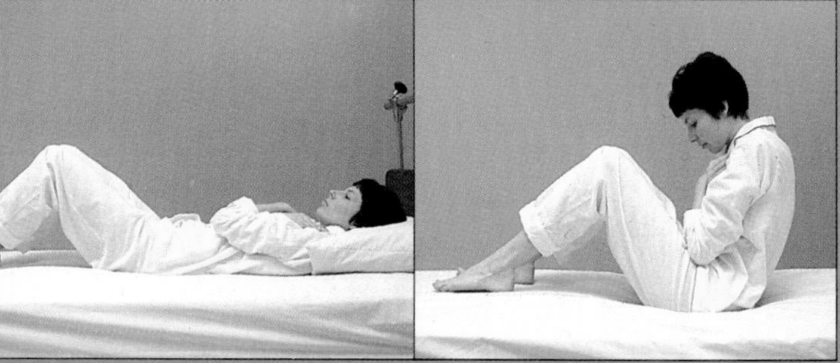

If your patient's going to be using crutches, a walker, or cane, the doctor may order bent leg sit-ups to strengthen her abdominal muscles. Here's how to teach your patient to do this exercise: Tell her to lie flat in bed, bend her knees and cross her arms on her chest. Instruct her to sit up as far as possible and then return to a flat position on the bed.

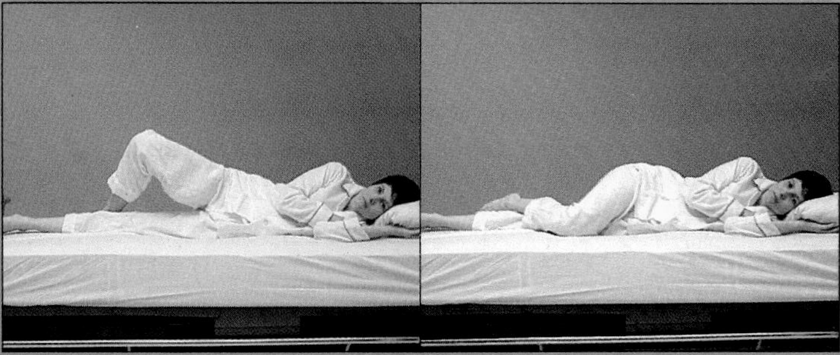

Suppose the doctor wants your patient to strengthen her hips. To perform an abduction/adduction exercise with the leg in flexion, position your patient on her side. Instruct her to fully flex her knee and hip closest to the ceiling. Then, have her move her knee first toward the ceiling, and then toward the mattress, as the patient's doing here.

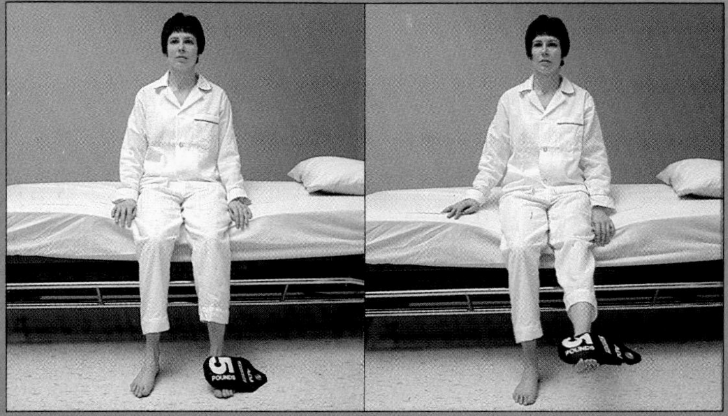

Let's say your patient has had surgery on her right leg. The doctor wants her to build strength in her left leg, for weight-bearing during crutch-walking. He may suggest the patient do leg raises with a 5-pound sandbag placed on the anterior surface of her foot, at ankle level. Have your patient sit at the edge of the bed with her feet flat on the floor. Position the sandbag over her foot and tell her to raise her leg as high as possible without causing pain. Instruct her to return her leg to starting position.

Common complications

Reviewing commonly prescribed exercises continued

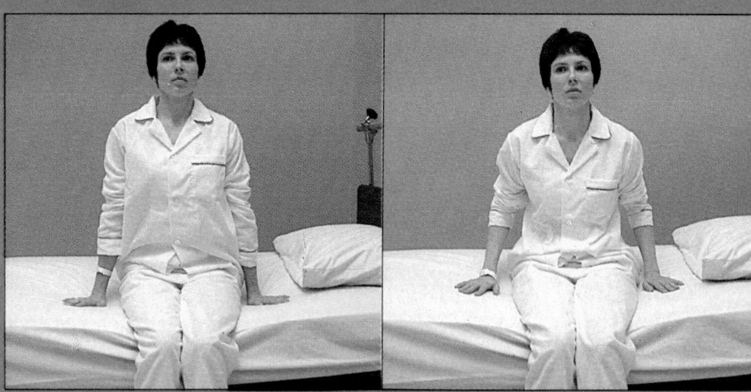

Your patient with special equipment such as crutches, a walker, cane, or wheelchair will also need to build arm strength. Have her sit on the edge of the bed with her back straight. Tell her to place her palms flat on the bed and lock her elbows. Now, encourage her to press down against her palms, gradually releasing pressure.

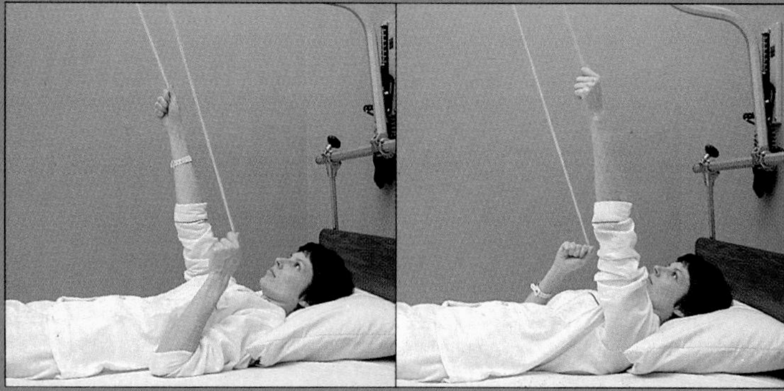

Here's another arm-strengthening exercise: Attach two pulleys on each end of a 36″ (91 cm) overhead bar. Thread the rope through the pulleys on the overhead bar. Make sure equal lengths extend on each side. Have your patient grasp both rope ends and alternately pull each downward.

Nursing tip: Tie a large knot or loop at each rope end. Doing so gives the patient something to grasp.

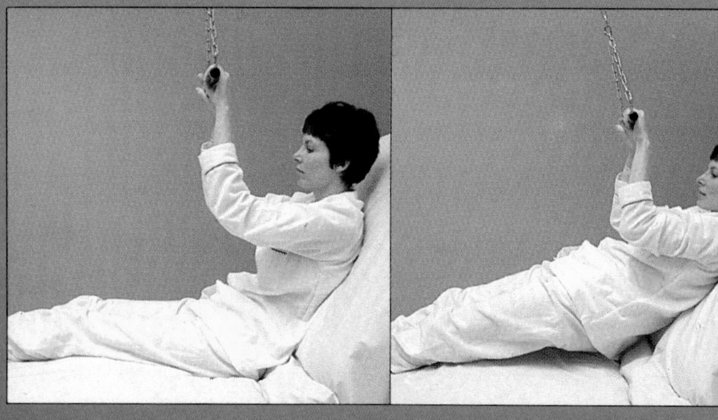

If the doctor wants your patient to use the overhead trapeze to strengthen her upper arm muscles, have her grasp the trapeze bar with both hands. Make sure the bed is in high Fowler's position. Then, tell her to pull herself up using the trapeze, until her buttocks are off the bed. Have her gradually lower herself back onto the bed.

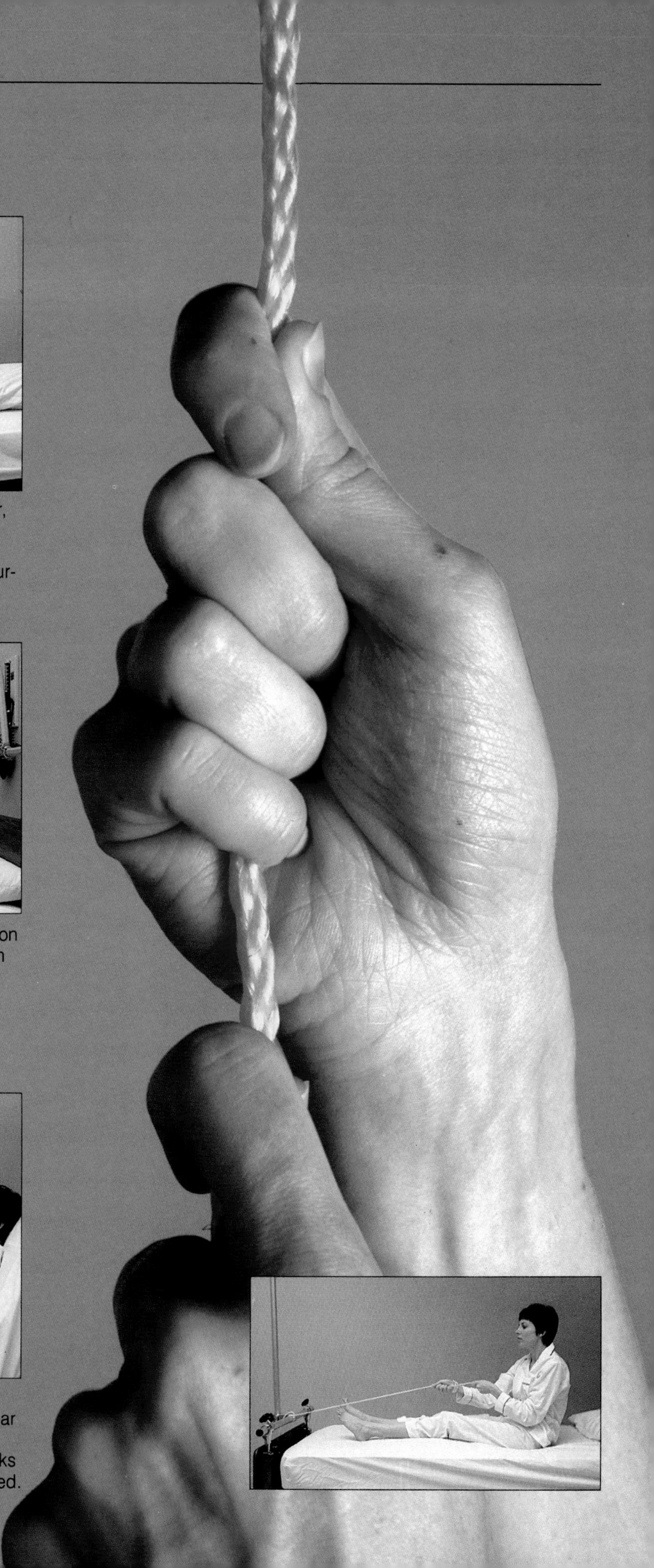

Pain control

Do you often worry about how to cope with an orthopedic patient's pain? A patient with arthritis may have such severe chronic pain that it restricts his mobility. A patient with a fractured femur probably has acute, agonizing pain, which may increase when the fracture's reduced. Either way, pain relief for the patient with an orthopedic problem is one of your top priorities as a nurse.

See the chart that follows for detailed information about commonly used pain-relief medications. Then, read the guidelines on pain assessment and noninvasive treatment alternatives. The next few pages could make a difference in how much pain your patient has to suffer.

Nurses' guide to pain control medications

If your patient with an orthopedic problem has muscle spasms, pre- and postoperative pain, or an inflammatory disorder, such as arthritis, the doctor may order a muscle relaxant, analgesic, or an anti-inflammatory agent. Of course, the drug, dose, and administration route the doctor chooses will depend on your patient's condition and past medical history.

For your reference, here's a list of commonly administered drugs. Read the indications to find out when each is used. Also, familiarize yourself with the special considerations for safe administration. For more information on these and other drugs, refer to the NURSING DRUG HANDBOOK™ or the NURSE'S GUIDE TO DRUGS™.

Meperidine hydrochloride

(Demerol*)
Narcotic analgesic

Indications and dosage

Moderate to severe pain
Adults: 50 to 150 mg P.O., I.M., or subcutaneously every 3 to 4 hours, as needed.
Preoperative
Adults: 50 to 100 mg I.M. or subcutaneously 30 to 90 minutes before surgery.

Side effects

Respiratory depression; dizziness; euphoria; lightheadedness; restlessness; transient hallucinations and disorientation; sedation; convulsions with high doses; tachycardia; bradycardia; palpitations; hypotension; shock; nausea; vomiting; dry mouth; constipation; biliary tract spasm; urinary retention; injection site pain; local tissue irritation and induration after subcutaneous injection; phlebitis after I.V. injection; pruritus; rash; urticaria; tolerance; sweating; weakness; physical and psychological dependence

Interactions

- MAO inhibitors and isoniazid (INH) cause increased central nervous system excitation or depression which may be severe or fatal. Don't use together.

Precautions

- Contraindicated if patient has used MAO inhibitors within 14 days.
- Use extreme caution if giving meperidine hydrochloride (Demerol*) with another narcotic analgesic; with a general anesthetic; a phenothiazine; a sedative; a hypnotic; a tricyclic antidepressant; or alcohol, as respiratory depression, hypotension, profound sedation, or coma may result. If drug combination's necessary, obtain an order to reduce meperidine hydrochloride dose. Closely monitor patient.
- Use cautiously in patients with increased intracranial pressure; increased cerebrospinal fluid (CSF) pressure or shock; central nervous system depression; head injury; asthma; chronic obstructive pulmonary disease (COPD); respiratory depression; supraventricular tachycardia; seizures; acute abdominal conditions; hepatic or renal disease; hypothyroidism; Addison's disease; urethral stricture; prostatic hypertrophy; alcoholism; and in children under 12 years old, or elderly or debilitated patients.

Nursing considerations

- Administer I.M. if possible. Oral dose less effective than parenteral dose. If changing from parenteral to P.O., increase dose, as ordered.

Nursing considerations continued

- If administering syrup P.O., give with a full glass of water, as syrup has local anesthetic effect.
- Avoid subcutaneous administration as drug may cause injection site pain, tissue irritation, or induration.
- Instruct ambulatory patients that drug causes drowsiness and they should avoid activities that require alertness and good psychomotor coordination, such as driving a vehicle.
- Monitor respiratory and cardiovascular status carefully. Don't administer drug if respirations are below 12 breaths per minute, or if you note any pupillary changes.
- Don't mix drug with a barbiturate (in the same syringe).
- Drug shouldn't be discontinued abruptly after long-term use. If drug is discontinued suddenly, observe for convulsions, tremors, abdominal and muscle cramps, vomiting, and sweating.
- Warn patient not to combine drug with alcohol or other depressants.

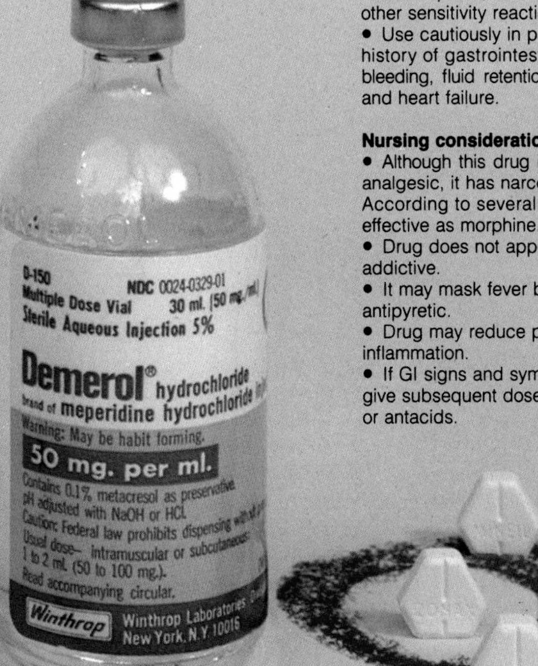

Zomepirac sodium

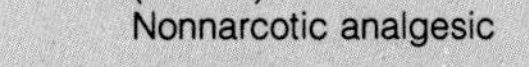

(Zomax)
Nonnarcotic analgesic

Indications and dosage

For mild to moderately severe pain
Adults: 100 mg P.O every 4 to 6 hours as needed, up to a maximum of 600 mg per day. (For mild pain, 50 mg every 4 to 6 hours may be sufficient.)

Side effects

Tinnitus; taste change; drowsiness; dizziness; insomnia; paresthesia; nervousness; edema; hypertension; cardiac irregularity; palpitations; nausea; vomiting; diarrhea; dyspepsia; constipation; flatulence; anorexia; urinary frequency; elevated blood urea nitrogen (BUN) and creatinine levels; urinary tract infection; vaginitis; rash; pruritus; chills

Interactions

- Aspirin may decrease zomepirac sodium's efficacy.

Precautions

- Contraindicated for patients in whom aspirin and other nonsteroidal anti-inflammatory drugs induce bronchospasm, rhinitis, urticaria, or other sensitivity reactions.
- Use cautiously in patients with a history of gastrointestinal (GI) bleeding, fluid retention, hypertension, and heart failure.

Nursing considerations

- Although this drug is a nonnarcotic analgesic, it has narcotic potency. According to several studies, it's as effective as morphine.
- Drug does not appear to be addictive.
- It may mask fever because it's antipyretic.
- Drug may reduce pain caused by inflammation.
- If GI signs and symptoms occur, give subsequent doses with food or antacids.

*Available in both the United States and in Canada

Pain control

Nurses' guide to pain control medications continued

Aspirin

(Empirin, Ecotrin*, A.S.A.)
Nonnarcotic analgesic

Indications and dosage

Arthritis (drug has anti-inflammatory effect)
Adults: 2.6 to 5.2 g P.O. daily in divided doses.
Mild pain or fever
Adults: 325 to 650 mg P.O. or rectally every 4 hours, as needed.
Thromboembolic disorders
Adults: 325 to 650 mg P.O. daily or b.i.d.

Side effects

Prolonged bleeding time; tinnitus and hearing loss (first sign of overdose or toxicosis); occult blood loss; nausea; vomiting; gastritis; ulcer; bleeding; hypersensitivity reactions, such as urticaria or anaphylaxis

Interactions

- Oral anticoagulants cause increased bleeding risk. If possible, avoid using together.
- Ammonium chloride (and other urine acidifiers) cause increased blood levels of aspirin products. Assess and monitor patient for aspirin toxicosis.
- Antacids (and other urine alkalinizers) cause decreased level of aspirin products. Monitor for decreased aspirin effect.

Precautions

- Contraindicated in GI ulcer, GI bleeding, and aspirin hypersensitivity.
- Use cautiously in patients with hypoprothrombinemia, vitamin K deficiency, bleeding disorders, asthma (may cause severe bronchospasm), and Hodgkin's disease (may cause profound hypothermia).

Nursing considerations

- Administer with food, milk, antacids, or a large glass of water to reduce GI side effects.
- Avoid giving enteric-coated (Ecotrin*) or timed-release preparations for chronic therapy as these drugs are absorbed erratically.
- Warn patient to check with his doctor or pharmacist before taking over-the-counter combinations containing aspirin.
- Slightly elevated serum salicylate level (20 to 30 mg/100 ml) may be noted in patients with arthritis.
- Instruct patient to avoid alcohol while taking aspirin, as it may increase GI irritation.

Ibuprofen

(Motrin*)
Nonnarcotic analgesic

Indications and dosage

Rheumatoid and osteoarthritis
Mild pain (drug is nonsteroidal and has anti-inflammatory effect)
Adults: 300 to 600 mg P.O. q.i.d. Maximum 2.4 g daily.

Side effects

- Prolonged bleeding time; headache; dizziness; nervousness; drowsiness; insomnia; depression; edema; hypertension; tinnitus; blurred vision; bronchospasm; anorexia; nausea; vomiting; constipation; diarrhea; flatus; hemorrhage; melena; peptic ulcer; heartburn; pruritus; rash; urticaria

Interactions

- None significant

Precautions

- Contraindicated in asthmatics with nasal polyps
- Use cautiously in patients with GI disorders; allergy to other noncorticosteroid anti-inflammatory drugs; hepatic or renal disease; cardiac decompensation; and aspirin hypersensitivity (may cause anaphylactoid reaction).

Nursing considerations

- Administer with food, milk, antacid, or a large glass of water to reduce GI side effects.
- Tell patient to notify the doctor immediately if he has any of the following signs or symptoms: anorexia, nausea, vomiting, diarrhea, constipation, flatus, heartburn, visual disturbances, rash, weight gain or edema, bloody or tar-like stools.
- Monitor renal and hepatic function periodically in long-term therapy. If abnormalities are present, discontinue drug immediately.

Sulindac

(Clinoril)
Nonnarcotic analgesic

Indications and dosage

Osteoarthritis, rheumatoid arthritis, ankylosing spondylitis (drug is nonsteroidal and has an anti-inflammatory effect)
Adults: 150 mg P.O. b.i.d. initially; may increase to 200 mg P.O. b.i.d.
Acute subacromial bursitis or supraspinatus tendinitis, acute gouty arthritis
Adults: 200 mg P.O. b.i.d. for 7 to 14 days. Dose may be reduced as signs and symptoms subside.

Side effects

Prolonged bleeding time, aplastic anemia; dizziness; headache; nervousness; tinnitus; epigastric distress; occult blood loss; nausea; rash; pruritus; edema

Interactions

- None significant

Precautions

- Contraindicated in acute asthmatics whose signs and symptoms are precipitated by aspirin or other nonsteroidal anti-inflammatory agents; and patients with active GI ulcers and GI bleeding.
- Use cautiously in patients with history of GI ulcers and GI bleeding; renal dysfunction; compromised cardiac function; and hypertension.

Nursing considerations

- Tell patient to notify the doctor *immediately* if GI bleeding occurs.
- To reduce GI side effects, give with food, milk, or antacids.
- Instruct patient to notify the doctor and have a complete visual exam if he experiences any visual disturbances.
- Drug causes sodium retention. Closely monitor patient for increasing edema.

Diazepam

(Valium*)
Tranquilizer/muscle relaxant

Indications and dosage

Tension and anxiety that may accompany skeletal muscle spasm
Adults: 2 to 10 mg P.O., t.i.d., or q.i.d.

Side effects

Fatigue, drowsiness, ataxia; dizziness; fainting; lethargy; headache; dysarthria; slurred speech; tremor; transient hypotension; bradycardia; cardiovascular collapse; diplopia; blurred vision; nystagmus; nausea; constipation; change in salivation; incontinence; urinary retention; pain; phlebitis at injection site; rash; urticaria

Interactions

- Phenothiazines, narcotics, barbiturates, MAO inhibitors, and other antidepressants potentiate action of diazepam (Valium*).
- Cimetidine (Tagamet*) causes increased sedation. Monitor patient carefully.

Precautions

- Contraindicated in shock; psychosis; coma; acute alcohol intoxication with depression of vital signs; acute narrow-angle glaucoma unless on treatment regime; and during first trimester of pregnancy.
- Use cautiously in elderly or debilitated patients, in patients with limited pulmonary reserve, and in patients in whom a blood pressure drop might cause cardiovascular complications. Also use cautiously in patients with history of anxiety and suicidal tendencies, blood dyscrasia, hepatic or renal damage; open-angle glaucoma, and alcoholism.

Nursing considerations

- Reduce dosage, as ordered, in elderly or debilitated patients.
- Drug should not be discontinued abruptly. If drug is discontinued, observe for vomiting and sweating, abdominal and muscle cramps, tremors, and convulsions.
- Warn patient to avoid any activities that require alertness and good psychomotor coordination until response to drug is determined.
- Instruct patient not to combine drug with alcohol or other depressants.
- Caution patient against giving medication to others.

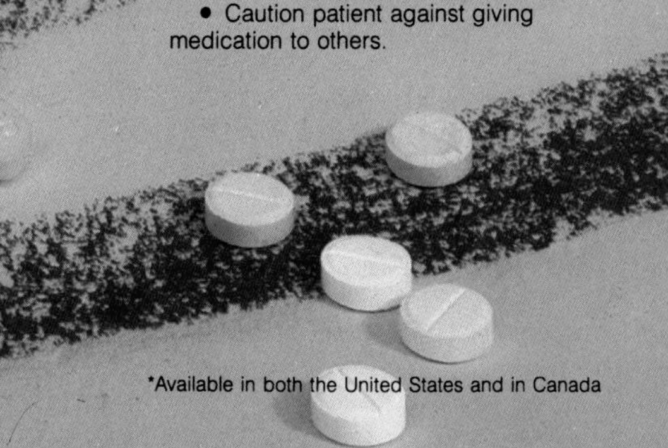

*Available in both the United States and in Canada

Assessing pain

Of course, you know that pain is one of the primary symptoms of a physical problem. When your orthopedic patient has a compound fracture, you can be sure he'll have some pain. However, the experience of pain is very subjective.

Pain intensity varies according to your patient's ability to cope with discomfort. One patient will request medication every few hours to relieve his pain. Another may refuse to admit his discomfort. You'll detect such a patient's pain only by careful assessment.

Also, the *type* of pain patients feel differs, depending on the cause. Common types of pain include:

- *acute pain.* Intense discomfort that usually accompanies an injury or inflammation; may immobilize the patient
- *chronic pain.* Continuous discomfort; may accompany many orthopedic conditions such as rheumatoid arthritis or osteoarthritis
- *superficial pain.* Localized discomfort occurring on or near the body surface
- *deep pain.* Discomfort arising from below the skin surface; accompanies inflammatory conditions or increased pressure affecting a large area
- *referred pain.* Superficial manifestation of a deeper pain. It's felt on the patient's skin away from the pain's actual source. For instance, a patient may feel splenic pain in his right shoulder.
- *phantom pain.* Sensory *perception* of pain. May occur in an amputated limb as part of a patient's attempt to cope with loss of his limb.

To treat and assess your patient's pain effectively, you'll need accurate data about his pain threshold and his response to pain. One way of assessing pain is to conduct a short interview with your patient.

Note: If your patient can't or won't talk, observe him for indications of pain such as restlessness, grimacing, or groaning.

In your assessment, try to determine the following:

Pain location. If a patient says he has pain, don't assume you know where it is. Ask him to point to the pain site. Or, provide him with an anatomical drawing on a sheet of paper, so he can mark the pain's location for you.

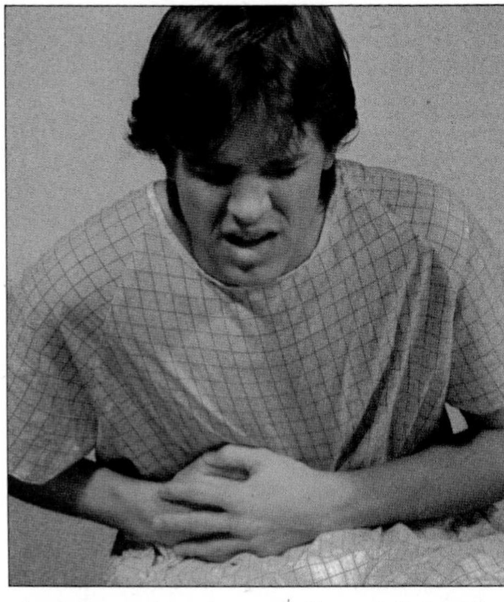

Pain quality. Ask your patient to describe the type of pain in detail. Is it sharp or tingling? Does it throb or ache? Let *him* describe the pain. Avoid putting words in his mouth.

Pain intensity. Ask your patient to rate the pain on a scale of 0 to 10 (with 0 for no pain and 10 for severe pain). Also, determine if any pattern in pain intensity exists. Find out how your patient feels before receiving medication. Then assess how much the pain decreases after he receives medication. Ask your patient what procedures or positions help, aggravate, or have no effect on his pain. Do any additional signs and symptoms, such as nausea and vomiting, accompany the pain? Relieving these may reduce the pain as well.

Pain onset. Find out when your patient first experienced his pain. What was he doing at the time? What were the pain's characteristics then? Is the pain different now? Do any signs precede its onset?

Setting goals. Suppose your patient experiences chronic pain; for example, from arthritis. Help him define some pain goals. What is his pain preventing him from doing? What does he think can relieve his pain? How would his life change if the pain were eliminated?

Carefully document all the information you've gathered. Then use it to help determine the effectiveness of the pain relief measures ordered. For the first 48 hours after trauma or surgery, the doctor may order narcotic injections. Subsequently, as your patient's pain subsides, the doctor may have you give oral nonnarcotic medication. For chronic pain, your patient may take anti-inflammatory medication. In addition, for a patient with either acute or chronic pain, consider implementing the noninvasive measures listed in the box below.

You probably won't be able to completely *eliminate* your patient's pain from an orthopedic problem. But understanding his tolerance and how the pain affects him will help you greatly in managing it.

SPECIAL CONSIDERATIONS

Understanding noninvasive pain-control techniques

Relieving your patient's pain doesn't always mean giving medication. You have a range of noninvasive techniques to choose from as well. These techniques work because they stimulate production of endorphins, the body's own opiate-like substances. Like narcotics, endorphins relieve pain by altering the patient's perception of it.

Are you familiar with these techniques? Noninvasive pain-control measures include:

- offering reassurance and support by spending extra time with the patient
- increasing comfort through frequent position changes and proper use of pillows
- providing a serene environment, by dimming harsh lighting, reducing noise volume, and maintaining a comfortable room temperature
- giving the patient a back rub, or applying a cool cloth to his head
- distracting the patient by having him sing, listen to music, or perform rhythmic breathing when he feels pain
- inducing relaxation, by breathing exercises, meditation, self-hypnosis, or biofeedback
- performing cutaneous stimulation, such as applying warm or cold packs, or menthol ointments.

For more detailed information on noninvasive pain-control techniques, see the NURSING PHOTOBOOK CARING FOR SURGICAL PATIENTS.

Positioning aids

No doubt you're aware how special mattresses, positioning aids, and beds help prevent immobility complications. You probably use some of this equipment as part of your nursing routine.

But, how familiar are you with specific pieces of equipment? For example, do you know when not to use a sheepskin pad? Or, how to use equipment on hand to prevent footdrop?

If you're uncertain, read the following section. We'll explain possible applications for this equipment, and review special considerations you'll want to know. In addition, we'll tell you the advantages of using the Stryker® frame, Roto Rest® and Clinitron® beds, and Egerton Stoke Mandeville Tilting and Turning Bed.

Nurses' guide to common pressure relief aids

Pressure relief aids vary in type and style. Depending on your hospital's policy, you may be expected to choose the aid best suited to your patient's needs. Before making a selection, consider your patient's age, present condition, possible complications that may develop, and the equipment your hospital has available. Keep in mind that pressure relief aids are always recommended for immobile, elderly, thin, debilitated, or obese patients as well as patients with poor skin tone and circulation.

Study this chart to learn how pressure relief aids differ. All the aids listed fit over a standard bed mattress.

Remember, these aids do not take the place of frequent turning, proper body positioning, and skin care.

Note: In some hospitals, you'll need a doctor's order before obtaining specific pressure relief aids.

Egg-crate mattress (Posey™ Convoluted Cushion)

Description
A foam rubber mattress with egg-carton-like bumps which allow for air circulation

Function
- Reduces contact pressure

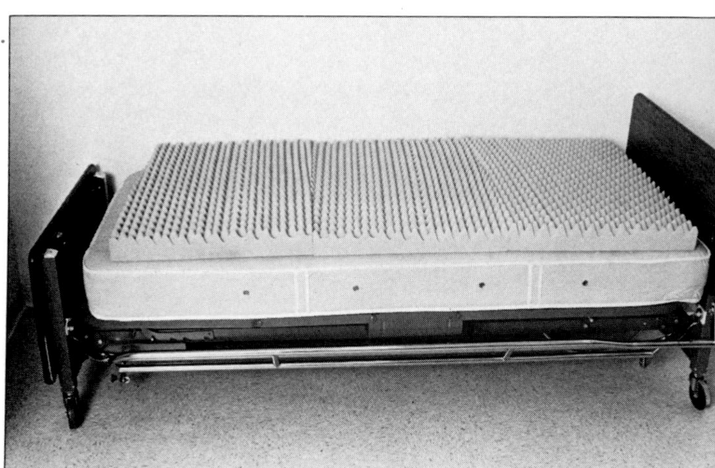

Flotation pad

A plastic-covered pad filled with a gelatinlike substance that fits into a foam rubber mattress

Functions
- Reduces contact pressure
- Provides support by conforming to body contours

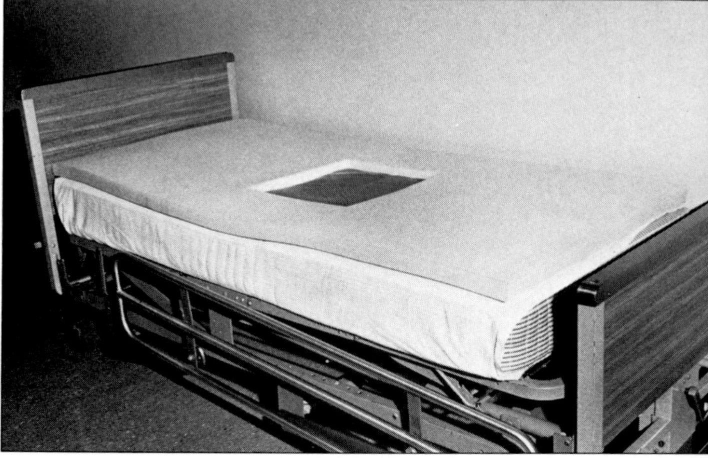

Sheepskin pad (Posey™ Decubitus Pad)

Description
A synthetic furlike pad that's positioned under patient's bony prominences

Function
- Reduces contact pressure

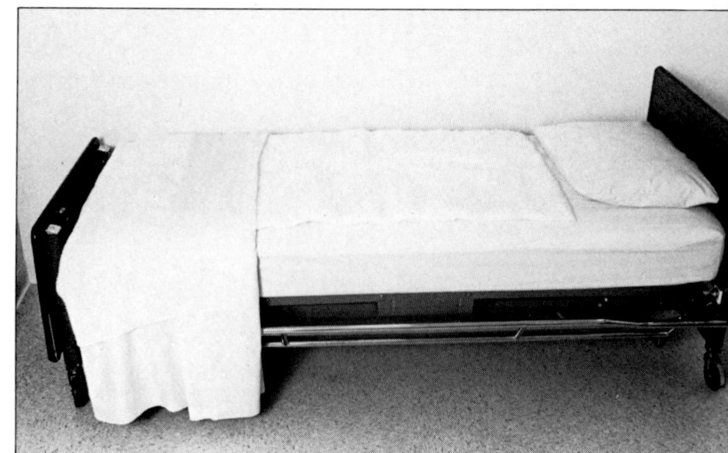

Nursing considerations
• If mattress becomes wet or soiled, rinse it with water and wring it dry. Make sure patient is not lying on wet area.
• If patient's incontinent, cover mattress with the provided plastic sleeve.
• Place a single flat sheet over mattress for positioning or transfer.
• Discard mattress after one use, or send it home with the patient.

Nursing considerations
• Place sheet over mattress.
• Cover pad with the special cover provided, or with a pillow case.
• Never use a sheepskin pad with a flotation pad, because it reduces effectiveness.
• During patient use, clean pad with an antiseptic solution.
• Pad is reusable; disinfect between patients. Foam mattress is not reusable.

Nursing considerations
• Pad's available in small, medium, and large sizes.
• Position sheepskin pad under patient's bony prominences such as his ankles, back, and sacrum.
• Make sure sheepskin pad is laundered daily, or as needed.
• If patient's incontinent, place bed-saver pad over sheepskin pad.
• Sheepskin pad may cause patient to perspire.

Water flotation mattress (Lotus™ Health Care Products)

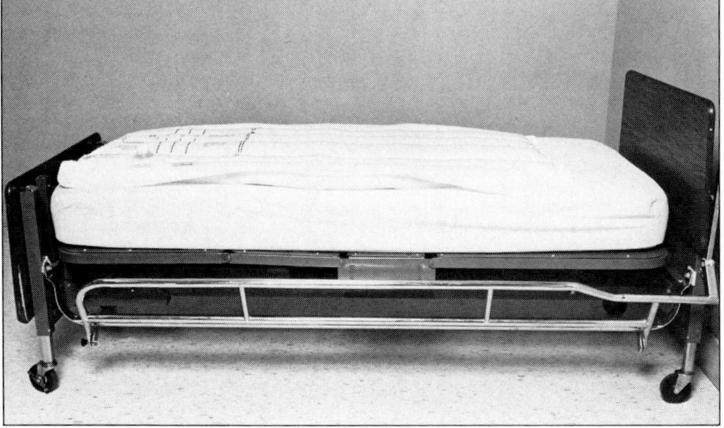

Description
A plastic water-filled mattress

Functions
• Reduces contact pressure by constantly shifting body weight
• Maintains patient in contact with a cooled surface, which he should find relaxing

Nursing considerations
• Follow manufacturer's instructions when filling mattress. Do not overfill.
• If patient can't adjust to water motion, discontinue use.
• To prevent mattress puncture or tears, never use pins or other sharp objects during care. Post a sign above your patient's bed alerting co-workers to this precaution.
• If your patient has a cardiac arrest, transfer him to a more solid foundation (such as the floor).
• If mattress begins to leak, fix it immediately with a specially designed patch kit. Patient may remain on mattress while you do this.
• Place a single flat sheet over the mattress for positioning and transfers.
• Place a hyper- hypothermia blanket under the flotation mattress, to lower or raise patient's temperature; also, place a second hyper- hypothermia blanket over the patient.
• During patient use, clean mattress daily with an antiseptic solution.
• Mattress is reusable; disinfect it between patients, according to hospital policy.

Alternating air pressure mattress

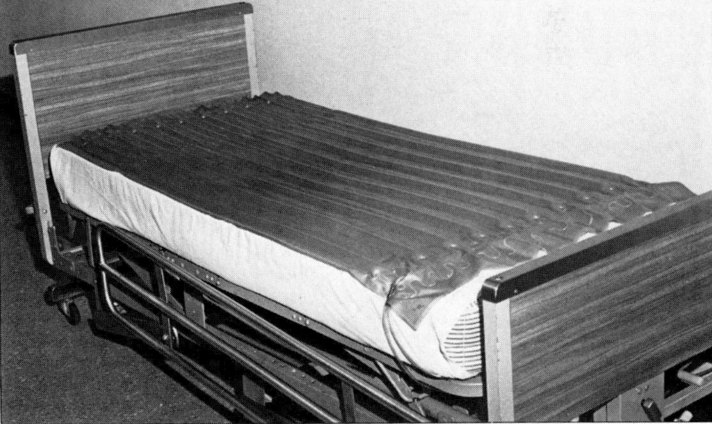

Description
Plastic air-filled mattress with longitudinal cylinders which are alternately inflated and deflated by an electrically driven air pump

Function
• Reduces contact pressure by constantly alternating mattress pressure

Nursing considerations
• To avoid reducing air flow, never sharply elevate bed.
• Make sure mattress is alternately inflating and deflating properly. If it is, you'll be able to indent the inflated plastic approximately ½" (1.3 cm) with your finger.
• Avoid using sheepskin or a drawsheet with the air mattress because they reduce its effectiveness.
• Make sure all connections are secure and the air pump is grounded.
• Place a single flat sheet over mattress for positioning and transfers. To avoid an air-flow interruption, tuck sheet loosely under mattress.
• During patient use, clean mattress with an antiseptic solution.
• Turn mattress air pump off when performing cardiopulmonary resuscitation.
• Keep air pump in an out-of-the-way location; for example, the bedside table. Doing so will prevent injury to personnel or damage to the pump itself.
• If the mattress is reusable, disinfect between patients, according to hospital policy.

Positioning aids

Learning about positioning aids

Has it been some time since you've reviewed positioning aids? As you know, positioning aids help keep your patient's body in proper alignment—no matter what position she's in. Proper alignment also helps ensure bone and tissue healing, preventing complications.

Learn which positioning aids your hospital has available, so you'll know when you can use the ones they have available, and when you must improvise.

The following chart shows some commercially available positioning aids in the top row of photos. In the bottom row, we show you how to improvise each aid.

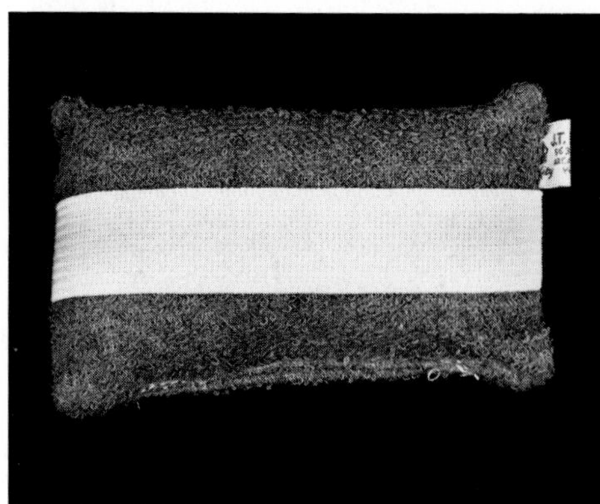

Posey Palm grip (Hand roll)

Possible application

- Keeps hand in functional position

How to improvise

- Place a rolled washcloth in patient's hand, so patient's fingers are wrapped around roll and her thumb is in opposition to her fingers.

Nursing considerations

- Make sure hand roll's large enough to prevent extreme finger flexion and to keep thumb in opposition.
- If hand roll slips out of place, secure it to the patient's hand with a gauze wrap. Fasten gauze with tape.
- Remove hand roll at least once every 4 hours for 1 hour. Clean skin and allow air to circulate. Inspect skin for signs of pressure or breakdown.

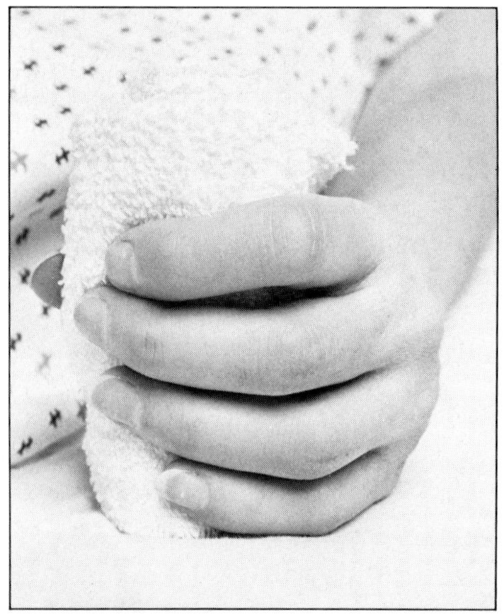

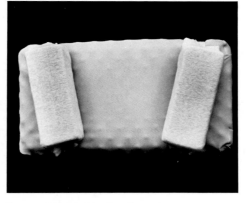

Posey Adjustable Footboard

Possible applications

- Prevents footdrop by keeping feet in upright position
- Addition of antirotation blocks helps prevent external hip rotation

How to improvise

- Put a sandbag inside a cardboard box. Then, pad the outside of box with a towel or bath blanket. Position the box on the bed so the ball of your patient's foot rests firmly against it. Place a folded bath blanket under your patient's lower legs so her heels extend over the blanket's edge.

Nursing considerations

- If the footboard isn't padded, pad it with a towel or bath blanket.
- Apply heel protectors, if necessary.
- Even if your patient is restless, a footboard will be effective.

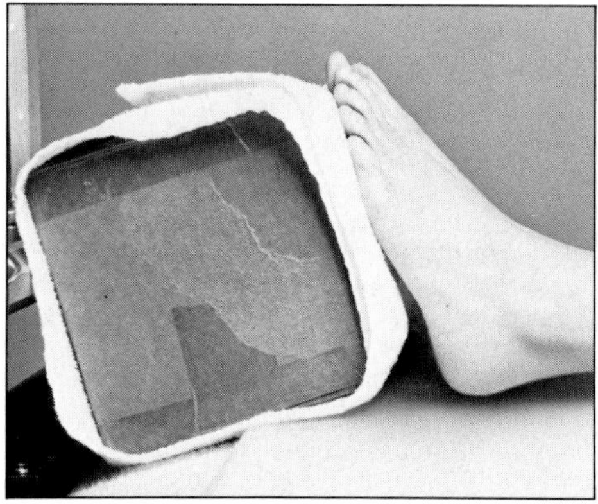

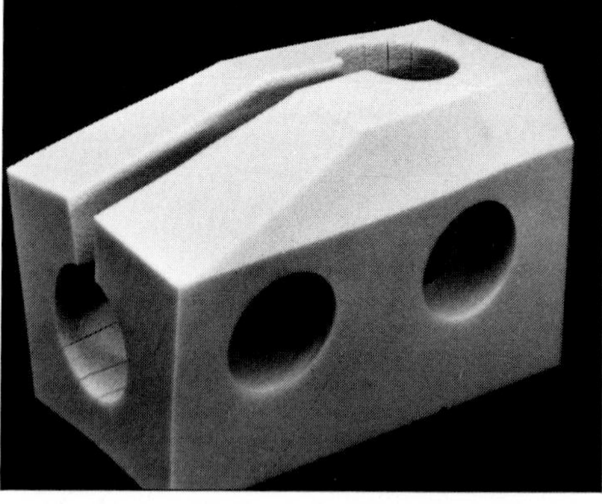

Span + Aids Deluxe-Cut Cradle Boot

Possible applications

- Decreases pressure on heel and ankle
- Helps prevent footdrop by keeping patient's foot upright. May be used on flaccid extremities.
- Helps eliminate foot rotation
- Prevents hip abduction
- Can be used with traction
- Can be used to elevate forearms, keeping the elbow off the mattress

How to improvise

- Place socks and shoes, preferably sneakers with some ankle support, on your patient's feet. Make sure they're tied properly.

Nursing considerations

- Remove boots or sneakers for 1 hour at least once every 4 hours. Check pressure areas. Keep patient's heels off bed.
- Boots' openings allow frequent skin checks.
- Patient may be positioned on side with one boot in place.

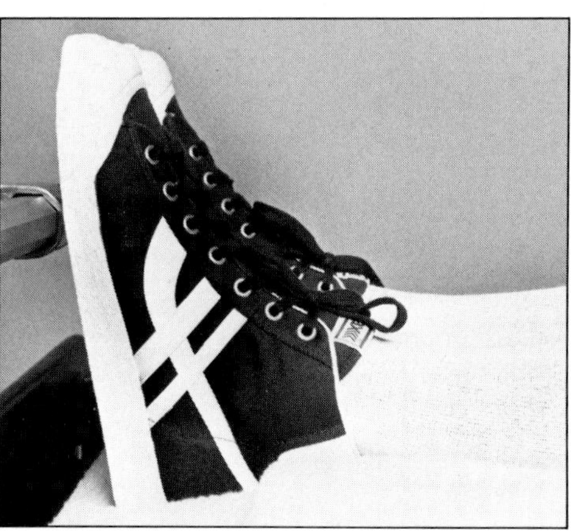

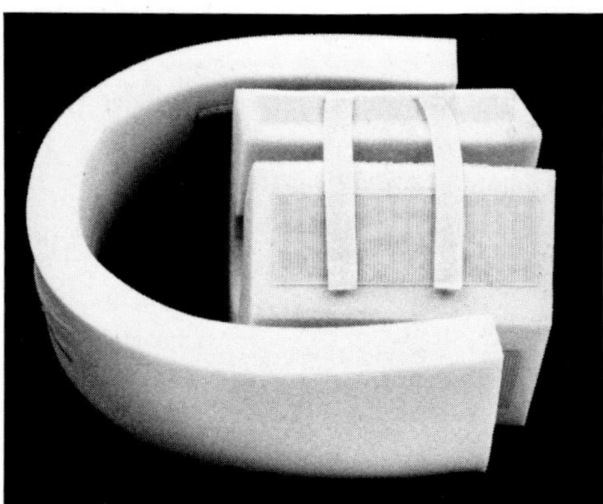

Span + Aids Footdrop Stop

Possible applications
- Maintains foot in functional position. May be used with spastic extremities.
- Helps prevent mattress pressure on patient's heel by elevating it
- Helps prevent foot rotation and footdrop

How to improvise
- Improvise footboard as described at left.
- Place a folded towel in a pillowcase and position around the patient's dorsiflexed foot. Secure pillowcase to patient's foot with gauze wrap. Place a bath blanket under both legs. Follow the same procedure on the patient's other foot.

Nursing considerations
- Patient may be placed in supine, side-lying, or prone position.
- Remove the footdrop stop for 1 hour at least once every 4 hours to check for possible pressure areas.

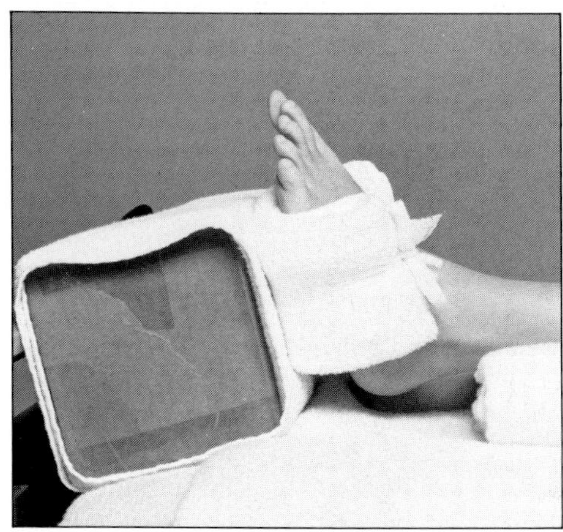

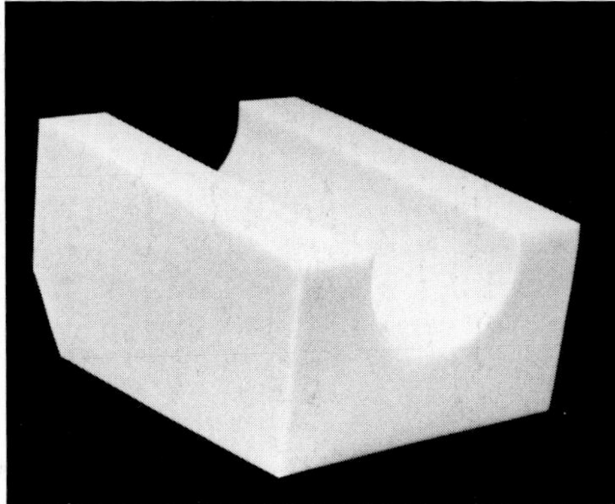

Span + Aids Cast Elevator

Possible applications
- Prevents mattress pressure on patient's cast by elevating it
- Helps prevent internal or external leg rotation
- Maintains constant elevation and position because elevator doesn't slide on linens
- Absorbs excess moisture from wet cast
- When used between legs in a side-lying position (along with body aligner at patient's back), helps prevent pressure between legs and allows blood circulation in legs

How to improvise
- Place two pillows covered with bed-saver pad under patient's cast.

Nursing considerations
- Patient may be placed in a supine, side-lying, or prone position.
- Keep knee flexed by positioning elevator's thicker end proximal to inner torso.
- When patient's in a side-lying position, place elevator's cradle portion over patient's lower leg; rest her leg on cradle's flat surface.
- Remove cast elevator at least once every 4 hours to check for pressure areas.
- Elevator may be used as an arm cradle for a patient with an I.V. line.

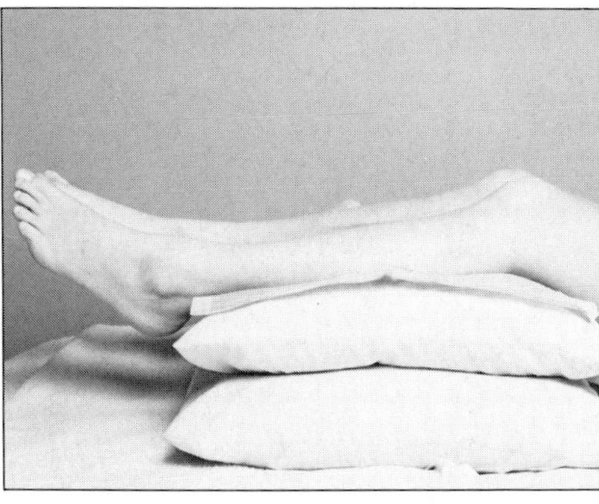

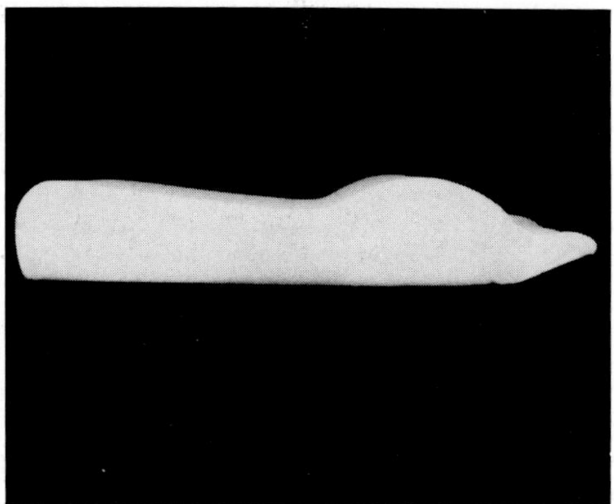

Span + Aids Popliteal Pillow

Possible applications
- Decreases mattress pressure on patient's lower legs
- Supports lower legs in proper alignment
- Reduces strain on lower back muscles. May be used for laminectomy patients.
- Helps prevent mattress pressure on heels by elevating them

How to improvise
- Fold two bath blankets in quarters lengthwise. Roll up ⅔ of one bath blanket. Back it with the second blanket, so that the roll is even with the top edge of the bottom bath blanket. Place the rolled portion under your patient's popliteal space and extend the flat portions of both blankets down under the patient's calf to just above her Achilles tendon.

Nursing considerations
- Place patient in supine position for best results.
- Check to be sure patient's knees, calves, and heels correspond to pillow's markings.
- Position patient's heels over pillow edge.
- Remove pillow or blankets at least once every 4 hours to check for pressure areas.

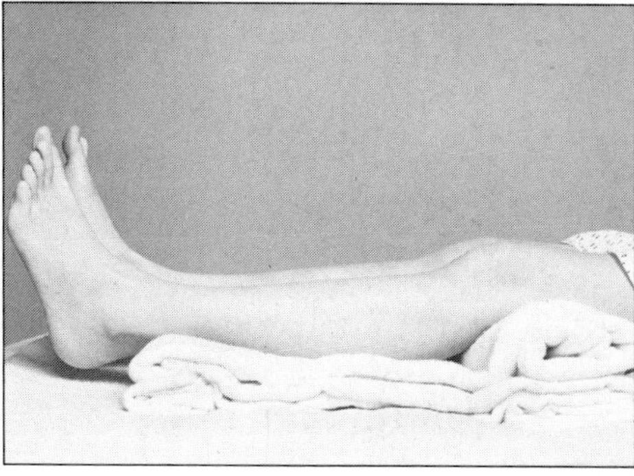

Positioning aids

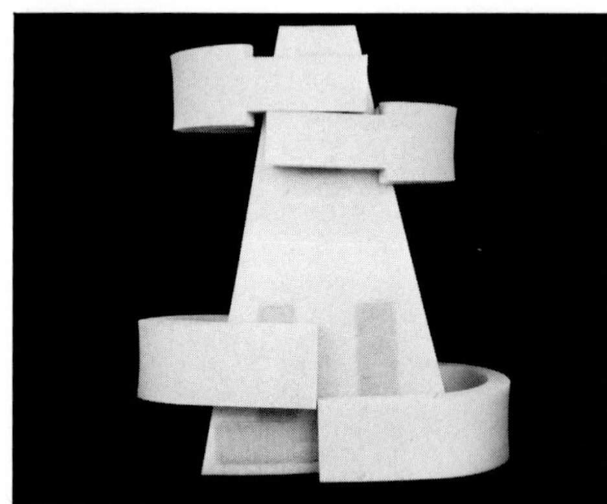

Span + Aids Schafer Abduction Pillow

Possible applications
- Maintains hip abduction. Usually used after surgical repair of hip.
- Immobilizes hip joint

How to improvise
- Place large pillow lengthwise between patient's legs. Place trochanter roll along outer thighs and calf areas.

Nursing considerations
- Check pillow strap tightness by slipping one finger between the strap and your patient's skin. Also, check her pedal pulses. Adjust strap, if necessary.
- When the pillow straps are in place, your patient may be turned on her side, or seated in a chair with her legs elevated and supported.
- Loosen and remove straps, and check skin surfaces for pressure areas every 2 hours, or when turning your patient.
- If you're improvising this aid, check pillows and trochanter rolls routinely to be sure they're in proper position.

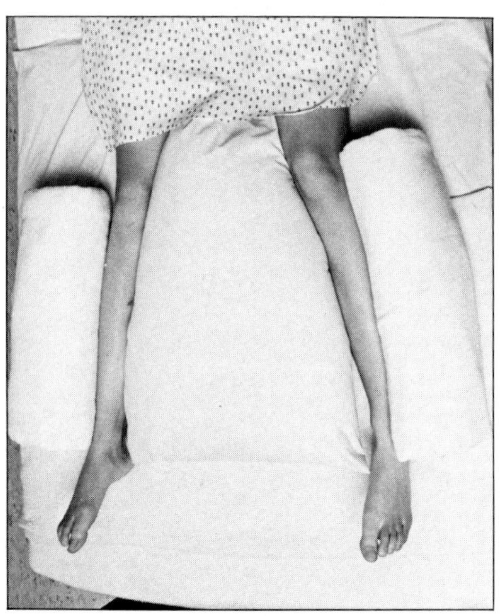

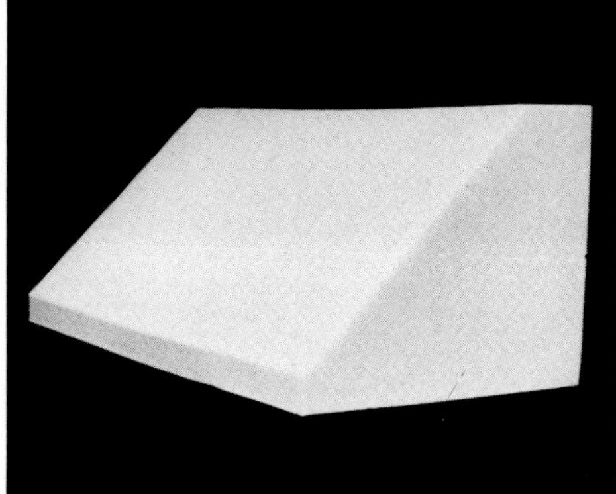

Span + Aids Body Aligner

Possible Applications
- Supports patient in a side-lying position, to help maintain proper hip placement and body alignment
- When patient's supine, aligner may be used as a footboard, to prevent footdrop
- When used as a bed cradle, keeps bed linens off patient's toes
- Can be used with pelvic traction under the patient's knees or against her buttocks

How to improvise
- To support patient in a side-lying position, place pillows behind patient's neck, shoulders, back, buttocks, chest, and stomach.

Nursing considerations
- When using as a footboard, rest patient's feet against slanted edge, for good elevation. Keep patient's heels *off* mattress.
- Maintains proper position because foam adheres to bed. Does not require checking to see if pillow has slipped out of place.
- If patient's in a side-lying position, tuck aligner along spine between shoulders and buttocks. Extend a second aligner from patient's chest to upper thighs. Rest patient's upper arm on aligner. You may place pillows or another positioning aid between her legs.
- Cut foam to provide air circulation and eliminate pressure on susceptible body parts, such as her scapula and her coccyx.

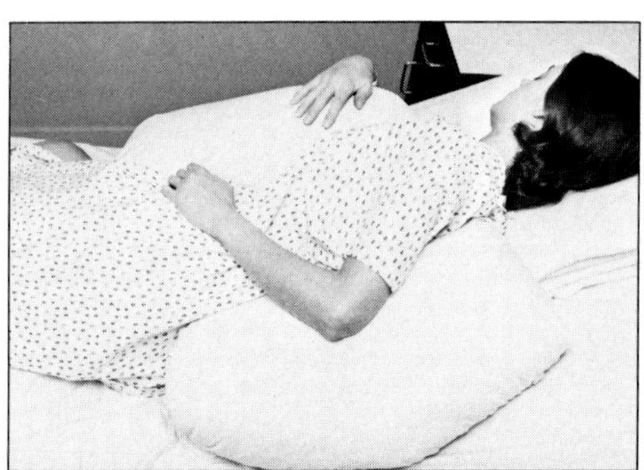

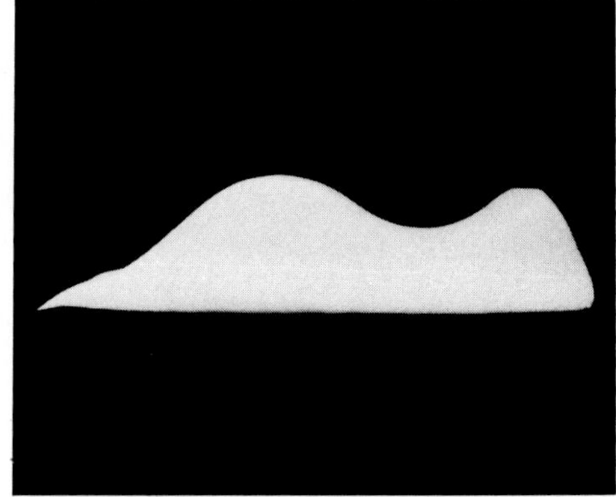

Span + Aids Dorsocervical Pillow

Possible applications
- Supports and aligns patient's head, neck, and shoulders
- Helps control neck flexion and hyperextension
- Decreases mattress pressure on head, neck, and shoulders

How to improvise
- Fold a bath blanket in quarters lengthwise. Then, fold it in half widthwise. Roll up one-half halfway, and place the roll underneath your patient's neck, so that the flat portions extend under her head and shoulders.

Nursing considerations
- Patient may be placed in supine or side-lying position.
- Position pillow under patient's head, neck, and shoulders.
- Check to be sure patient's head, neck, and shoulders correspond to pillow's markings (arrows on side of pillow).
- Remove at least every 4 hours to check for pressure areas.

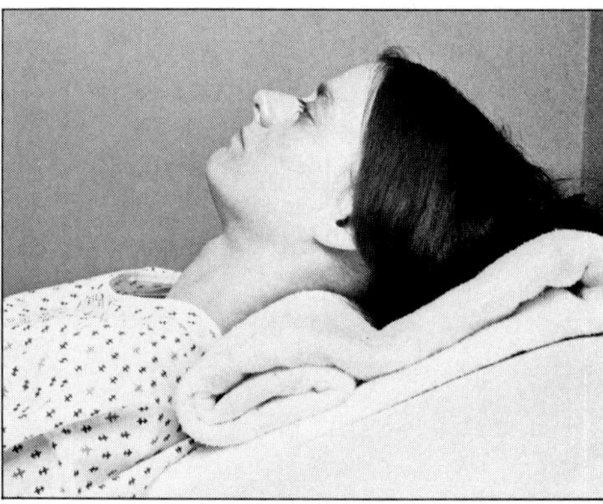

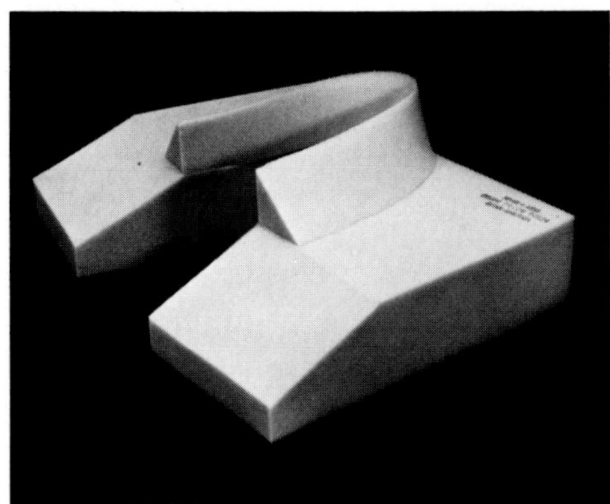

Span + Aids Prone Pillow

Possible application
- Supports prone patient's head and shoulder without hyperextending her neck, allowing her head to turn to the side

How to improvise
- Place a small pillow under your patient's chest crosswise. Fold a small bath blanket up so it's 1' (30 cm) square. Place the lower edge under your patient's forehead. Fold a second small bath blanket into quarters. Then roll it widthwise tightly. Place one end under the chest pillow on one side. Then, curve the roll up along your patient's cheek, under her forehead (on top of the folded bath blanket), and back down her other cheek. Tuck the roll's end under the chest pillow.

Nursing considerations
- Reassure your patient that the pillow won't suffocate her.
- Make sure your patient's breathing isn't obstructed.
- Initially, use the pillow for only a short time, and stay with your patient until she becomes comfortable with it.

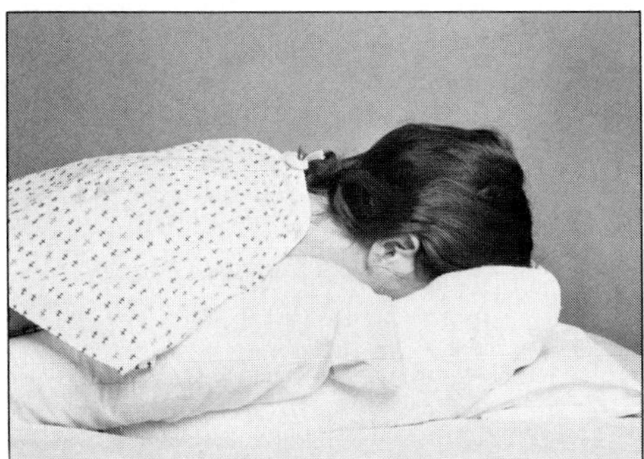

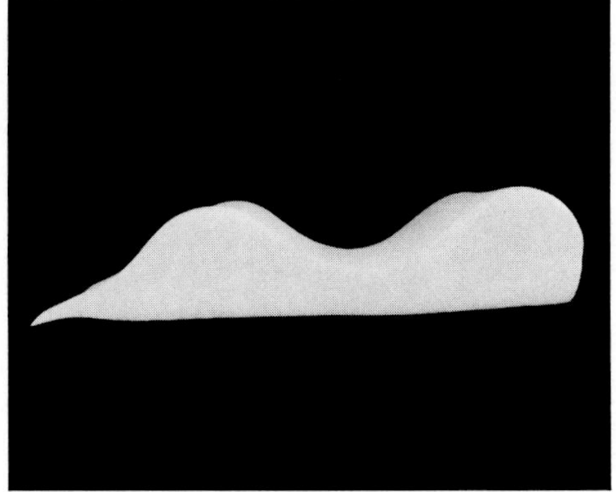

Span + Aids Dorsolumbar Pillow

Possible applications
- Decreases mattress pressure on lower back and buttocks
- Supports lumbar region to reduce muscle strain and help induce pelvic tilt

How to improvise
- Fold a bath blanket in quarters lengthwise. Then, fold it in half widthwise. Roll up one-half halfway, and place the roll underneath your patient's lumbar area, so that the flat portions extend under her waist and to her upper thigh.

Nursing considerations
- Available in medium and firm densities.
- To protect pillow, cover with a pillowcase or bed-saver pad.
- Check to be sure patient's back and buttocks correspond to pillow's markings. Adjust pillow according to patient comfort.
- Remove pillow at least once every 4 hours to check pressure areas.

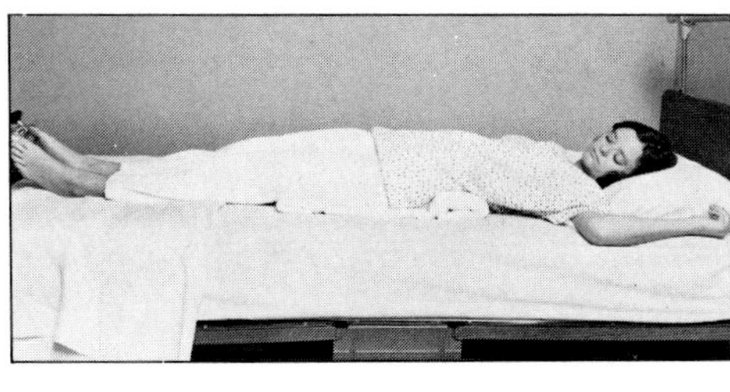

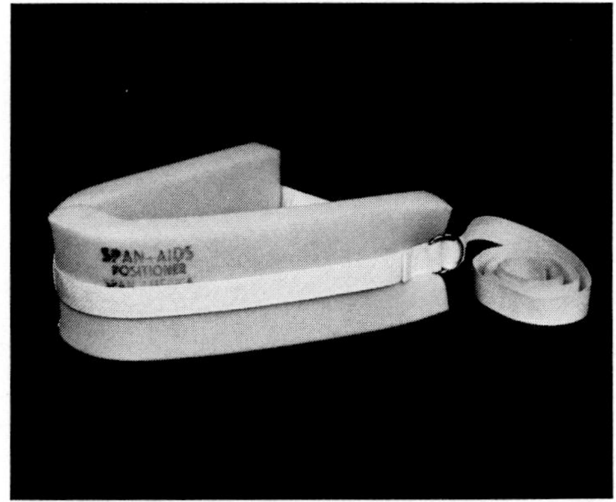

Span + Aids Positioner

Possible application
- Supports patient in a sitting position

How to improvise
- Wrap a rolled sheet or bath blanket around patient's chest, under her arms, and around the back of a chair. Tie the ends to each other and the chair.

Nursing considerations
- If your patient's positioned in a chair, make sure positioner fits comfortably under her underarms.
- Remove at least every 4 hours to check for pressure areas.

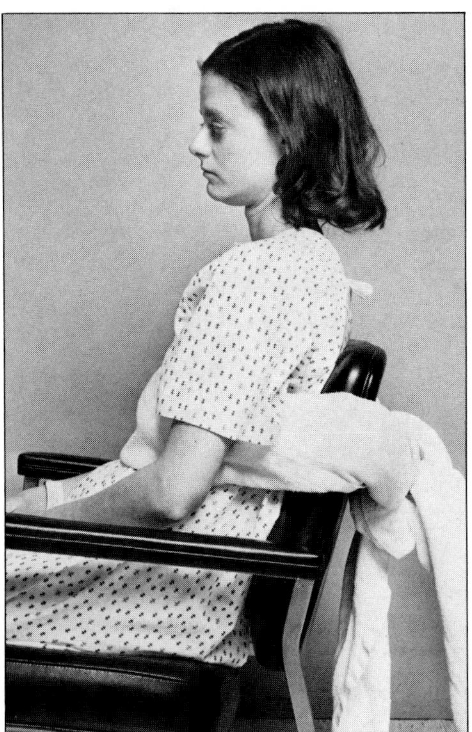

Positioning aids

Learning about special beds

Regardless of your patient's orthopedic disorder, you'll need to turn and position him every few hours. Doing so minimizes pressure on his bony prominences, decreases venous stasis (which causes deep vein thrombosis,) and in other ways helps prevent immobility complications. Consider using a specially designed bed to help you do this with greater ease and less patient discomfort. Familiarize yourself with the four special beds shown here. *Important:* For each bed, also learn the manufacturer's recommended procedure for performing cardiopulmonary resuscitation (CPR).

Which bed is best for your patient? That depends on his condition and what your hospital has available. Suggest to the doctor which bed you think best meets your patient's needs.

Stryker® frame	Description	Functions
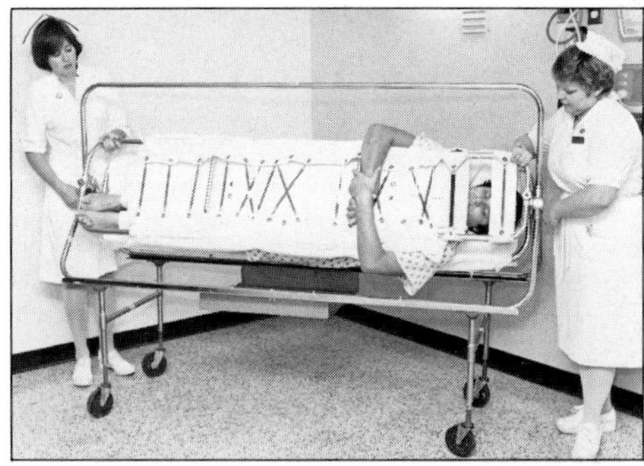	Two frames (one anterior and one posterior), with canvas covers and thin padding over each, support the patient between them during turning. The frames, which are mounted on a movable cart, have a pivot apparatus at each end.	• Allows changing a patient's position to either prone or supine, while maintaining body alignment and immobilization • Maintains vertebral traction during turning
Clinitron®		
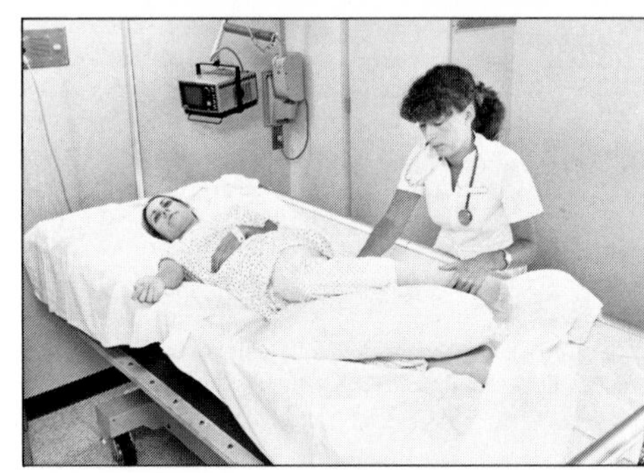	This air-fluidized support system is made up of a rectangular frame containing 1,600 pounds of silicone-coated glass beads (microspheres) covered with a closely woven monofilament polyester sheet. The beads are fluidized by a flow of warm pressurized air, which floats the polyester cover. The patient is positioned on the cover. Bed is designed for use with traction.	• Provides a clean, controlled environment • Reduces contact pressure
Roto Rest®		
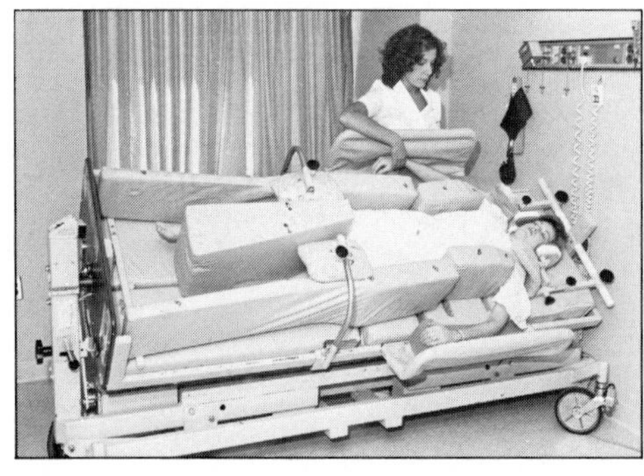	Bed is equipped with supportive packs and straps that keep patient's body in proper alignment while continuously but slowly rotating him 180° in either direction. Designed for use with vertebral or long-bone traction.	• Minimizes patient discomfort by eliminating manipulation involved in turning and repositioning • Reduces risk of fecal impaction and constipation, as continuous motion stimulates peristalsis • Stimulates comatose patient through constant movement by affecting the vestibular system • Immobilizes vertebral column even though patient's limbs are continually moving • Helps decrease spasticity and resulting contractures
Egerton Stoke Mandeville Tilting and Turning Bed		
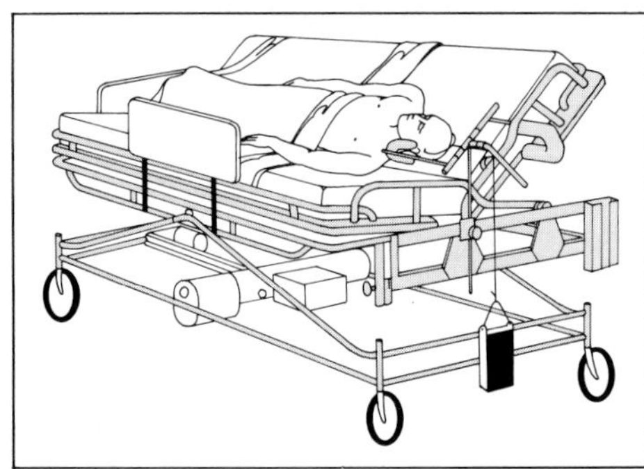	Specially designed metal hinged frame moves mattress sides from flat to 90° angle. Bed is equipped with supportive pads and traction equipment that keep the patient's vertebrae in proper alignment.	• Maintains vertebral and long-bone traction while turning or tilting patient • Allows positioning patient supine or side-lying while maintaining vertebral alignment and immobilization

Nursing considerations

- Turn and position patient every 2 hours, or as ordered.
- Always follow your hospital's specific procedures when turning your patient. During the turn, have a co-worker positioned at the patient's head to check pulleys and weights. Never turn patient without co-worker's help.
- Before beginning the turning procedure, provide additional patient comfort by placing a foam mattress or sheepskin next to your patient. Also, secure any equipment he may have, such as an I.V. line, indwelling (Foley) catheter, or respirator tubing, so it won't be displaced. Be sure the patient is strapped securely to frame, and have him fold his arms around the frame, if possible.
- After turning, gently rock frame to be sure it's locked into place.
- Always remove top frame after turning.
- To prevent misalignment, check the equipment periodically, and tighten the canvas lacing.
- When patient's prone, check chin and forehead straps often for slippage.
- Add armrest wings to frame at a level comfortable for your patient. These permit him to rest his arms and maintain proper body alignment.
- For meals and giving oral medication, place patient prone.
- When your patient's prone, monitor him closely for signs of respiratory problems, such as dyspnea. This position may impair breathing.
- For elimination, place patient supine, with bedpan under opening in canvas.
- Teach patient to use the overhead bar to improve arm muscle tone.
- Never use this bed if patient: can be positioned on his sides; is broader than external frame, over 6 feet tall, or over 200 pounds; is immobilized and hyperextended without skull tongs after cervical cord injury; has thoracic or lumbar spine compression fractures reduced by hyperextension; can't adjust emotionally to turning.

- If necessary, patient may be positioned directly on her wound or skin grafts.
- If patient has excessive wound drainage, place a porous dressing over her wound. Keep the dressing as small as possible.
- Put a regular hospital flat sheet over the filter sheet for positioning and transfer.
- If you use petroleum-based or silver compounds on patient's skin, place an impervious covering over the filter sheet. Doing so prevents these compounds from seeping into the bed's microspheres.
- To prevent tears in filter sheet, make sure patient has no pins or clamps on her dressing.
- For accurate assessment, check the patient frequently for draining blood, perspiration, and urine. Because the double-permeable filter sheet allows body fluids to filter through the microspheres, infrequent checks could mislead you about actual drainage amounts.
- Keep patient's room at 75° for maximal system efficiency.
- Select system's temperature according to patient comfort.
- For elimination, roll patient away from you and push bedpan into the microspheres. Reposition patient on bedpan. Afterward, defluidize the system. Remove bedpan by holding it flat as you roll patient away from you with your other hand. Clean patient as usual. Fluidize the system and reposition patient.
- Be sure the microspheres are sieved once a month, as well as between patients.
- If the microspheres leak onto floor, wipe up immediately with damp cloth.
- Make sure the filter is checked monthly and changed as needed.
- Special decontamination procedure between patients requires 24 hours.

- Make sure cycle gauge registers at least 45 cycles per 8 hours.
- Before activating turning mechanism, secure straps and replace all packs. Secure any equipment the patient may have, such as an I.V. line or indwelling (Foley) catheter, to be sure it'll move easily with her.
- Bed can be locked into lateral or supine positions for patient care.
- Routinely check patient's bony prominences for pressure signs and symptoms.
- Because patient lies directly on bed covering, without any sheets, make sure you rinse soap residue from her body and support packs after bathing her.
- For elimination, place bedpan under opening in bed. *Note:* Because of constant motion, diarrhea is common.
- When using mechanical ventilation, do not tape patient's connecting hose to head packs.
- Perform endotracheal suctioning frequently in the first 24 to 48 hours, as continuous movement provides postural drainage and thereby increases secretions.
- Apply foot supporters every 8 hours for 2 to 4 hours. Perform range-of-motion exercises when you remove them.
- If patient has skull tongs in place, routinely check that tongs and head pads are not in contact with each other.
- If your patient's in vertebral traction, check her shoulders frequently for pressure areas. To prevent excess pressure, periodically tilt bed into reverse Trendelenberg position.
- To help prevent patient isolation and provide additional visual stimulation, attach a television to the side of the bed.
- In case of power failure or motor malfunction, turn bed manually and lock in lateral or central position every 2 hours.

- Before turning patient, check that mattress center fits securely in frame's well.
- When tilting or turning patient, first raise the side of the bed the patient's turning onto about 20 degrees. Free any equipment, such as an I.V. line, to be sure it won't be displaced. Position yourself on the side of the bed your patient's turning toward.
- Make sure both head support pads are in place when turning patient. Remove pad on upward side after turn to prevent claustrophobia.
- Allows you to maintain eye contact with your patient as you turn him.
- Provide visual stimulation during use since range of vision is limited.
- Position patient at least 70 degrees laterally, before feeding him or administering oral medication.
- For elimination, face patient and raise opposite side of bed. Support patient in a side-lying position as you lower the bed's opposite side and a co-worker positions the bedpan under him. Afterward, reverse these steps to remove the bedpan.
- Keep all removable bed parts in designated areas—either attached to end of bed or at bedside.
- In the event of power failure or motor malfunction, operate bed manually.

Ambulation aids

Has the doctor ordered a walker, cane, crutches, or other ambulation aid for your patient with an orthopedic condition? In this section, we'll tell you how to teach your patient to use these ambulation aids properly.

Specifically, we'll show you:

- how to teach your patient who's had a below-the-knee amputation to walk with a pneumatic prosthesis system and an ambulatory aid.
- how to teach your patient to walk with a quad cane.
- how to teach your patient to walk with crutches, as well as get in and out of a chair, pick up objects, and go up and down stairs.

You'll also find important guidelines on determining weight-bearing differences, selecting proper crutch size, and assessing your patient's discharge needs.

Applying a pneumatic prosthesis

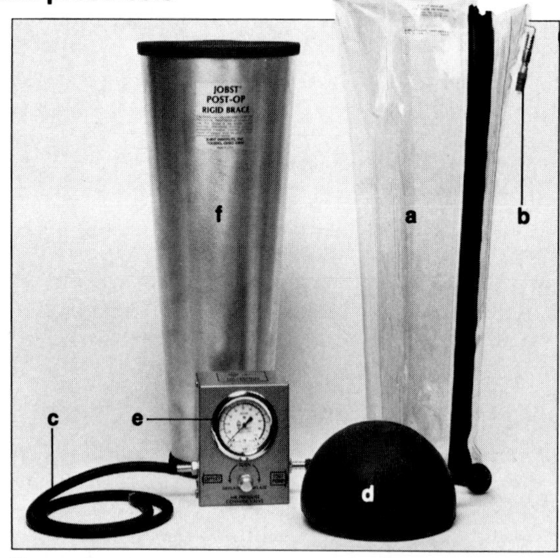

1 *Your patient, 52-year-old Tom McLaughlin, has had his right leg amputated below the knee. The doctor orders application of the Jobst postoperative pneumatic prosthesis system to control edema and allow early ambulation. The system's components include: (a) pneumatic prosthesis, (b) prosthesis air stem, (c) connecting tubing, (d) footpump, (e) pressure control unit, (f) postop rigid brace.*

You'll usually apply the prosthesis within 24 hours following surgery, to help control edema. The prosthesis will also help control superficial bleeding. It permits visual inspection of the stump, when the patient's not wearing the rigid brace necessary for ambulation.

Caution: Avoid using the prosthesis for patients with a cardiac or neurologic disability, or as an ambulation aid for a patient unable to control his balance. Use it with caution on a patient whose amputation resulted from diabetes. Also, never use the prosthesis alone for weight-bearing ambulation. Supplement it with a Jobst postop rigid brace and an ambulation aid such as a walker.

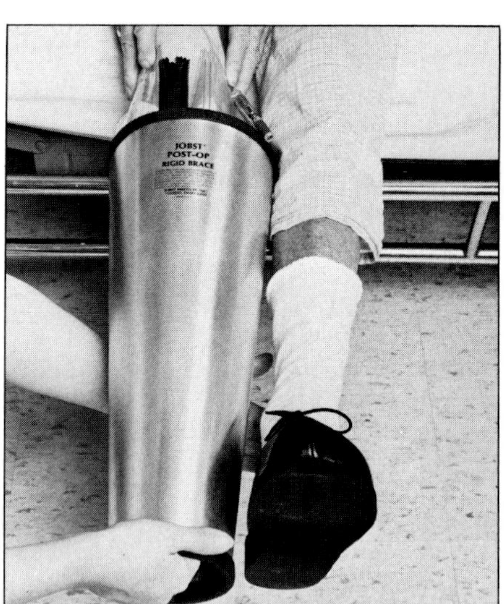

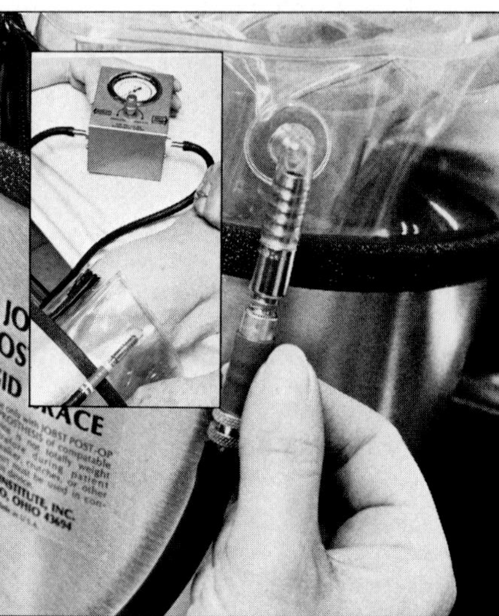

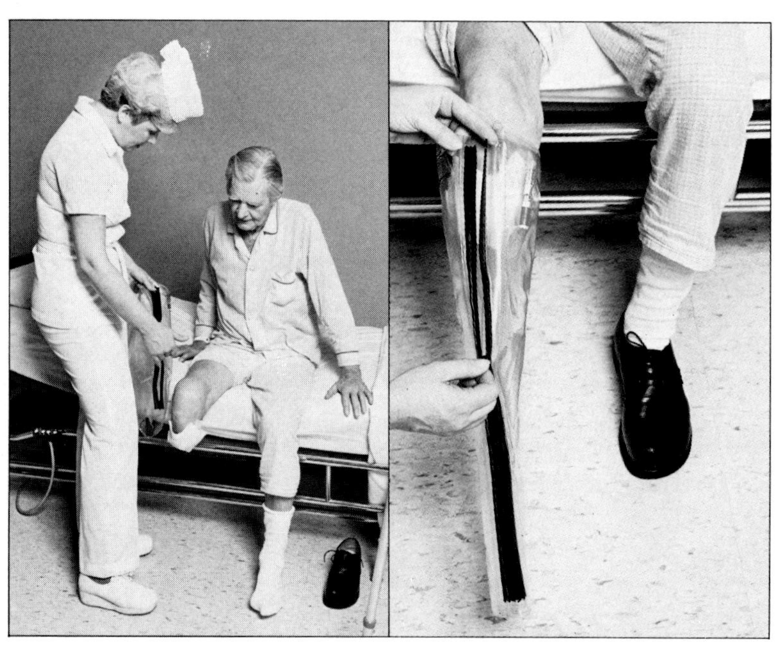

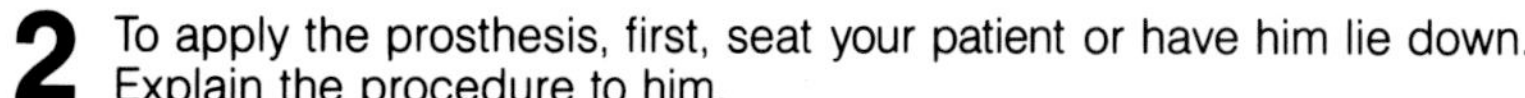

2 To apply the prosthesis, first, seat your patient or have him lie down. Explain the procedure to him.

Now, unzip the prosthesis and carefully slide it around the stump just below the knee. Position the zipper over the front of the stump (see right photo). Then, zip the prosthesis completely closed, making sure your patient can bend his knee. Put a shoe on his unaffected foot.

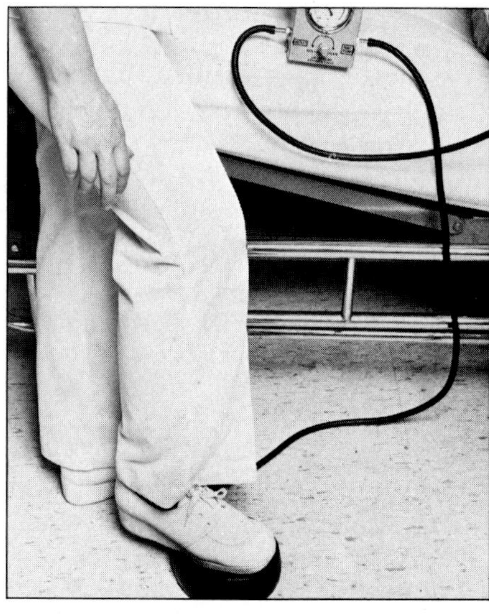

3 Next, open the inflation valve, located on the prosthesis air stem, by turning it counterclockwise approximately three times, until you feel resistance. If your patient will be bearing weight, you should now put on the postop rigid brace. Carefully slip the brace over the prosthesis, as shown, making sure brace length approximately equals prosthesis length. Then, adjust both to match the length of the patient's unaffected leg. The prosthesis should extend approximately 4" (10.2 cm) above the brace's top edge.

Caution: Never allow the prosthesis to extend below the bottom of the brace.

Remember to place Mr. McLaughlin's affected leg and brace on a chair or stool for support during inflation.

4 Next, attach the inflation pump tubing to the fitting marked FOOTPUMP on the pressure control unit. Then, attach the end of the connecting tubing without the metal slip connector to the other side of the pressure unit, marked OUTLET. Take the opposite end of the connecting tubing and attach it to the prosthesis air stem by pushing the halves together, until tight, as the nurse has done here. [Inset] The system will appear as shown when you've completed the setup.

Now, prepare to inflate the prosthesis by turning the air pressure control valve knob clockwise, until it's tight.

Note: For some models, set the valve knob pointer to the AIR IN position.

5 Then, with the inflation valve on the prosthesis air stem still open, use the footpump to inflate the prosthesis, as shown. Monitor the air pressure gauge and continue inflating the prosthesis until you reach the desired pressure.

Important: Inflate the prosthesis until the air pressure gauge reads between 20 and 25 mmHg, if your patient's in bed or not ambulating. If your patient will be ambulating, the gauge should read 25 to 50 mmHg. The exact level depends on your patient's comfort. Never inflate the prosthesis above 50 mmHg, which may cause premature failure or sudden prosthesis breakage.

Now, close the inflation valve on the prosthesis by turning the valve end clockwise approximately three times, until you feel resistance.

Then, detach the connecting hose from the air stem by twisting the two halves in opposite directions, while pulling them apart.

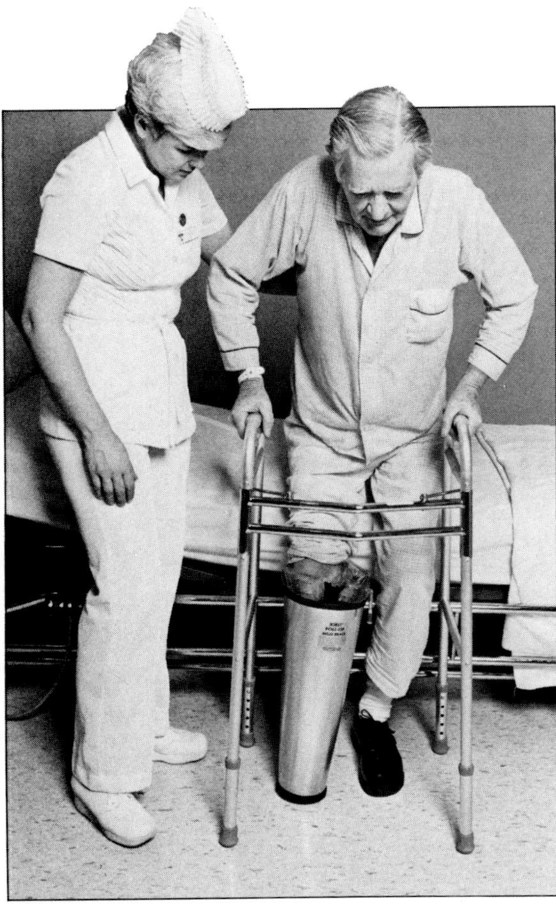

6 Now, position a walker, crutches, or a cane close to the bed. Assist your patient to his feet and give him one of the ambulatory aids for support. During each ambulation period, inspect the affected limb periodically for any signs of restricted circulation. Ask your patient to tell you if he becomes uncomfortable or experiences numbness or tingling.

If you detect signs or symptoms of circulatory impairment, or if your patient's ready to return to bed, readjust the air pressure to relieve tightness. First, have your patient sit or lie down. Then, remove the brace.

Assemble the inflation system, open the valve on the prosthesis air stem, and gradually turn the air pressure control valve knob counterclockwise toward the DEFLATE position. *Note:* For some models, turn the knob toward the AIR OUT position. When you've reached the desired pressure, return the valve knob to the INFLATE position, close the inflation valve on the air stem, and disconnect the inflation system.

However, if your patient cannot tolerate the prosthesis or you want to remove it for any other reason, slowly allow it to deflate until the pressure gauge indicates zero. Disconnect the inflation system. Then unzip and remove the prosthesis. Next, gently squeeze any remaining air from the prosthesis. Now, inspect the skin and dressing on your patient's affected limb. Clean the prosthesis, following manufacturer's instructions. Finally, document the procedure, and how your patient tolerated it, in your nurses' notes.

Understanding weight-bearing differences

Is your patient using an ambulation aid? If so, the doctor will prescribe a non-weight-bearing, partial-weight-bearing, or total-weight-bearing gait for your patient. Do you know these gaits differ from each other? Study the information below for the answers.

Non-weight-bearing gait

Requires patient to support his weight on the ambulation aid and his unaffected leg.

Nursing considerations

- Instruct your patient to keep his affected leg off the floor at all times.

Partial-weight-bearing gait

Allows patient to support 25% to 50% of his weight on his affected leg. The rest of his weight is divided between his unaffected leg and the ambulation aid.

Nursing considerations

- Instruct patient to distribute his weight between his unaffected leg, the ball of his affected foot, and his ambulation aid. Tell him to keep the heel of his affected foot off the floor.

Total-weight-bearing gait

Allows patient to support full weight on his affected leg (unless it causes excessive pain), his unaffected leg, and the ambulation aid.

Nursing considerations

- Instruct patient to try to distribute equal weight between each leg. Tell him to place minimal weight on his ambulation aid.
- When he puts full weight on his affected leg, patient should touch walking surface first with his heel and then with the ball of his foot.

Ambulation aids

How to select the proper crutches for your patient

Anthony Giordano, a 28-year-old schoolteacher, sprained his right ankle playing basketball. An elastic bandage supports his ankle. Now, you must fit him for crutches. You know how important it is for your patient to use properly fitting crutches. But do you know how to evaluate their size and safety? If not, read the following.

First, check the safety features of Mr. Giordano's crutches. Make sure the crutches have rubber pads at the top, and rubber tips at the bottom, to prevent them from slipping. Then, ask your patient if he wants the hand supports padded.

Select the proper crutch size for your patient by asking him to stand and position the crutch tips 2" (5.1 cm) in front of and 6" (15.2 cm) to the side of his feet. Make sure the tops of the crutches are about 1" to 1½" (2.5 to 3.8 cm) below his underarms.

If they're too long or short, adjust them accordingly. Then, remeasure them for proper fitting.

Nursing tip: If your patient can't stand up yet, measure him as he lies supine. Measure from his underarms to 4" (10.2 cm) lateral to his heel.

Check the hand supports to make sure they're positioned correctly. To do this, ask your patient to grasp the supports. His arms should be slightly flexed; never straight. Readjust the supports, if needed.

Important: Remind him to support his weight on his hands, not his underarms. Tell him to immediately report any tingling or numbness in his arms, which could mean the crutches are the wrong size, or that he's using them incorrectly.

Finally, document the fitting, in your nurses' notes.

SPECIAL CONSIDERATIONS

Suggestions to give your patient using an ambulation aid

Will your patient be ambulating with crutches, a cane, or a walker? If so, here are some suggestions to remember:

- When possible, teach your patient how to use his ambulation aid before he needs it; for example, before surgery.
- For ambulation, make sure he wears a supportive, nonskid shoe (or shoes) with a tie or buckle.
- Make sure the surface your patient will be walking on is uncluttered, flat, dry, and well lighted.
- Teach your patient always to check the rubber tips on the bottom of his ambulation aid before use. He should make sure they're wearing evenly, have no cracks or tears, and fit snugly.
- For added psychological support, place a transfer or walking belt around your patient's waist. Have one hand prepared to grasp the transfer belt. *Note:* Always grasp the belt from above, not from underneath it.
- To prevent falls, stay with your patient as he's learning the procedure. Stand slightly behind him on his affected side. By doing this, you can support him if he loses his balance.
- To begin ambulation, have your patient *slowly* rise from a seated position and stand for several minutes with his crutches, cane, or walker, until he can maintain his balance. Instruct him to take deep, slow breaths and look straight ahead. Remind him that some temporary dizziness is normal. However, if he seems excessively dizzy, lower him back onto a bed or chair and try again when he seems to have recovered.
- Instruct your patient to look ahead when walking, not at his feet. If possible, have him walk close to a wall (on his unaffected side) for support.

Crutch-walking: Teaching your patient the three-point gait (non-weight-bearing)

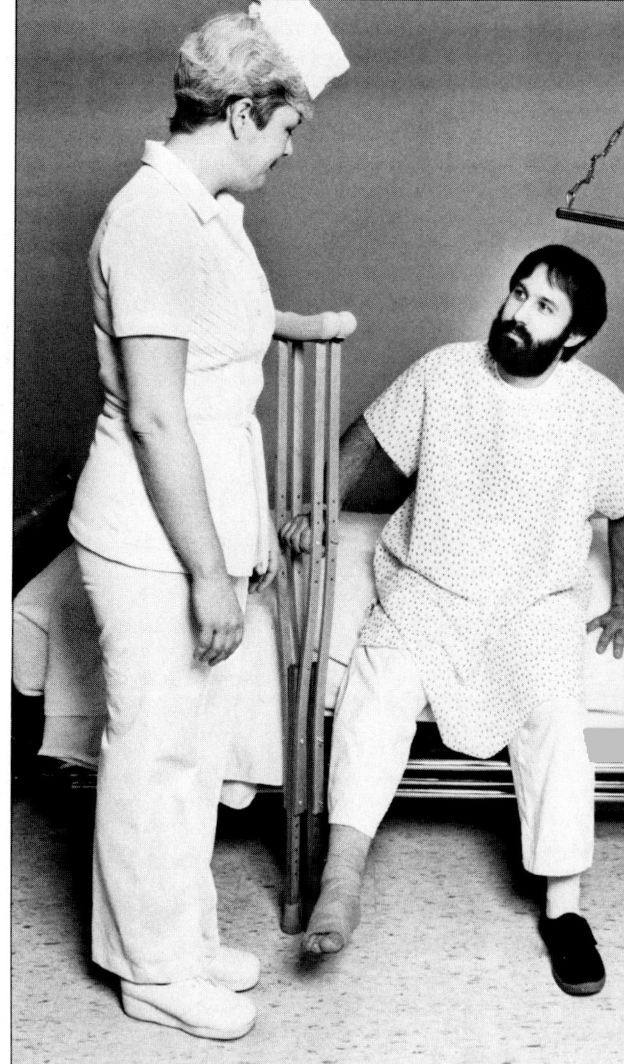

1 *Anthony Giordano has been fitted with crutches. Now, you'll want to teach him how to ambulate correctly, using his crutches and a three-point gait.*

First, explain the procedure to him. Instruct Mr. Giordano to avoid putting any weight on his affected limb while standing and walking. Remind him to place all his weight on his unaffected limb and his crutches. Then, put a supportive, nonskid shoe on his unaffected limb. Position yourself slightly in front of him, on his affected side, in case he loses his balance. *Remember:* You must remain on his affected side throughout the procedure.

Now, have him sit on the edge of the bed and hold both crutches in his right hand. Tell him to lean forward and bring his left foot slightly ahead of his right foot. Then, have him place his left hand on the side of the bed and push himself up, using his left hand and the crutches for support, as shown here. Make sure he doesn't place any weight on his affected foot.

2 After Mr. Giordano is standing, position yourself behind him, slightly to his right side. Instruct him to transfer one crutch to his left side and grasp it firmly. Have him position his left foot so it's even with the crutch tips. Make sure his right knee is slightly flexed and his right foot is off the floor. Remind him to put pressure on the hand supports when he ambulates, not on the crutch tops.

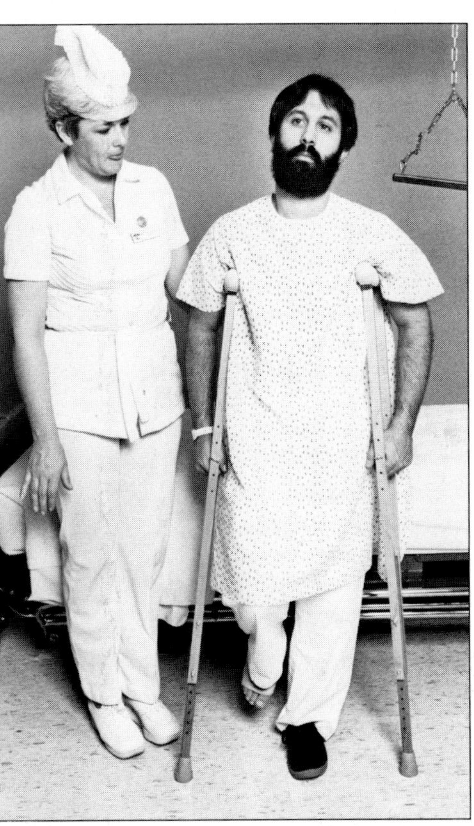

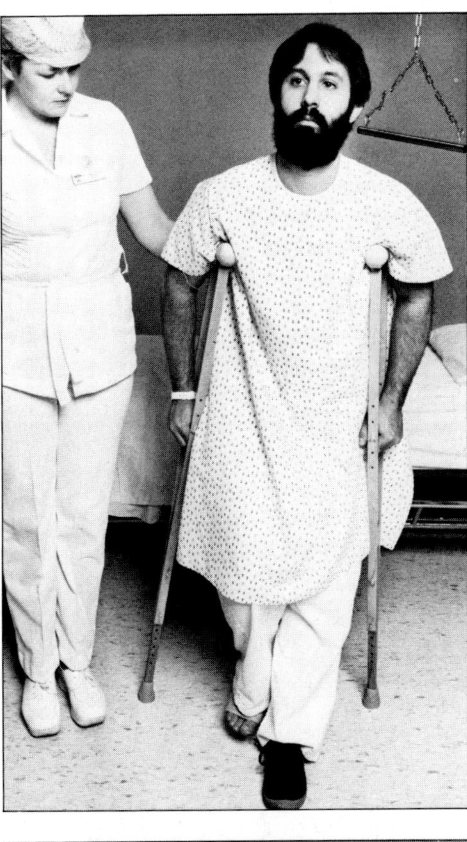

4 Now, have your patient balance his weight on both crutches as he swings his left foot forward, as shown here.

Then, have him move both crutches and his right foot forward and repeat the procedure.

3 Then, with his balance maintained, instruct him to lean his body slightly forward, supporting his weight on his left foot and crutches.

Ask him to put all his weight on his left leg, maintain his balance, and move both crutches forward. Next, he'll swing his right leg forward, keeping all weight off his right foot.

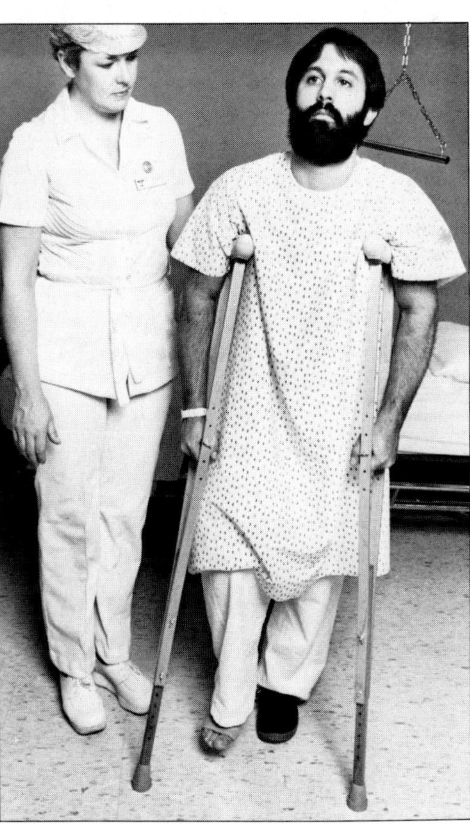

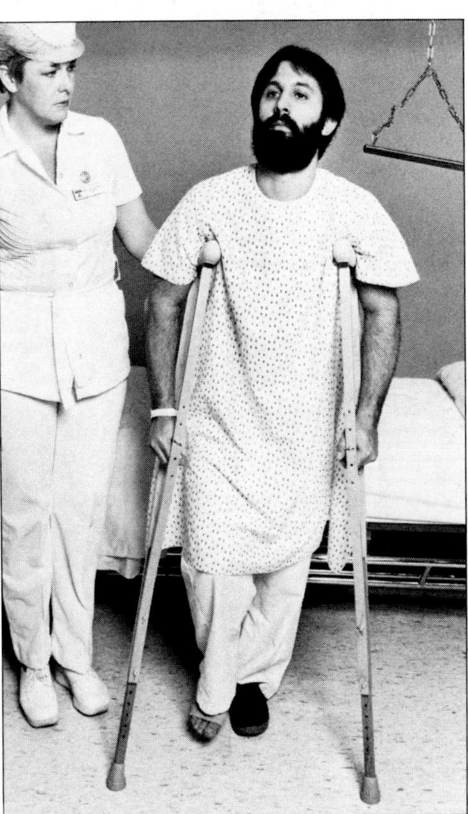

5 As your patient's balance and strength improve, teach him the swing-through three-point gait. To do this, instruct him to advance his left foot beyond the crutches. Then he'll advance both crutches and his right leg past his left foot, as shown here. Have him repeat the procedure.

Document all patient teaching in your nurses' notes.

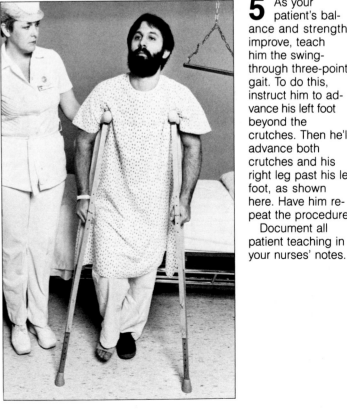

Ambulation aids

Teaching your patient to get in and out of a chair

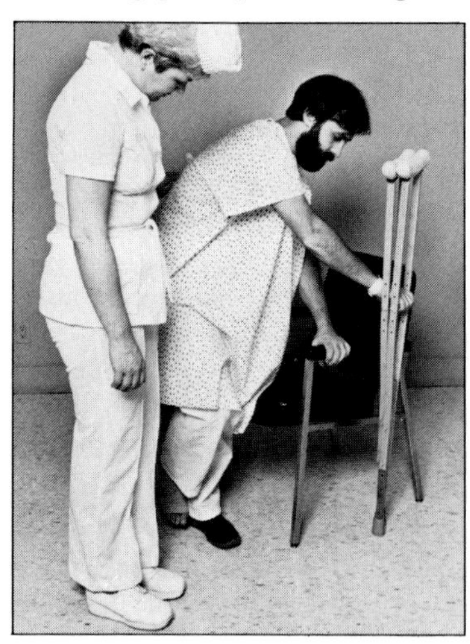

1 *After Mr. Giordano has learned the three-point gait, you'll want to teach him how to get in and out of a chair. First, explain the procedure to him.*

Then, have him approach the chair so his left leg's close to the front of the chair seat. Tell him to grasp both crutches, using his right hand.

Next, tell him to put his left hand on the left arm of the chair. Have him place the crutches against the chair's armrest, as shown here.

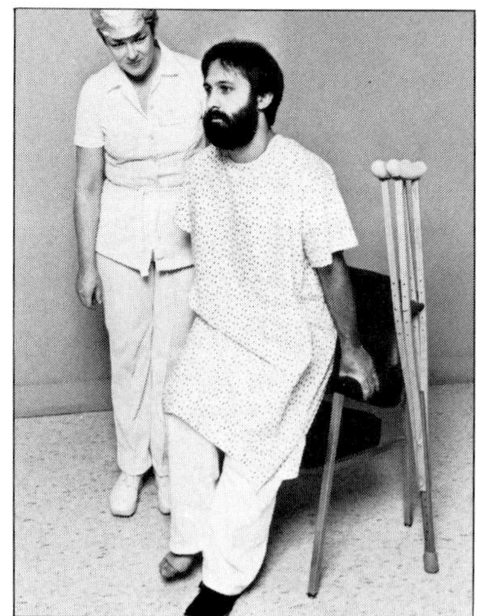

2 Now, instruct your patient to pivot on his left foot until the back of his left leg is against the seat of the chair. Ask him to place his right hand on the right arm of the chair.

Then, as he supports his weight with his hands, have him lower himself into the chair, keeping his weight off his affected foot, as shown here.

Teaching your patient to pick up objects

1 *Mr. Giordano is walking with crutches. As he walks into the room, you see him drop the shaving case he was carrying. Show him the proper way to pick up the shaving case from the floor. Here's how:*

First, carefully explain the procedure to him. Then, instruct him to look around the room for a low piece of furniture; for example, a chair. Now, have him push the case over to the chair with his left crutch, as shown here.

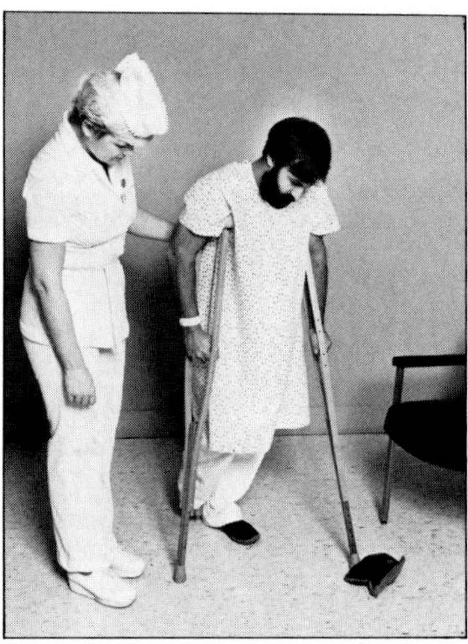

2 Tell your patient to shift his crutches to his right hand and place them against the armrest, as shown here. Then, have him sit down in the chair, following the procedure described above.

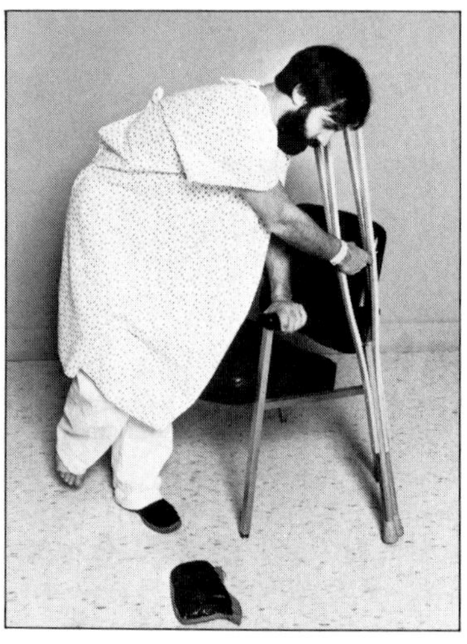

Teaching your patient to go up and down stairs

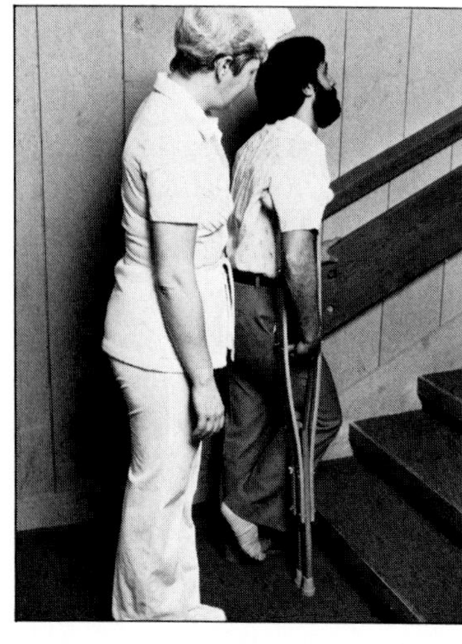

1 *Now that Mr. Giordano has learned crutch-walking and getting in and out of a chair, you're ready to teach him how to walk up and down stairs.*

First, explain the procedure, and have him stand at the bottom of the stairs. Stand behind him, slightly to his right. Then, instruct Mr. Giordano to shift his left crutch to his right hand and grasp the banister with his left hand. Have him support his weight on both crutches and his left leg.

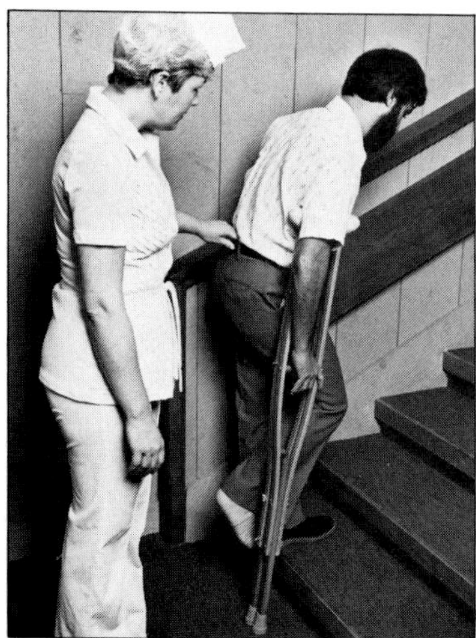

2 Then, tell your patient to push down on his crutches and hop onto the first step with his left foot. His other leg will move up onto the step at the same time, as shown here.

Next, have your patient swing his crutches up onto the next step, alongside his feet. Ask him to hop onto the second step with his left leg.

Encourage your patient to repeat this procedure, advancing his left leg first, until he reaches the top of the stairs.

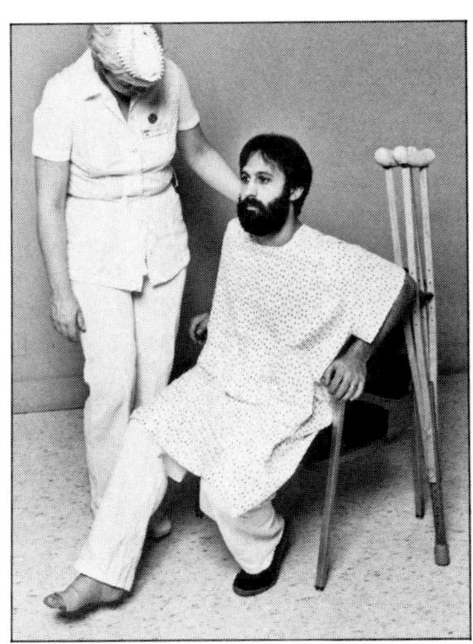

3 Now, let's suppose he wants to get out of the chair. Tell Mr. Giordano to slide forward, keeping his left foot slightly under the chair. Remind him not to put any weight on his right foot. Have him press down on the armrests.

Then, instruct him to support his weight on his hands and left foot as he lifts himself out of the chair, as shown here.

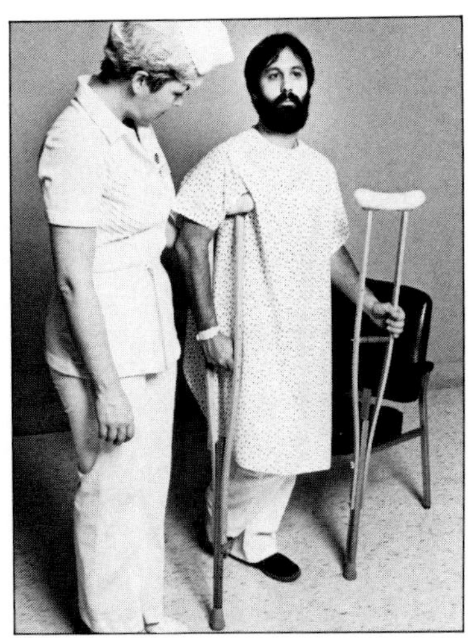

4 Next, ask Mr. Giordano to pivot on his left foot, while grasping the armrest with his left hand. With his right hand, he'll grasp the crutches.

Then, tell him to place both crutches under his right arm. As soon as he feels steady, have him shift one crutch to his left arm, as shown. Your patient is now ready to walk.

Document all patient teaching in your nurses' notes.

3 Next, tell him to lean forward in the chair, reach down, and pick up the case with his left hand.

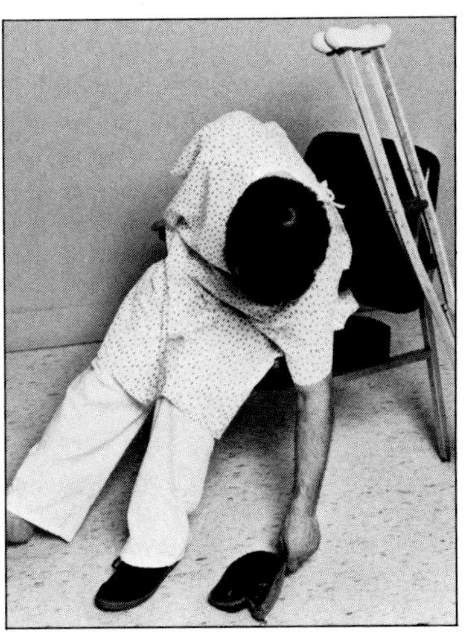

4 Now, as he grasps the crutches with his right hand, instruct him to push himself off the chair with his left hand, while holding onto the case.

Finally, tell him to transfer one crutch to his left hand (which is holding the case) after he rises and has balanced himself.

Document all patient teaching in your nurses' notes.

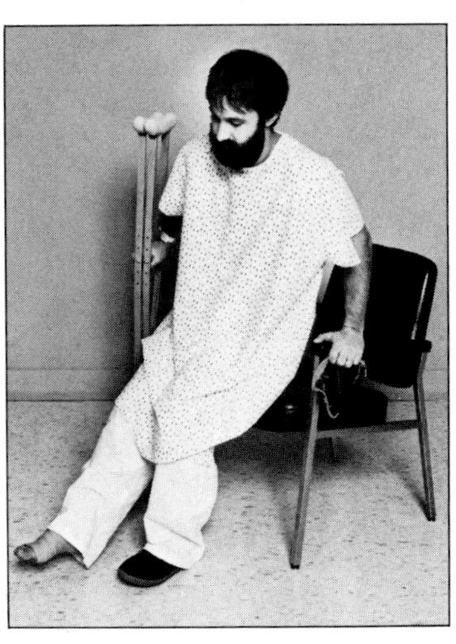

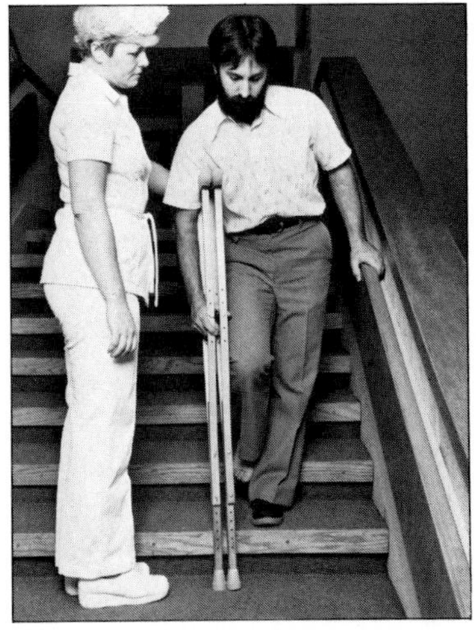

3 Now you're ready to show him how to get down the stairs. Make sure your patient's unaffected leg is closest to the banister, and that you're positioned one step below him, on his affected side. He should shift his left crutch to his right hand, and then grasp the banister. Now, ask him to lower his crutches to the step below him, as he's doing here.

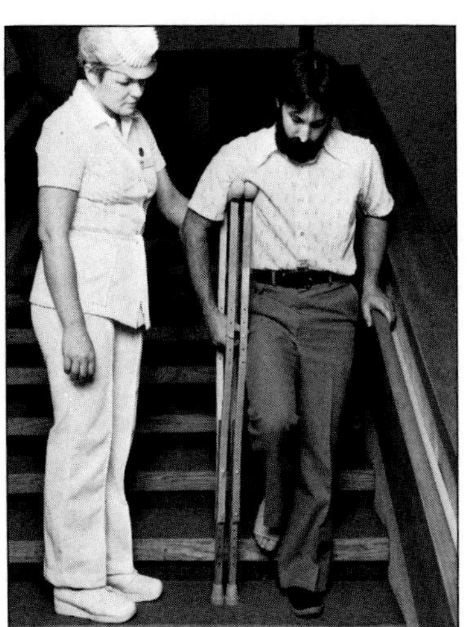

4 Then, tell him to lower his left foot onto the next step. As he does, his other leg will follow, as shown.

Have him repeat this procedure, advancing the crutches first.

Document your teaching in your nurses' notes.

Ambulation aids

Teaching your patient to walk with a quad cane

1 *Zelda McPherson, a 54-year-old archaeologist, is recovering from a total hip replacement. She's able to bear full weight on her affected left leg during ambulation. She's progressed from using a walker to using two quad canes. Now you'll teach her how to use a single quad cane.*

Note: In this photostory, Ms. McPherson will be using a Guardian Quadripoise® cane.

Begin by reviewing cane-walking with your patient. Remind her to divide most of her weight between both feet, and put only minimal weight on the cane. Then, check that she's wearing nonskid, flat-soled, supportive shoes. Also, check that the canes rubber tips are intact and fit securely.

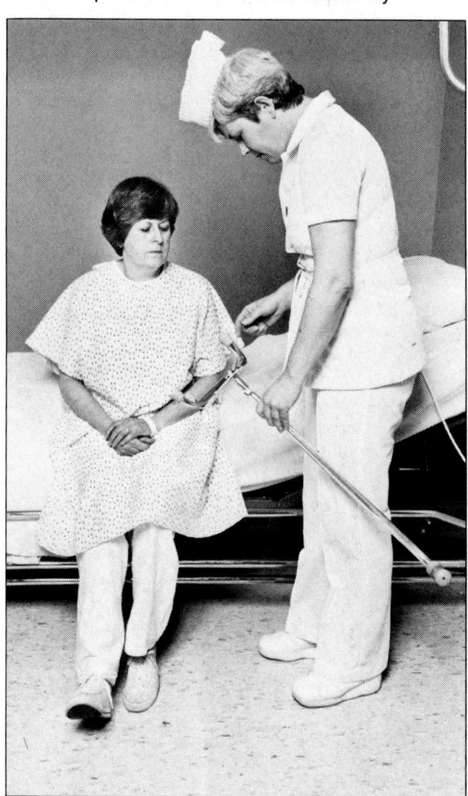

2 Lower the bed, if necessary. Have Ms. McPherson sit on the edge of the bed with her feet flat on the floor, 6" (15.2 cm) apart.

Nursing tip: For added security, consider putting a transfer belt around the waist of a weak or apprehensive patient.

Then, assist your patient into a standing position, as the nurse is doing here. Place the cane in her right hand. Tell her to position it about 4" (10.2 cm) to the side of her right foot. Stand to her left side and slightly behind her.

Remember: Always position yourself at your patient's affected or weakened side.

[Inset] Before your patient begins to walk, check that her cane is the proper height. If it is, the cane will extend from her hip joint to the floor. As she holds it, her elbow should be flexed at a 30° angle.

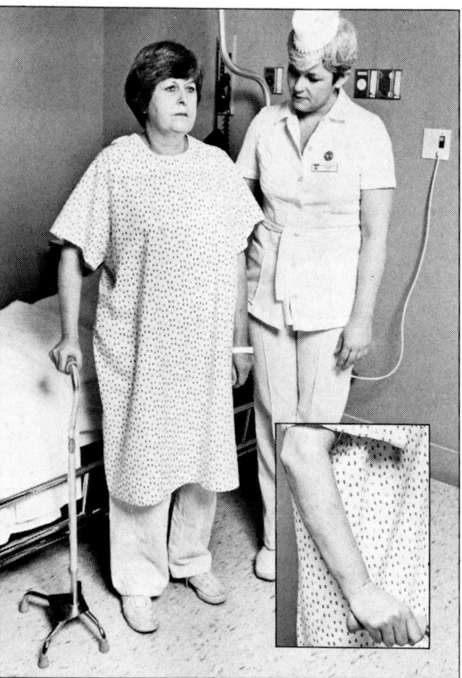

3 Tell Ms. McPherson to look ahead when she walks instead of looking at her feet. Have her shift her weight to her right leg as she moves the cane forward about 4" (10.2 cm).

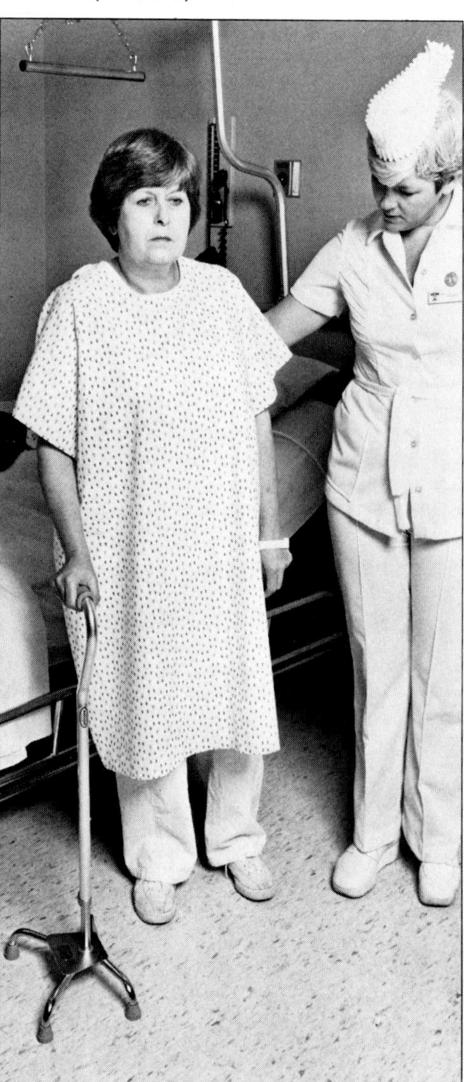

Assessing your patient's discharge needs

Let's say you're caring for a patient who's ready to return home. Before he leaves the hospital, you'll need to assess—and help provide for—his daily living needs. Be sure to consider the points covered in these guidelines:

- *Does your patient live alone?* If he does, you may want to refer him (and a family member) to the hospital's social service department, or to outside agencies and programs, such as the Visiting Nurse Association, Meals on Wheels, and Homemaker Services. If agencies and programs like these are inaccessible to your patient, recommend that he and his family consider a boarding home, a rehabilitation hospital, or a nursing home.
- *Can he ride in a car?* If not, contact an ambulance to transport him home.
- *Does your patient need an ambulation aid?* If he does, determine approximately how long he'll need the aid. If he'll need the aid for only a short time, suggest he rent it from an equipment agency (if possible), instead of purchasing it.
- *Does he need a special bed or mattress at home?* If so, do one of the following: contact a rental agency and arrange for him to rent the equipment; give the family a list of rental agencies; or have a representative from your hospital's social service department arrange for the rental. Of course, if the special mattress your patient

4 Tell her to support her weight on both her right leg and the cane as she moves her left foot forward parallel with the cane.

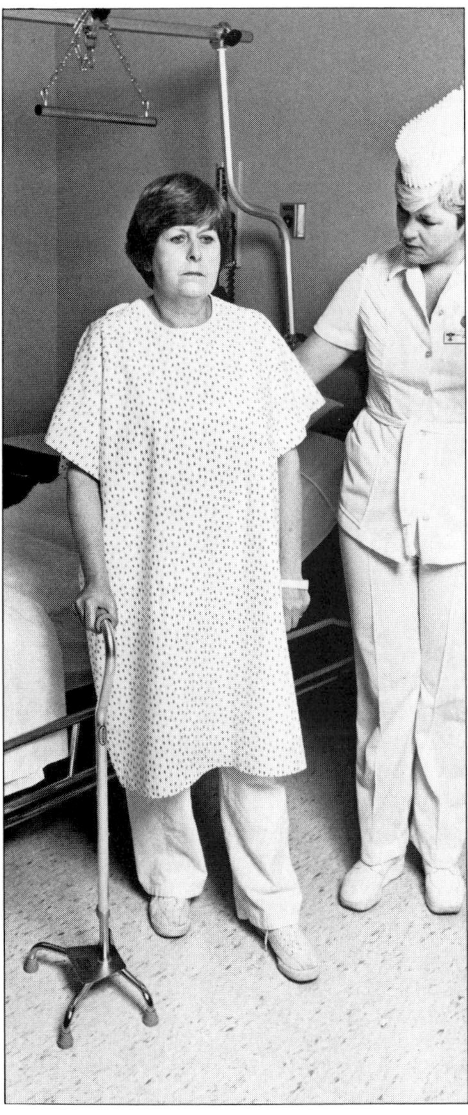

5 Instruct Ms. McPherson to shift her weight to her left leg and the cane, and then move her right leg forward ahead of the cane. If she does this correctly, her heel will be slightly beyond the tip of the cane.

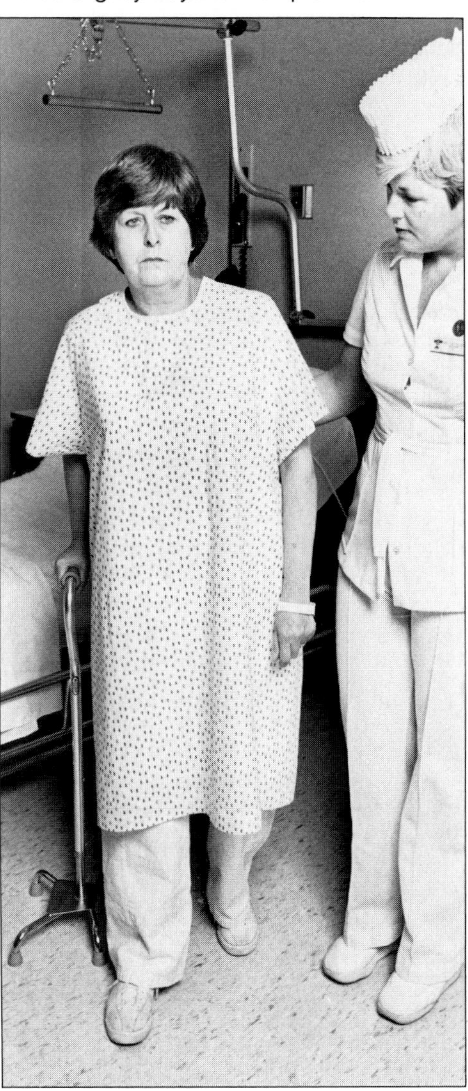

6 Now, have her move her left foot forward so it's even with her right foot. Then, tell her to move her cane forward as instructed in step 3.

Guide her through the entire procedure several times until you both think she's ready to try it alone. Stay with her while she tries it by herself.

Finally, document all patient teaching in your nurses' notes.

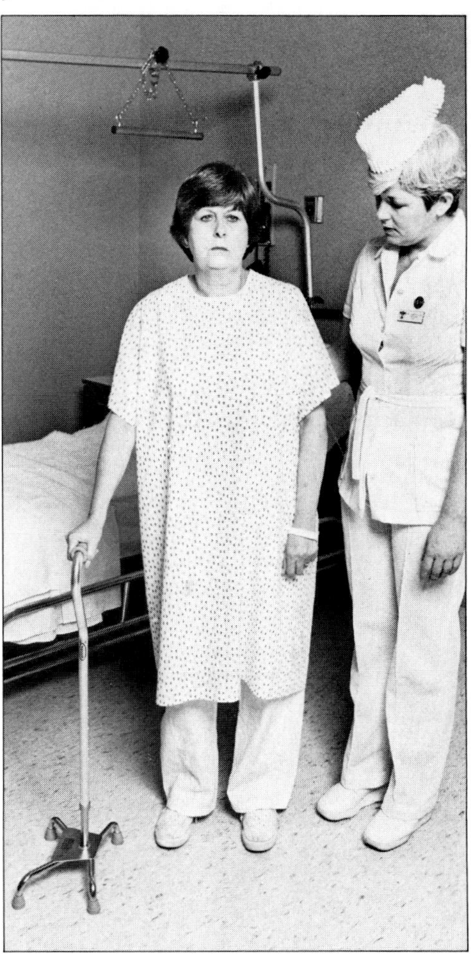

used in the hospital is intended for only one patient's use, be sure to send it home with him.

• *Is your patient's house or apartment on one floor?* If it is, he should be able to move easily from the bedroom to the bathroom and kitchen. But, if your patient's dwelling has more than one floor and he isn't allowed to walk up and down stairs, suggest that he convert one of the rooms on the first floor into a bedroom. If the bathroom's on the second floor, recommend that he rent a portable commode chair for the first floor. However, if the bathroom's on the first floor, he may need to obtain an elevated toilet seat.

• *Does your patient know how to adapt his home to his needs?* Suggest these possible adaptations: telephones in easy-to-reach locations with cords out of walkways; safety rails on the bed; grab bars around the toilet and bathtub; handrails along all halls and stairways.

• *Is your patient going home with any special instructions or home care aids?* If he is, make sure he—and his family—understand the instructions completely. Answer any questions they may have.

If your patient can't meet all his discharge expenses, refer him to the hospital social service department or another agency. Depending on hospital policy, this referral may require a doctor's order.

Ambulation aids

Home care

Going home with a cane

1 Dear Patient:
Your doctor says you're ready to return home. But he wants you to use a cane, to help you put full weight on your affected leg as you walk. Following we give guidelines for a person with an affected *left* leg. If your *right* leg is affected, start with the cane on your left side, and adapt the instructions. You may want to draw the patterns for yourself.

Before you begin, be sure you have nonskid, flat-soled, supportive shoes on, and check that they're buckled or tied securely. Avoid wearing slip-on shoes, such as loafers or clogs, as they don't support your weight properly. In addition, check your cane's rubber tip to be sure it's without cracks or tears, and is wearing evenly. Also, make sure the tip fits securely on the cane's end.

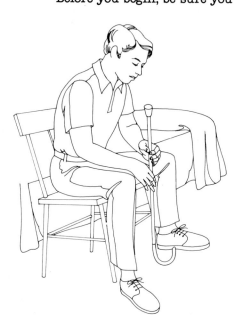

If possible, remove throw rugs and avoid walking on slippery, wet, or waxed floors, or gravel driveways. Also, try to walk close to a wall, so you have something to lean against if you drop your cane.

2 Now, position the cane about 4″ (10 cm) to the side of your unaffected leg, as shown in this illustration. Distribute your weight between your feet and your cane.

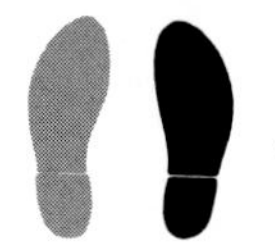

3 Next, shift your weight to your unaffected leg and move the cane about 4″ (10 cm) in front of you.

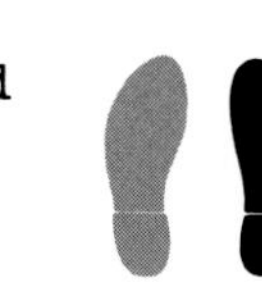

4 Now, you're ready to move your affected foot forward so it's parallel with the cane.

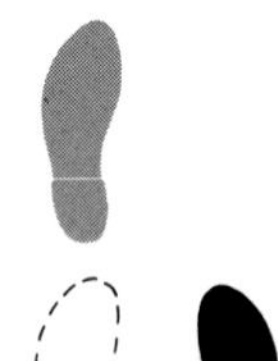

5 Shift your weight to your affected leg and the cane. Now, move your unaffected leg forward, ahead of the cane. If you've done this step correctly, your heel will be slightly beyond the tip of the cane.

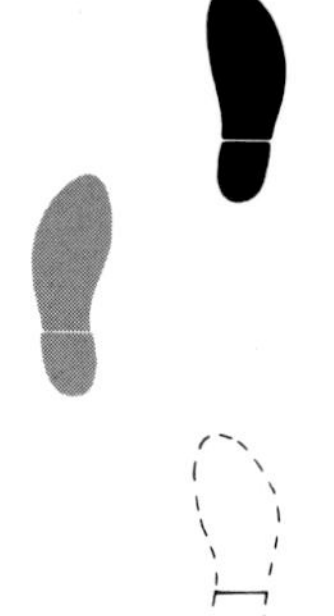

6 Next, move your affected foot forward, so it's even with your unaffected foot. Then, move your cane in front of you about 4″ (10 cm).

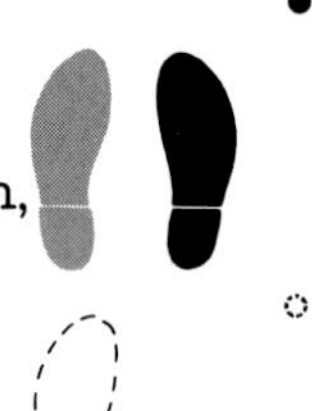

Repeat these steps. As you proceed, remember to keep your head erect, shoulders back, back straight, abdomen in, and knees slightly flexed.

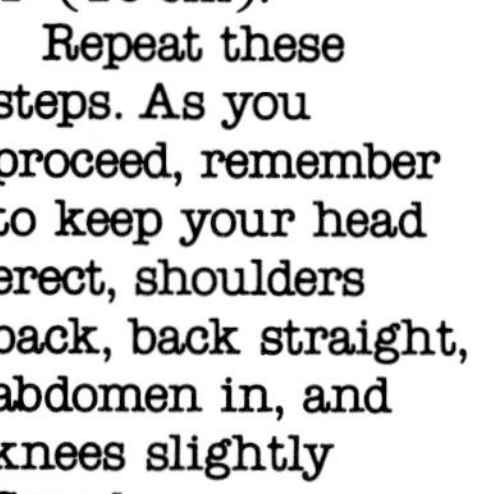

PATIENT TEACHING

Sending your patient home with an ambulation aid

When your patient with an orthopedic condition is ready to go home, the doctor may want him to use a walker, cane, or crutches. If so, you'll need to prepare your patient properly. *Note:* Try to include a family member in your teaching sessions.

Explain to your patient why he's using the ambulation aid chosen for him. Then, teach him how to walk with it. Stay with your patient until you're both confident he can walk with it alone.

In addition to teaching your patient how to use his ambulation aid, help him anticipate the specific problems he may confront in his home environment. For example, does your patient have thick shag wall-to-wall carpeting in his home? If so, tell him the carpeting may adversely affect his balance. Suggest that he be especially careful when walking on it.

Advise the patient that hardwood, tile, and lineolum floors provide the best walking surfaces for using an ambulation aid. And remind him to avoid walking on slippery, waxed, or wet floors, or on uneven surfaces, such as gravel or dirt-covered driveways.

Note: If your patient will be using a cane when he returns home, photocopy the home care aid on the opposite page and give it to him. In addition, be sure he understands how the instructions apply to his affected leg. That way, you'll personalize the aid for your patient.

If your patient's orthopedic condition is temporary, recommend he rent the ambulation aid he'll need. Or, suggest he buy a less expensive model, since he'll use it for only a short time.

For other helpful discharge recommendations you can make to your patient, see pages 152 and 153. *Remember:* He may need help from social services.

Remember to document all patient teaching in your nurses' notes.

Acknowledgements

We'd like to thank the following people and companies for their help with this PHOTOBOOK:

ACCURATE MEDICAL SERVICE
Willow Grove, Pa.
Chuck Hepler, Manager

ALL ORTHOPEDIC APPLIANCES (AOA)
Greenwood, S.C.
George Rosselle, Product Manager

THE JOBST INSTITUTE, INC.
Toledo, Ohio

JOHNSON & JOHNSON PRODUCTS INC.
Patient Care Division
New Brunswick, N.J.

KARL STORZ ENDOSCOPY-AMERICA, INC.
Culver City, Calif.

LOTUS HEALTH CARE PRODUCTS
Division Connecticut Artcraft Corporation
Naugatuck, Conn.

MW ORTHOPAEDICS INCORPORATED
Bala Cynwyd, Pa.

J.T. POSEY CO.
Arcadia, Calif.

RICHARDS MANUFACTURING COMPANY, INC.
Memphis, Tenn.

SPAN-AMERICA, INC.
Greenville, S.C.
Donald C. Spann, President

FLEETWOOD VOLUNTEER AMBULANCE CORPS
Leon Bergstresser
Fleetwood, Pa.

Maureen Hamilton, RN
Staff Development Coordinator
Chestnut Hill Hospital
Philadelphia, Pa.

John Esterhai, MD, (Bone stimulation)
Michael Fried, MD, (Hyperbaric oxygen chamber)
Hospital of The University of Pennsylvania
Philadelphia, Pa.

Margaret A. Cianci, RN
Richard Nutt, MD
William H. Spellman, MD
Lansdale Medical Group—Orthopedic Group
Lansdale, Pa.

Sister St. Gregory
St. Joseph's Villa
Flourtown, Pa.

Also the staffs of:

BERKS VISITING NURSE HOME HEALTH AGENCY
Reading, Pa.

CHESTNUT HILL HOSPITAL
Philadelphia, Pa.

COMMUNITY GENERAL HOSPITAL
Reading, Pa.

HOSPITAL OF THE UNIVERSITY OF PENNSYLVANIA
Orthopedic Units

THOMAS JEFFERSON UNIVERSITY HOSPITAL
Philadelphia, Pa.

VISITING NURSE ASSOCIATION OF EASTERN MONTGOMERY COUNTY INC.
Abington, Pa.

Selected references

Books

Aguilera, Donna C., and Janice M. Messick. CRISIS INTERVENTION: THEORY AND METHODOLOGY, 3rd ed. St. Louis: C.V. Mosby Co., 1978.

Bates, Barbara. A GUIDE TO PHYSICAL EXAMINATION, 2nd ed. Philadelphia: J.B. Lippincott Co., 1979.

Berci, George, ed. ENDOSCOPY. New York: Appleton-Century-Crofts, 1976.

Blauvelt, Carolyn T., and Fred R. Nelson. A MANUAL OF ORTHOPEDIC TERMINOLOGY, 2nd ed. St. Louis: C.V. Mosby Co., 1977.

Brashear, H. Robert, and R. Beverly Raney. SHAND'S HANDBOOK OF ORTHOPAEDIC SURGERY, 9th ed. St. Louis: C.V. Mosby Co., 1978.

Brunner, Lillian S., and Doris S. Suddarth. TEXTBOOK OF MEDICAL-SURGICAL NURSING, 4th ed. Philadelphia: J.B. Lippincott Co., 1980.

CARING FOR SURGICAL PATIENTS. Nursing Photobook™ Series. Springhouse, Pa.: Intermed Communications, Inc., 1982.

Carini, Geraldine K., and Jacqueline Birmingham. TRACTION MADE MANAGEABLE: A SELF LEARNING MODULE. New York: McGraw-Hill Book Co., 1979.

COPING WITH NEUROLOGIC DISORDERS. Nursing Photobook™ Series. Springhouse, Pa.: Intermed Communications, Inc., 1981.

Delp, Mahlon H., and Robert T. Manning, eds. MAJOR'S PHYSICAL DIAGNOSIS, 8th ed. Philadelphia: W.B. Saunders Co., 1975.

Dison, Norma. CLINICAL NURSING TECHNIQUES, 4th ed. St. Louis: C.V. Mosby Co., 1979.

Dunphy, J. Englebert, and Lawrence W. Way, eds. CURRENT SURGICAL DIAGNOSIS AND TREATMENT, 4th ed. Los Altos, Calif.: Lange Medical Publications, 1979.

Farrell, Jane. ILLUSTRATED GUIDE TO ORTHOPEDIC NURSING. Philadelphia: J.B. Lippincott Co., 1977.

Gartland, John. FUNDAMENTALS OF ORTHOPEDICS, 3rd ed. Philadelphia: W.B. Saunders Co., 1979.

Goss, Charles M., ed. GRAY'S ANATOMY OF THE HUMAN BODY, 29th ed. Philadelphia: Lea and Febiger, 1973.

Guyton, Arthur C. TEXTBOOK OF MEDICAL PHYSIOLOGY, 6th ed. Philadelphia: W.B. Saunders Co., 1981.

Hilt, Nancy E., and Shirley B. Cogburn. MANUAL OF ORTHOPEDICS. St. Louis: C.V. Mosby Co., 1979.

Hollinshead, W. Henry. FUNCTIONAL ANATOMY OF THE LIMBS AND BACK, 4th ed. Philadelphia: W.B. Saunders Co., 1976.

Hoppenfeld, S. PHYSICAL EXAMINATION OF THE SPINE AND EXTREMITIES. New York: Appleton-Century-Crofts, 1976.

Jones, Dorothy, et al. MEDICAL SURGICAL NURSING: A CONCEPTUAL APPROACH. New York: McGraw-Hill Book Co., 1978.

Judge, Richard, and George D. Zuidema, eds. METHODS OF CLINICAL EXAMINATION: A PHYSIOLOGIC APPROACH, 3rd ed. Boston: Little, Brown, and Co., 1974.

Krupp, Marcus A., and Milton J. Chatton, eds. CURRENT MEDICAL DIAGNOSIS AND TREATMENT. Los Altos, Calif.: Lange Medical Publications, 1980.

Larson, Carroll B., and Marjorie Gould. ORTHOPEDIC NURSING, 9th ed. St. Louis: C.V. Mosby Co., 1978.

LeMaitre, George D., and Janet A. Finnegan. THE PATIENT IN SURGERY, 4th ed. Philadelphia: W.B. Saunders Co., 1980.

Luckmann, Joan, and Karen C. Sorenson. MEDICAL-SURGICAL NURSING: A PSYCHOPHYSIOLOGIC APPROACH, 2nd ed. Philadelphia: W.B. Saunders Co., 1980.

Miller, Marjorie A., et al. KIMBER-GRAY-STACKPOLE'S ANATOMY AND PHYSIOLOGY, 17th ed. New York: Macmillan Pub. Co., Inc., 1977.

Mourad, Leona. NURSING CARE OF ADULTS WITH ORTHOPEDIC CONDITIONS. New York: John Wiley and Sons, Inc., 1980.

PROVIDING EARLY MOBILITY. Nursing Photobook™ Series. Springhouse, Pa.: Intermed Communications, Inc., 1980.

Rosse, Cornelius, and D. Kay Clawson. INTRODUCTION TO THE MUSCULOSKELETAL SYSTEM. New York: Harper and Row Pubs., Inc., 1970.

Sorenson, Karen C., and Joan Luckmann. BASIC NURSING: A PSYCHOPHYSIOLOGIC APPROACH. Philadelphia: W.B. Saunders Co., 1979.

Stewart, J.D. TRACTION AND ORTHOPAEDIC APPLIANCES. New York: Churchill-Livingstone, Inc., 1975.

Turek, Samuel L. ORTHOPAEDICS: PRINCIPLES AND THEIR APPLICATION, 3rd ed. Philadelphia: J.B. Lippincott Co., 1977.

Periodicals

Anderson, M.G. *Basic Biomechanics of Orthopedic Traction,* ONA JOURNAL, 3:267-269, September 1976.

Bass, L. *More Fiber—Less Constipation,* AMERICAN JOURNAL OF NURSING, 77:254-255, February 1977.

Berecek, K.H. *Etiology of Decubitus Ulcers,* NURSING CLINICS OF NORTH AMERICA, 10:157-170, March 1975.

Ciuca, Rudy, et al. *Range of Motion Exercises, Active and Passive: A Handbook,* NURSING73, 3:25-37, December 1973.

Cohen, S. *Nursing Care of a Patient in Traction,* AMERICAN JOURNAL OF NURSING, 79:1771-1798, October 1979.

Cohen, S. *Programmed Instruction: Patient Assessment: Examining Joints of the Upper and Lower Extremities,* AMERICAN JOURNAL OF NURSING, 81:763-786, April 1981.

Cooper, S.B. *Motivation of the Immobilized Orthopedic Patient,* ONA JOURNAL, 3:191-193, June 1976.

Duncan, C. *The Nurse and the Patient in Pain,* ONA JOURNAL, 6:242-244, June 1979.

Hirschberg, G.G., et al. *Promoting Patient Mobility and Other Ways to Prevent Secondary Disabilities,* NURSING77, 7:42-47, May 1977.

Hogberg A. *Orthopedic Nursing, Preventing Orthopedic Complications, Part 2,* RN, 38:34-37, March 1975.

Jacox, A.K. *Assessing Pain,* AMERICAN JOURNAL OF NURSING, 79:895-900, May 1979.

Johnson, M. *Pain: How Do You Know It's There and What Do You Do?* NURSING76, 6:48-50, September 1976.

Jungreis, S. *Exercises for Expediting Mobility and Decreasing Disability in Bedridden Patients,* NURSING77, 7:47-51, August 1977.

Kryschyshen, Patt L., and David A. Fischer. *External Fixation for Complicated Fractures,* AMERICAN JOURNAL OF NURSING, 80:256-259, February 1980.

McCaffery M., and L. Hart. *Undertreatment of Acute pain with Narcotics,* AMERICAN JOURNAL OF NURSING, 76:1586-1591, October 1976.

Mikulic, M.A. *Treatment of Pressure Ulcers,* AMERICAN JOURNAL OF NURSING, 80:1125-1128, June 1980.

Moyer, K.W. *Put the Patient's Leg on Ice?* RN, 44:44-45, May 1981.

Pace, J.B. *Helping Patients Overcome the Disabling Effects of Chronic Pain,* NURSING77, 7:38-43, July 1977.

Perdue, Patricia. *Abdominal Injuries and Dangerous Fractures, Part 4,* RN, 44:34-37, July 1981.

Perdue, Patricia. *Urgent Priorities in Severe Trauma. Life-Threatening Respiratory Injuries, Part 1,* RN, 44:26-33, April 1981.

Ryan, R. *Thrombophlebitis: Assessment and Prevention,* AMERICAN JOURNAL OF NURSING, 76:1634-1636, October 1976.

Stewart E. *To Lessen Pain: Relaxation and Rhythmic Breathing,* AMERICAN JOURNAL OF NURSING, 76:958-959, June 1976.

Sutcliffe, S.A. *Comprehensive Nursing Care: The Patient with a Ruptured Lumbar Disc,* JOURNAL OF NEUROSURGICAL NURSING, 10:86-91, September 1978.

Twedt, B. *Skeletal Traction for Supracondylar Fractures of the Humerus,* ONA JOURNAL, 4:9, January 1977.

West, B. Anne. *Understanding Endorphins: Our Natural Pain Relief System,* NURSING81, 11:50-53, February 1981.

Wyper, M. *Pulmonary Embolism: Fighting the Silent Killer,* NURSING75, 5:30-38, October 1975.

Index

Index